Diagnosis and Treatment of Gastrointestinal Cancers

Editors

RAQUEL E. DAVILA
MARTA L. DAVILA

GASTROENTEROLOGY CLINICS OF NORTH AMERICA

www.gastro.theclinics.com

Consulting Editor
ALAN L. BUCHMAN

September 2022 • Volume 51 • Number 3

ELSEVIER

1600 John F. Kennedy Boulevard • Suite 1800 • Philadelphia, Pennsylvania, 19103-2899
http://www.theclinics.com

GASTROENTEROLOGY CLINICS OF NORTH AMERICA Volume 51, Number 3
September 2022 ISSN 0889-8553, ISBN-13: 978-0-323-85011-7

Editor: Kerry Holland
Developmental Editor: Hannah Almira Lopez

Gastroenterology Clinics of North America (ISSN 0889-8553) is published quarterly by Elsevier Inc., 360 Park Avenue South, New York, NY 10010-1710. Months of issue are March, June, September, and December. Business and Editorial Offices: 1600 John F. Kennedy Blvd., Suite 1800, Philadelphia, PA 19103-2899. Customer Service Office: 6277 Sea Harbor Drive, Orlando, FL 32887-4800. Periodicals postage paid at New York, NY and additional mailing offices. Subscription prices are $368.00 per year (US individuals), $100.00 per year (US students), $973.00 per year (US institutions), $395.00 per year (Canadian individuals), $100.00 per year (Canadian students), $1002.00 per year (Canadian institutions), $468.00 per year (international individuals), $220.00 per year (international students), and $1002.00 per year (international institutions). Foreign air speed delivery is included in all *Clinics* subscription prices. All prices are subject to change without notice. **POSTMASTER**: Send address changes to *Gastroenterology Clinics of North America*, Elsevier Health Sciences Division, Subscription Customer Service, 3251 Riverport Lane, Maryland Heights, MO 63043. **Telephone: 1-800-654-2452 (U.S. and Canada); 314-447-8871 (outside U.S. and Canada). Fax: 314-447-8029. E-mail: journalscustomerservice-usa@elsevier.com (for print support); journalsonlinesupport-usa@elsevier.com (for online support).**

Reprints. For copies of 100 or more, of articles in this publication, please contact the Commercial Reprints Department, Elsevier Inc., 360 Part Avenue South, New York, New York 10010-1710. Tel. 212-633-3874, Fax: 212-633-3820, E-mail: reprints@elsevier.com.

Gastroenterology Clinics of North America is also published in Italian by Il Pensiero Scientifico Editore, Rome, Italy; and in Portuguese by Interlivros Edicoes Ltda., Rua Commandante Coelho 1085, 21250 Cordovil, Rio de Janeiro, Brazil.

Gastroenterology Clinics of North America is covered in *MEDLINE/PubMed (Index Medicus)*, *Excerpta Medica, Current Contents/Clinical Medicine, Science Citation Index, ISI/BIOMED*, and *BIOSIS*.

Contributors

CONSULTING EDITOR

ALAN L. BUCHMAN, MD, MSPH, FACP, FACN, FACG, AGAF
Professor of Clinical Surgery, Medical Director, Intestinal Rehabilitation and Transplant Center, The University of Illinois at Chicago/UI Health, Chicago, Illinois, USA

EDITORS

RAQUEL E. DAVILA, MD, FACP, AGAF, FACG, FASGE
Associate Professor, The University of Texas at Dallas, Dallas, Texas, USA

MARTA L. DAVILA, MD, AGAF, FACG, FASGE
Professor, Department of Gastroenterology, Hepatology, and Nutrition, Division of Internal Medicine, Department of Clinical Cancer Prevention, Division of Cancer Prevention and Population Sciences, The University of Texas MD Anderson Cancer Center, Houston, Texas, USA

AUTHORS

JORDAN E. AXELRAD, MD, MPH
Director of Clinical and Translational Research, Inflammatory Bowel Disease Center at NYU Langone Health, Assistant Professor, Division of Gastroenterology, Department of Medicine, NYU Grossman School of Medicine, New York, New York, USA

VEROUSHKA BALLESTER, MD, MSc
University of Puerto Rico Comprehensive Cancer Center, Rio Piedras, Puerto Rico, USA; Assistant Professor, Department of Medicine, Biochemistry and Surgery, University of Puerto Rico Medical Sciences Campus, San Juan, Puerto Rico, USA

OMER BASAR, MD
Gastroenterology Fellow, The University of Missouri, Department of Gastroenterology, Columbia, Missouri, USA

ROBERT S. BRESALIER, MD
Department of Gastroenterology, Hepatology and Nutrition, Professor of Medicine, Distinguished Professor in Gastrointestinal Oncology, The University of Texas MD Anderson Cancer Center, Houston, Texas, USA

WILLIAM R. BRUGGE, MD
Professor in Medicine, Harvard Medical School, Chief, Mount Auburn Hospital, Department of Gastroenterology, Cambridge, Massachusetts, USA

SAHIN COBAN, MD
Research Coordinator, Mount Auburn Hospital, Department of Gastroenterology, Cambridge, Massachusetts, USA

D. CHAMIL CODIPILLY, MD
Fellow Physician, Division of Gastroenterology and Hepatology, Mayo Clinic, Rochester, Minnesota, USA

CARY C. COTTON, MD, MPH
Department of Medicine, Division of Gastroenterology and Hepatology, Center for Esophageal Diseases and Swallowing, The University of North Carolina at Chapel Hill, Chapel Hill, North Carolina, USA

MARCIA CRUZ-CORREA, MD, PhD
University of Puerto Rico Comprehensive Cancer Center, Rio Piedras, Puerto Rico, USA; Professor, Department of Medicine, Biochemistry and Surgery, University of Puerto Rico Medical Sciences Campus, San Juan, Puerto Rico, USA

ROHIT DAS, MD
Division of Gastroenterology, Hepatology and Nutrition, University of Pittsburgh Medical Center, Pittsburgh, Pennsylvania, USA

RAQUEL E. DAVILA, MD, FACP, AGAF, FACG, FASGE
Associate Professor, The University of Texas at Dallas, Dallas, Texas, USA

RICARDO L. DOMINGUEZ, MD
Western Honduras Gastric Cancer Prevention Initiative, Copan Region Ministry of Health, Honduras

JENNIFER R. EADS, MD
Division of Hematology/Oncology, Department of Medicine, Perelman School of Medicine, University of Pennsylvania, Philadelphia, Pennsylvania, USA

SWATHI ELURI, MD, MPH
Department of Medicine, Division of Gastroenterology and Hepatology, Center for Esophageal Diseases and Swallowing, The University of North Carolina at Chapel Hill, Chapel Hill, North Carolina, USA

ADAM S. FAYE, MD, MS
Assistant Professor, Division of Gastroenterology, Department of Medicine, NYU Grossman School of Medicine, Inflammatory Bowel Disease Center at NYU Langone Health, New York, New York, USA

CONRAD J. FERNANDES, MD
Department of Medicine, Hospital of the University of Pennsylvania, Philadelphia, Pennsylvania, USA

MICHAEL GOGGINS, MD
Departments of Pathology, Medicine, and Oncology, Bloomberg School of Public Health, The Sol Goldman Pancreatic Cancer Research Center, Johns Hopkins Medical Institutions, Baltimore, Maryland, USA

ARIELA K. HOLMER, MD
Assistant Professor, Division of Gastroenterology, Department of Medicine, NYU Grossman School of Medicine, Inflammatory Bowel Disease Center at NYU Langone Health, New York, New York, USA

BRYSON W. KATONA, MD, PhD
Division of Gastroenterology and Hepatology, Department of Medicine, Perelman Center for Advanced Medicine, Perelman School of Medicine, University of Pennsylvania, Philadelphia, Pennsylvania, USA

GALEN LEUNG, MD
Division of Gastroenterology and Hepatology, Department of Medicine, Perelman School of Medicine, University of Pennsylvania, Philadelphia, Pennsylvania, USA

ELEAZAR E. MONTALVAN, MD
Western Honduras Gastric Cancer Prevention Initiative, Copan Region Ministry of Health, Honduras; Department of Medicine, Indiana University School of Medicine, Indianapolis, Indiana, USA

DOUGLAS R. MORGAN, MD, MPH
UAB Department of Medicine, The University of Alabama at Birmingham, Birmingham, Alabama, USA

DALTON A. NORWOOD, MD
UAB Department of Medicine, The University of Alabama at Birmingham, Birmingham, Alabama, USA; Western Honduras Gastric Cancer Prevention Initiative, Copan Region Ministry of Health, Honduras

HELENA SABA, MD
Post-Doctoral Fellow Michael Goggins, Professor of Pathology, Medicine, and Oncology, Department of Pathology, Johns Hopkins Medical Institutions, Baltimore, Maryland, USA

NICHOLAS J. SHAHEEN, MD, MPH
Department of Medicine, Division of Gastroenterology and Hepatology, Center for Esophageal Diseases and Swallowing, The University of North Carolina at Chapel Hill, Chapel Hill, North Carolina, USA

AATUR D. SINGHI, MD, PhD
Department of Pathology, University of Pittsburgh Medical Center, Pittsburgh, Pennsylvania, USA

ADAM SLIVKA, MD, PhD
Division of Gastroenterology, Hepatology and Nutrition, University of Pittsburgh Medical Center, Pittsburgh, Pennsylvania, USA

KENNETH K. WANG, MD
Professor of Medicine, Division of Gastroenterology and Hepatology, Mayo Clinic, Rochester, Minnesota, USA

JENNIFER A. WARGO, MD, MMSc
Professor, Departments of Genomic Medicine and Surgical Oncology, The University of Texas MD Anderson Cancer Center, Houston, Texas, USA

MICHAEL G. WHITE, MD, MSc
Department of Surgical Oncology, The University of Texas MD Anderson Cancer Center, Houston, Texas, USA

Contents

> Esophageal squamous cell carcinoma (ESCC) is common in the developing world with decreasing incidence in developed countries and carries significant morbidity and mortality. Major risk factors for ESCC development include significant use of alcohol and tobacco. Screening for ESCC can be recommended in high-risk populations living in highly endemic regions. The treatment of ESCC ranges from endoscopic resection therapy or surgery in localized disease to chemoradiotherapy in metastatic disease, and prognosis is directly related to the stage at diagnosis. New immunotherapies and molecular targeted therapies may improve the dismal survival outcomes in patients with metastatic ESCC.

> While patients with Barrett's esophagus without dysplasia may benefit from endoscopic surveillance, those with low-grade dysplasia may be managed with either endoscopic surveillance or endoscopic eradication. Patients with Barrett's esophagus with high-grade dysplasia and/or intramucosal adenocarcinoma will generally require endoscopic eradication therapy. The management of Barrett's esophagus with dysplasia and early esophageal adenocarcinoma is predominantly endoscopic, with multiple effective methods available for the resection of raised neoplasia and ablation of flat neoplasia. High-dose proton-pump inhibitor therapy is advised during the treatment of Barrett's esophagus with dysplasia and early esophageal adenocarcinoma. After the endoscopic eradication of Barrett's esophagus and associated neoplasia, surveillance is required for the diagnosis and retreatment of recurrence or progression.

> Gastric adenocarcinoma (GC) is the fourth leading cause of global cancer mortality, and the leading infection-associated cancer. Helicobacter pylori is the dominant risk factor for GC and classified as an IARC class I carcinogen. Surveillance of gastric premalignant conditions is now indicated in high-risk patients. Upper endoscopy is the gold standard for GC diagnosis, and image-enhanced endoscopy increases the detection of gastric premalignant conditions and early gastric cancer (EGC). Clinical staging is crucial for treatment approach, defining early gastric cancer, operable

locoregional disease, and advanced GC. Endoscopic submucosal dissection is the treatment of choice for most EGC. Targeted therapies are rapidly evolving, based on biomarkers including MSI/dMMR, HER2, and PD-L1. These advancements in surveillance, diagnostic and therapeutic strategies are expected to improve GC survival rates in the near term.

The human microbiome has been recognized as increasingly important to health and disease. This is especially prescient in the development of various cancers, their progression, and the microbiome's modulation of various anticancer therapeutics. Mechanisms behind these interactions have been increasingly well described through modulation of the host immune system as well as induction of genetic changes and local inactivation of cancer therapeutics. Here, we review these associations for a variety of gastrointestinal malignancies as well as contemporary strategies proposed to leverage these associations to improve cancer treatment outcomes.

GASTROENTEROLOGY
CLINICS OF NORTH AMERICA

SERIES OF RELATED INTEREST

Clinics in Liver Disease
(Available at: http://www.liver.theclinics.com/)
Gastrointestinal Endoscopy Clinics of North America
(Available at: http://www.www.giendo.theclinics.com/)

THE CLINICS ARE AVAILABLE ONLINE!
Access your subscription at:
www.theclinics.com

GASTROENTEROLOGY
CLINICS OF NORTH AMERICA

FORTHCOMING ISSUES

December 2022
Psychogastroenterology
Laurie Keefer, Editor

March 2023
Covid-19 and Gastroenterology
Mitchell S. Cappell, Editor

June 2023
Management of Obesity, Part 1: Overview
and Basic Mechanisms
Lee M. Kaplan, Editor

RECENT ISSUES

June 2022
Medical and Surgical Management of
Crohn's Disease
Sunanda V. Kane, Editor

March 2022
Pelvic Floor Disorders
Darren M. Brenner, Editor

December 2021
Diseases of the Esophagus
John O. Clarke, Editor

SERIES OF RELATED INTEREST

Clinics in Liver Disease
(Available at: https://www.liver.theclinics.com)
Gastrointestinal Endoscopy Clinics of North America
(Available at: http://www.giendo.theclinics.com)

THE CLINICS ARE AVAILABLE ONLINE!
Access your subscription at:
www.theclinics.com

Preface

Recent Advancements in the Diagnosis and Treatment of Gastrointestinal Cancers

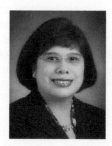
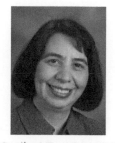

Raquel E. Davila, MD, FACP, AGAF, FACG, FASGE   Marta L. Davila, MD, AGAF, FACG, FASGE

Editors

Approximately 19.3 million new cases of cancer were diagnosed worldwide in 2020, of which 5 million were cancers of the gastrointestinal (GI) tract. Furthermore, GI cancers were the cause of more than one-third of all cancer-related deaths.[1] In 2022, the estimated incidence of cancers of the digestive system (343,040) in the United States will surpass the incidence of breast cancers (290,560) and cancers of the respiratory system (254,850).[2] Although recent trends in incidence and mortality rates have been encouraging for cancers of the colorectum and stomach, no improvements have been observed in cancers of the esophagus, liver and intrahepatic bile ducts, and pancreas. Subsequently, the early detection, diagnosis, and accurate staging of GI cancers have become essential to gastroenterologists in the care of these patients. Newer strategies for screening and surveillance have led to the detection of GI cancers at an earlier stage and in a younger patient population. The availability of enhanced endoscopic imaging techniques, endoscopic tissue acquisition, endoscopic resection, and new ablative therapies has completely revolutionized our approach to GI cancer patients in the past two decades while avoiding the morbidity and mortality associated with surgery. A greater understanding of GI tumors at the molecular level has ultimately led to the development of new treatment modalities including tyrosine kinase inhibitors, immune checkpoint inhibitors, and anti-angiogenesis therapies that target key aspects of carcinogenesis.

In this issue of *Gastroenterology Clinics of North America*, you will find an exhaustive review of the latest topics in GI cancer by distinguished authors recognized internationally as leading authorities in the field. We want to express our deepest gratitude to the authors, who dedicated their valuable time and efforts to this important endeavor. We

https://doi.org/10.1016/j.gtc.2022.07.009
0889-8553/22/© 2022 Published by Elsevier Inc.

gastro.theclinics.com

hope this issue serves as an essential resource and guidance to practicing gastroenterologists worldwide.

Raquel E. Davila, MD, FACP, AGAF, FACG, FASGE
The University of Texas at Dallas
4500 S. Lancaster Road
Dallas, TX 75216-7167, USA

Marta L. Davila, MD, AGAF, FACG, FASGE
Department of Gastroenterology
Hepatology and Nutrition
Division of Internal Medicine
Department of Clinical Cancer Prevention
Division of Cancer Prevention and Population Sciences
The University of Texas MD Anderson Cancer Center
1515 Holcombe Boulevard, Unit 1466
Houston, TX, 77030, USA

E-mail addresses:
rdavila.1996@gmail.com (R.E. Davila)
mdavila@mdanderson.org (M.L. Davila)

REFERENCES

1. Sung H, Ferlay J, Siegel RL, et al. Global cancer statistics 2020: GLOBOCAN estimates of incidence and mortality worldwide for 36 cancers in 185 countries. CA Cancer J Clin 2021;71:209–49.
2. Siegel RL, Miller KD, Fuchs HE, et al. Cancer statistics, 2022. CA Cancer J Clin 2022;72:7–33.

Squamous Cell Carcinoma of the Esophagus

D. Chamil Codipilly, MD, Kenneth K. Wang, MD*

KEYWORDS

- Esophageal squamous cell carcinoma • Epidemiology • Prognosis
- Endoscopic eradication therapy • Neoadjuvant chemoradiotherapy

KEY POINTS

- Risk factors for esophageal squamous cell carcinoma (ESCC) include alcohol and tobacco use.
- Screening for ESCC may be warranted in endemic regions in high-risk populations.
- Therapy for ESCC may include endoscopic resection, surgery, and chemoradiotherapy.
- Immunomodulatory and molecular targeted therapies may herald a new paradigm in the treatment of ESCC.

EPIDEMIOLOGY

Esophageal cancer is the 9th most common incident cancer worldwide and contributes to the 6th highest number of deaths.[1] In the United States, esophageal cancer is the 6th most commonly diagnosed gastrointestinal malignancy but contributes the 4th highest number of deaths.[2] Well over three-quarters of this morbidity and mortality affect men. Esophageal cancer has 2 major histologic subtypes: esophageal adenocarcinoma, which is prevalent in developed Western nations, and esophageal squamous cell carcinoma (ESCC), which is prevalent in developing nations.[3] Well more than 80% to 90% of esophageal cancer diagnosed globally is ESCC.[3] Despite the elevated prevalence in developing countries, in developed nations ESCC is seen disproportionately in minority racial subgroups including Africans, Hispanics, and Native Americans.

The burden of ESCC disproportionately affects nations and regions along 2 "ESCC belts"; one which stretches from Eastern Asia through Central Asia to the Caspian Sea, and the other extending south into sub-Saharan Africa along the eastern coast of the African continent (**Fig. 1**).[1,4] Within these areas, certain regions, such as the North Central Taigun Mountain Range of China, have incidence rates of ESCC

Division of Gastroenterology and Hepatology, Mayo Clinic, SMH Campus, 6 Alfred GI Unit, 200 1st Street South West, Rochester MN 55905, USA
* Corresponding author.
E-mail address: Wang.kenneth@mayo.edu

Gastroenterol Clin N Am 51 (2022) 457–484
https://doi.org/10.1016/j.gtc.2022.06.005
0889-8553/22/© 2022 Elsevier Inc. All rights reserved.

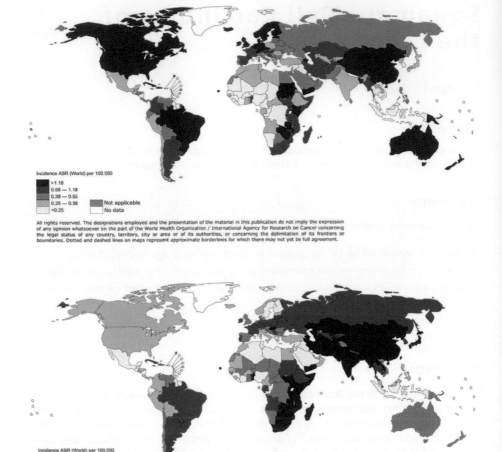

Incidence ASR (World) per 100,000
- ■ >1.18
- ■ 0.55 — 1.18
- ■ 0.38 — 0.55
- ■ 0.25 — 0.38
- □ <0.25
- ■ Not applicable
- □ No data

Incidence ASR (World) per 100,000
- ■ >3.5
- ■ 2.1 — 3.5
- ■ 1.3 — 2.1
- ■ 0.8 — 1.3
- □ <0.8
- ■ Not applicable
- □ No data

Fig. 1. Incidence of esophageal squamous cell carcinoma. (WHO 2019. All rights reserved.)

exceeding 125/100,000.[5] For perspective, from 2014 to 2018, the incidence of esophageal adenocarcinoma in the United States was 4.2/100,000.[2] In these high incidence areas, the epidemiology of the disease also changes becoming more evenly divided between genders and less related to environmental exposures such alcohol or tobacco use.

Mortality outcomes for ESCC are quite bleak, with 5-year mortality rates well less than 20% (and likely significantly lower in developing nations whereby the burden of ESCC is disproportionately high).[6] Five-year survival rates exceed 50% in early-stage disease, but unfortunately, more than 75% of ESCC is diagnosed at either stage III or IV.[7]

Risk factors for ESCC are distinct from those for adenocarcinoma (**Table 1**). Traditional risk factors include tobacco use and alcohol, though in several regions whereby the ESCC incidence is high, these substances are rarely used due to cultural and

Table 1	
Risk factor for esophageal squamous cell carcinoma	
Risk Factor	**Increase in Risk (Compared with General Population)**
Alcohol	2-9x
Tobacco	2-4x
Consumption of Hot Beverages	1.5–2.5x
Low Fruit Intake	2x
High Pickled Vegetable Intake	2x
Low Socioeconomic Status	2-4x
Esophageal Lichen Planus	Up to 6.1% of all affected
Tylosis	Up to 80% of all affected

religious beliefs. Regardless, the development of squamous cell carcinoma precursor lesions has been associated with a smoking history of greater than 20 years (odds ratio: 1.48), alcohol use of more than 30 years (odds ratio: 1.40), and daily alcohol intake of greater than 100 cc (odds ratio: 1.44).[8] Former and current smoking tobacco use is associated with a 2- to 4-fold increased risk of ESCC compared with never smokers,[9] while alcohol use results in a 2- to 9-fold increased risk of ESCC compared with nondrinkers.[10,11]

The intake of scalding hot beverages has been postulated to induce inflammatory processes in the esophagus stimulating the endogenous formation of reactive nitrogen species, causing specific TP53 mutations that have been found in patients with ESCC.[12,13] Furthermore, thermal injury may result in loss of the esophageal barrier function permitting increased exposure of carcinogenic substances.[14] Consequently, population-based studies have demonstrated increased ESCC risk in patients who consume hot tea, coffee, and mate.[12] The effects of multiple risk factors are likely synergistic. A prospective cohort study based on 10 geographic regions in China demonstrated that patients with greater than 15 g of alcohol intake and daily "burning" hot tea had 5 times the odds of ESCC development compared with those without increased alcohol or hot tea intake.[15] Mate is composed of a significant amount of polycyclic aromatic hydrocarbons which may also increase the risk of ESCC.[16,17]

The association of nitrosamines to the development of ESCC has also been found in populations with endemic pickled vegetable intake. Due to fermentation, a relatively high percentage of nitrosamines are formed during the pickling process. A meta-analysis of 34 studies incorporating data from more than 225,000 patients demonstrated an odds ratio of 2.08 for those with excess pickled vegetable intake compared with those with lower intake.[18] Low fruit intake may also be associated with ESCC.[19,20] Oxidative stress mediated via iron overload, also known as African iron overload, or Bantu siderosis may play a role in carcinogenesis as this condition has been associated with ESCC in sub-Saharan Africa.[21]

Unskilled laborers were found to have a 2.1-fold increased risk of ESCC compared with skilled professionals in a Swedish population-based database, highlighting the increased risk of ESCC in those from lower socioeconomic backgrounds.[22] Furthermore, those without a life partner were found to have doubled the risk of ESCC in this same cohort.[22] Less well-established risk factors for the development of ESCC include radiation and agrochemical exposure, excess fried food intake, sedentary lifestyle, and low fiber intake.[23]

Other medical conditions may increase the risk of ESCC, likely through chronic inflammatory pathways. Esophageal lichen planus is associated with the development of ESCC in up to 6.1% of patients.[24] Tylosis or hyperkeratosis palmaris et plantaris is a rare but autosomal dominant genetic disease marked by aberrations of the RHBDF2 gene resulting in a significant risk of ESCC of at least 80% in a small kindred.[25,26] Human papillomavirus has also been associated with the development of ESCC.[27]

PATHOGENESIS

The dysplasia-carcinoma sequence is believed to mediate the transition from normal esophageal squamous epithelium to ESCC. Squamous dysplasia is associated with nuclear atypia, loss of normal cell polarity, and abnormal tissue maturation without invasion through the basement membrane.[28] Although early retrospective studies suggested that esophagitis was a risk factor for ESCC, subsequent studies determined that esophageal squamous cell dysplasia was the only histopathologic factor associated with a high risk of ESCC.[29] Prospective studies further demonstrated that the risk of ESCC increased with higher grades of dysplasia (**Table 2**), and confirmed that dysplasia is the only known precursor lesion of ESCC.[30,31]

The stepwise progression from normal squamous epithelium to ESCC can be followed histologically from basal cell hyperplasia (BCH), to mild dysplasia, moderate dysplasia, severe dysplasia, carcinoma in situ (CIS), and invasive carcinoma. This scheme has subsequently been revised by the World Health Organization (WHO) with mild to moderate dysplasia classified as low-grade intraepithelial neoplasia (LGIEN), and severe dysplasia or CIS classified as high-grade intraepithelial neoplasia (HGIEN).[32]

A significant number of genetic markers have been identified that underlie the dysplasia-carcinoma sequence. High-level amplification of several oncogenes, including *CCND1, FGF3/4/19, SOX2,* and *EGFR* have been associated with malignant transformation, as well as homozygous deletions of tumor suppressor genes such as *CDKN2A* and *CDKN2B*.[33] Furthermore, sequence analysis of ESCC tumors have identified several significantly mutated genes that drive carcinogenesis, including the tumor suppressor genes *TP53* and *NOTCH1,* as well as the oncogene *NFE2L2*.[34–37] Indeed, mutations in *TP53* may be found in up to 80% of all ESCC.[38] Several genetic mutations may impart prognostic information, as alterations of *FAM135 B* and *TET2* are associated with poor survival.[34,39]

Epigenetic factors have also been extensively studied in the pathogenesis of ESCC. Several of the previously mentioned genes, including *CDKN2A* and *TFF1* may be hypermethylated in ESCC and may indicate early-stage disease. Epigenetic factors

Table 2
Risk of ESCC transformation based on the degree of dysplasia

Dysplasia Grade	WHO 2010 Classification	OR (95% CI) of ESCC
Basal Cell Hyperplasia	IEN	2.1 (0.4–9.8)
Mild Dysplasia	LGIEN	2.2 (0.7–7.5)
Moderate Dysplasia		15.8 (5.9–42.2)
Severe Dysplasia	HGIEN	72.6 (29.8–176.9)

IEN: intraepithelial neoplasia; low-grade intraepithelial neoplasia; high-grade intraepithelial neoplasia (also includes carcinoma *in situ*).

may also impart prognostication, as inactivation and methylation of the *CDKN2* tumor suppressor gene are associated with advanced-stage disease.[40,41]

The transformation of dysplasia to ESCC is likely mediated by a step-wise approach involving many of the above genetic and epigenetic aberrations (**Fig. 2**). Mutations in *TP53, NOTCH1, CDKN2A, EP300,* and *MLL2* are likely early mediators of the dysplasia sequence given their presence in basal cell hyperplasia and persistence in higher grades of dysplasia and cancer.[42] However, the true cascade of events (and exact pathogenesis) of ESCC development remains under intense study.

Risk factors for ESCC are likely implicated in the rapid development of genetic aberrations that can lead to malignancy. Alcohol is directly toxic to the epithelium which may allow for further direct toxic damage from persistent alcohol use, and exposure to other carcinogenic environmental factors.[43] Byproducts of alcohol metabolism, namely acetaldehyde, may further contribute to genetic abnormalities through DNA adduct formation, resulting in aberrant gene methylation.[44] Alcohol-associated methylation and inhibition of several key pathways, including *NOTCH, PI3K/AKT,* and *WNT* signaling pathways may then drive the pathogenesis of ESCC.[45] Variant copies of *ALDH2,* which are present in most East Asian populations, result in decreased metabolism of acetaldehyde and may partly explain the increased risk of ESCC noted in this region.[46]

Tobacco is associated with an increased risk of ESCC as previously mentioned and smoked tobacco is associated with at least 60 carcinogenic compounds.[47] The specific pathogenesis involved is likely multifactorial. Research has demonstrated that tobacco smoke increases the levels of acetaldehyde in saliva, and as previously

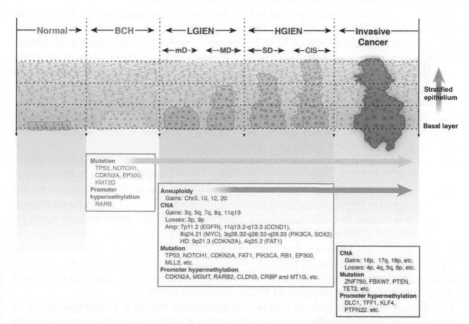

Fig. 2. Molecular progression of esophageal squamous precancerous lesions to ESCC. BCH, basal cell hyperplasia; HGIEN, high-grade intraepithelial neoplasia; LGIEN, low-grade intraepithelial neoplasia. (*From* Lin DC, Wang MR, Koeffler HP. Genomic and Epigenomic Aberrations in Esophageal Squamous Cell Carcinoma and Implications for Patients. Gastroenterology. 2018;154(2):374–389. https://doi.org/10.1053/j.gastro.2017.06.066; with permission)

demonstrated, this could result in downregulation of important cell signaling pathways that can lead to ESCC.[48] Tobacco smoke (particularly nicotine) may activate the *EGFR* tyrosine kinase in esophageal tissue resulting in diminished apoptosis, promotion of angiogenesis, and enhanced invasion capabilities.[49] DNA adduct formation can also occur with tobacco smoking resulting in the inactivation of the tumor suppressor *FHIT* gene, further promoting carcinogenesis.[50]

DIAGNOSIS

Patients may not have any symptoms when presenting with ESCC and may be diagnosed incidentally through testing conducted for other indications, or through screening programs in high-risk regions. However, patients with locally advanced disease may have dysphagia, initially with solid foods and progressing to liquids as tumor growth obliterates the esophageal lumen. Indeed, prediagnosis dysphagia is a reliable predictor of at least T3/T4 advanced disease.[51] Some patients may report heartburn, dyspepsia, or cough, though these symptoms are nonspecific. Hematemesis is an uncommon initial presenting sign of ESCC but may occur, and in some patients, occult or overt lower GI bleeding may be present. In rare cases, tumor ingrowth can lead to the formation of a tracheobronchial fistula.[52] Patients with metastatic disease may also exhibit significant weight loss, fatigue, low-grade fevers, and failure to thrive.

Barium esophagography may demonstrate an esophageal mass causing luminal obstruction or stricture. Computed tomography may show the presence of esophageal wall thickening or mass, and may provide staging information assessing for regional lymphadenopathy, as well as liver or lung metastases.

The gold standard for diagnosis of ESCC involves histopathologic confirmation of malignant tissue obtained typically during esophagogastroduodenoscopy (EGD). The endoscopic appearance of ESCC can vary markedly, from subtle nodularity that can easily be missed to large, friable, fungating masses completely obstructing the esophageal lumen. ESCC classically is found in the upper or mid-esophagus, in comparison to adenocarcinoma, which is typically found in the distal third. Bronchoscopy may be required for proximal tumors above the carina especially if there is suspicion of a tracheoesophageal fistula. Endoscopic ultrasound (EUS) can be used to assess for regional lymphadenopathy, and the use of a linear echoendoscope allows for tissue sampling of any suspicious lymph nodes.

Several techniques can be used to enhance the visual detection of abnormalities that are found in ESCC and squamous dysplasia. Narrow-band imaging (NBI) is an optical technique in which 3 specific wavelengths (under the blue light spectrum) are used to observe in detail the capillary system of tissues.[53] When coupled with magnification, irregularities in the intrapapillary capillary loop (IPCL) structure can highlight suspicious areas. Superficial carcinoma may demonstrate the dilation and elongation of IPCLs, and invasive disease has been associated with ectatic, irregularly branched IPCLs. These visual criteria on NBI are widely used in Japan in the initial staging of ESCC.[54] Studies have demonstrated sensitivity and specificity rates ranging from 75% to 100% in the identification of ESCC when using NBI.[55,56]

Lugol's solution composed of iodine and potassium iodide preferentially binds to glycogen in nonkeratinized tissue. Normal squamous epithelium of the esophagus absorbs the solution resulting in a dark-brown or black discoloration of the mucosa. Dysplastic or malignant cells have low levels of glycogen and will not have significant uptake of this solution. Use of Lugol's solution during endoscopy can help detect and demarcate areas of dysplasia and early ESCC allowing for targeted biopsies or endoscopic resection (**Fig. 3**).[57]

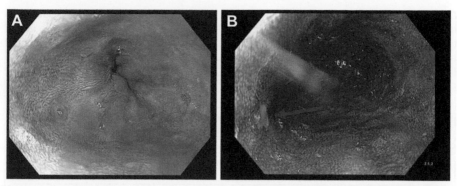

Fig. 3. Endoscopic images of Lugol's staining. (*A*) Lugol's solution was applied to the lower third of the esophagus highlighting uniform uptake. (*B*) An area of poor uptake, due to decreased glycogen in dysplastic cells, is identified. Biopsies from this region showed low-grade squamous dysplasia.

The sensitivity and specificity of chromoendoscopy with Lugol's is comparable to NBI and superior to high definition white light endoscopy (HD-WLE).[55] Importantly, false-positive Lugol's unstained lesions may be found in regenerative squamous tissue (for instance, tissue that may have previously undergone ablation) or in tissue with significant inflammation.[58]

Invasive ESCC is marked by tumor invasion into the lamina propria and deeper layers. Pathology hallmarks of ESCC include keratinization, and "tumor budding." Tumors can range from well to poorly differentiated histopathology based on nuclear atypia and basal cell layer abnormalities.[59] Characteristics of well-differentiated tumors include keratin pearls, individual cell keratinization, and intercellular bridges which are absent on poorly differentiated specimens.[60] Squamous dysplasia and/or carcinoma *in situ* may be found at the periphery of resected tumor specimens. Immunohistochemical staining for *P63, cytokeratin 5/6, MUC5AC,* and *AGH2* distinguish ESCC from esophageal adenocarcinoma.[61] A spindle-cell subtype of ESCC has been identified that is associated with grossly polypoid tissue, and has a slightly improved survival compared with traditional ESCC.[62] Other morphologic subtypes of ESCC include: basaloid ESCC (predominant basal cell layer changes including oval, hyperchromatic nuclei, scant cytoplasm, and solid nests with peripheral palisading); verrucous carcinoma (papillary tumor with mild cellular atypia in the basal cell layers, and may have a broad pushing front without significant metastatic potential); and carcinosarcoma (features of malignant spindle and epithelial cells with possible mesenchymal differentiation).[60]

Screening for ESCC has been suggested in high-risk regions and populations. This is discussed in the "Controversies" section of this article.

PROGNOSIS

Staging of ESCC is the most significant predictor of disease prognosis. Formal conventions following American Joint Committee on Cancer guidelines are typically used for staging (**Tables 3** and **4**) based on tumor invasion (T), lymph node involvement (N), and metastatic spread (M).[63] Staging may involve computed tomography, which is most helpful for identifying liver or lung metastases, but typically is completed with positron emission tomography (PET) to assess the distal spread of tumor. EUS

Table 3
Cancer staging categories for cancer of the esophagus and esophagogastric junction

Category	Criteria
T catorgory	
TX	Tumor cannot be assessed
T0	No evidence of primary tumor
Tis	High-grade dysplasia, defined as malignant cells confined by the basement membrane
T1	Tumor invades the lamina propria, muscularis mucosae, or submucosa
T1a[a]	Tumor invades the lamina propria or muscularis mucosae
T1b[a]	Tumor invades the submucosa
T2	Tumor invades the muscularis propria
T3	Tumor invades adventitia
T4	Tumor invades adjacent structures
T4a[a]	Tumor invades the pleura, pericardium, azygos vein, diaphragm, or peritoneum
T4b[a]	Tumor invades other adjacent structures, such as aorta, vertebral body, or trachea
N category	
NX	Regional lymph nodes cannot be assessed
N0	No regional lymph node metastasis
N1	Metastasis in 1–2 regional lymph nodes
N2	Metastasis in 3–6 regional lymph nodes
N3	Metastasis in 7 or more regional lymph nodes
M category	
M0	No distant metastasis
M1	Distant metastasis
Adenocarcinoma G Category	
GX	Differentiation cannot be assessed
G1	Well-differentiated.> 95% of tumor is composed of well-formed glands
G2	Moderately differentiated. 50% to 95% of tumor shows gland formation
G3[b]	Poorly differentiated. Tumors composed of nest and sheets of cells with <50% of tumor demonstrating glandular formation
Squamous cell carcinoma G category	
GX	Differentiation cannot be assessed
G1	Well-differentiated. Prominent keratinization with pearl formation and a minor component of nonkeratinizing basal-like cells. Tumor cells are arranged in sheets, and mitotic counts are low
G2	Moderately differentiated. Variable histologic features, ranging from parakeratotic to poorly keratinizing lesions. Generally, pearl formation is absent
G3[c]	Poorly differentiated. Consists predominantly of basal-like cells forming large and small nests with frequent central necrosis. The nests consist of sheets or pavement-like arrangements of tumor cells, and occasionally are punctuated by small numbers of parakeratotic or keratinizing cells
Squamous cell carcinoma L category[d]	
LX	Location unknown

(continued on next page)

Table 3 (continued)	
Category	**Criteria**
Upper	Cervical esophagus to lower border of azygos vein
Middle	Lower border of azygos vein to lower border of inferior pulmonary vein
Lower	Lower border of inferior pulmonary vein to stomach, including esophagogastric junction

[a] Subcategories.
[b] If further testing of "undifferentiated" cancers reveals a glandular component, categorize it as adenocarcinoma G3.
[c] If further testing of "undifferentiated" cancers reveals a squamous cell component, or if after further testing they remain undifferentiated, categorize as squamous cell carcinoma G3.
[d] Location is defined by the epicenter of esophageal tumor.

can determine the depth of tumor invasion and may assess regional lymphadenopathy if the distant spread is not apparent. Survival by stage of diagnosis is shown in **Table 5**. Five-year survival for patients with advanced-stage disease (stages III/IV) is less than 15%.[2,7] Risk factors associated with poor survival regardless of stage at

Table 4 AJCC clinical staging groups, 8th edition			
cStage Froup	**cT**	**cN**	**cM**
Squamous cell carcinoma			
0	Tis	N0	M0
I	T1	N0-1	M0
II	T2	N0-1	M0
	T3	N0	M0
III	T3	N1	M0
	T1-3	N2	M0
IVA	T4	N0-2	M0
	T1-4	N3	M0
IVB	T1-4	N0-3	M1
Adenocarcinoma			
0	Tis	N0	M0
I	T1	N0	M0
IIA	T1	N1	M0
IIB	T2	N0	M0
III	T2	N1	M0
	T3-4a	N0-1	M0
IVA	T1-4a	N2	M0
	T4b	N0-2	M0
	T1-4	N3	M0
IVB	T1-4	N0-3	M1

diagnosis include male gender, age more than 65 at diagnosis, and family history of esophageal cancer.[7,64] A significant difference between ESCC and esophageal adenocarcinoma is the finding that ESCC may skip adjacent lymph nodes and metastasize to more distant lymph nodes (nodal skip metastasis).[65]

CLINICAL MANAGEMENT
Early disease

Carcinoma *in situ* and T1a/T1b lesions without regional lymphadenopathy may be definitively treated via endoscopic techniques such as endoscopic mucosal resection (**Fig. 4**) or endoscopic submucosal dissection (**Fig. 5**). However, the role of endoscopic resection in the management of healthy patients with T1b lesions is somewhat controversial and will be discussed in greater detail in the "Controversies" section of this article. Patients undergoing endoscopic resection should be healthy enough to undergo general anesthesia. A staging endoscopic ultrasound is typically conducted to determine tumor depth of invasion and exclude deep involvement which would preclude endoscopic resection. Marking of the lesion of interest is conducted typically with argon plasma coagulation or a resection knife. This step assists the proceduralist in identifying the lesion during resection when viewing planes may be inhibited by bleeding and/or smoke, and to ensure clear margins. Typically, a solution of methylene blue or indigo carmine, combined with a viscous lifting agent is injected into the submucosa to assess whether the lesion "lifts," that is, separates the esophageal mucosa and submucosa from deeper layers. Evidence of poor lifting indicates a degree of invasion into the deeper layers of the esophageal wall and may preclude endoscopic resection. Poor lifting may also indicate fibrosis from prior extensive biopsies or resection, or history of previous radiation, which can result in a technically more difficult procedure with increased risk of bleeding and perforation.

Cap-assisted endoscopic mucosal resection (cEMR) uses a hard cap with a single-use snare seated on an inner ring on the distal aspect of the cap or a hard cap with a modified banding kit allowing for the multiband resection of larger lesions.

After the adequate lift, the lesion is suctioned into the hard cap, and in the single-use device the snare is closed. When using a multiband device, a band is deployed to capture the lesion, and the snare is usually closed below the band to allow a wider resection area. Electrosurgical current is then applied to resect the lesion. The resection bed is examined carefully, and removal of any residual tissue can then be performed.

Endoscopic submucosal dissection (ESD) is an alternative technique that allows for *en bloc* resection of lesions. ESD requires adequate lifting of the lesion of interest. Various electrosurgical knives may be used to dissect the submucosa and proceed

Table 5	
5-year overall survival by stage of diagnosis	
Stage 0	52.7%
Stage 1	44.2%
Stage 2	27.5%
Stage 3	15.6%
Stage 4	3.4%

Adapted from Cheng YF, Chen HS, Wu SC, et al. Esophageal squamous cell carcinoma and prognosis in Taiwan. Cancer Med. 2018;7(9):4193–4201. https://doi.org/10.1002/cam4.1499; with permission.

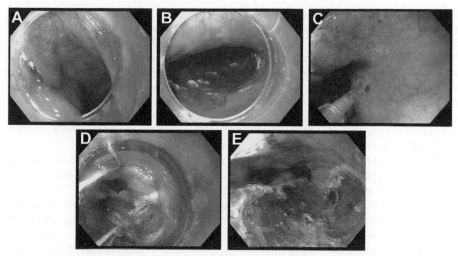

Fig. 4. Cap-assisted endoscopic mucosal resection. (*A*). An area of tissue suspicious for esophageal squamous cell cancer is identified on narrow-band imaging. (*B*). The area is marked with cautery. (*C*). Using a stained lifting agent, the mucosa is separated from the submucosa to prepare for resection. (*D*). The Duette Multiband Mucosectomy Device (Cook Medical, Bloomington, IN) is attached to the endoscope and resection proceeds with the removal of the entire suspicious area. Tissue is suctioned into the cap and a band is released, capturing the involved tissue, followed by the utilization of a snare with electrosurgical current to cut the banded tissue. (*E*). Resection bed following complete removal of lesion. Pathology demonstrated carcinoma-in-situ.

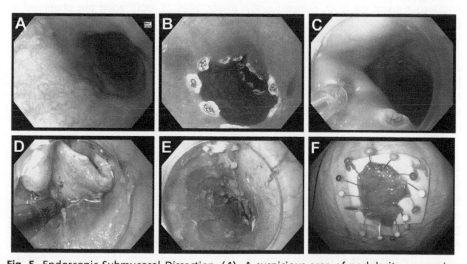

Fig. 5. Endoscopic Submucosal Dissection. (*A*). A suspicious area of nodularity concerning squamous cell carcinoma is identified. (*B*). The area is marked with cautery. (*C*). Using a stained lifting agent, the mucosa is separated from the submucosa to prepare for resection. (*D*). Dissection of the lesion proceeds using several electrosurgical knives. (*E*). The resection bed after complete removal of the lesion. (*F*) Final pinned specimen after removal of the lesion. Pathology revealed squamous cell carcinoma *in situ*.

with careful dissection of the mucosal and submucosal layers from the muscularis propria (see **Fig. 5**). Once the entire lesion has been removed, the resection bed is inspected, and hemostasis can be achieved via coagulation, clipping, or suturing.

Both cEMR and ESD may result in R0, curative resection of early-stage disease, and save patients from undergoing esophagectomy which carries its own morbidities and adverse outcomes. However, there are specific differences between these 2 techniques that must be carefully discussed between the proceduralist and patient. Of note, no head-to-head trials involving these techniques have been completed for the management of early-stage ESCC, but meta-analyses provide some indication of the efficacy and differences between these 2 techniques.

ESD is a technically challenging procedure and requires more extensive training compared with cEMR. Estimates of the number of procedures needed to achieve proficiency may be as high as 250 for ESD compared with 25 for cEMR.[66,67] The optimal paradigm for ESD training may include: practice in *ex vivo* porcine models, observerships in high volume ESD centers, experience in third space endoscopy and other advanced endoscopic techniques, and finally, hands-on training in human subjects.[68] In comparison, cEMR training is more widely available and may be accomplished during gastroenterology fellowship training.

ESD is associated with significantly longer procedure times compared with cEMR, with a weighted mean difference of approximately 45 minutes.[69] Overall rates of complications of both ESD and cEMR are rare, and occur in less than 5% of cases.[69,70] Rates of perforation appear to be approximately 2 times higher in ESD compared with cEMR. Rates of bleeding and stricture formation do not seem to differ between these techniques. Variations of ESD that use submucosal tunneling followed by circumferential dissection have been shown to decrease procedural time without increasing complications.

Overall, *en bloc* resection and R0 resection can be achieved at a significantly higher rate in ESD compared with cEMR.[69] This is likely due to the ability to resect broader and larger areas via ESD. Subsequently, lower rates of recurrence are observed in ESD compared with cEMR.[69] What is unclear at this time, however, is whether the differences in these outcomes result in improved cancer-free survival or morbidity.

It is important to note that, in a retrospective study of 171 cases of ESCC treated by cEMR or ESD, the rate of *en bloc* resection and local recurrence were equivalent for lesions measuring < 1.5 cm. cEMR, therefore, may be a reasonable alternative to ESD for the management of small lesions measuring < 1.5 cm.[71] ESD is recommended for larger lesions as it allows for *en bloc* resection and accurate histopathologic staging with the assessment of both lateral and deep margins, which improves the prognostication of cancer and may influence further management.

Locoregional disease

If the involvement of ESCC is beyond the submucosa, but without direct extension into the heart, great vessels, trachea, lungs, (T1b–T4a lesions) or evidence of metastatic disease, esophagectomy may be the procedure of choice for definitive management. Bulky lymphadenopathy may also preclude surgical management. Staging laparoscopy with peritoneal washings is typically recommended in patients with T3 or N+ disease as the presence of positive peritoneal cytology would confirm metastatic disease and preclude surgery. In patients who may require enteral feedings, surgical placement of a percutaneous jejunal feeding tube is recommended over endoscopic placement to prevent tumor seeding. Percutaneous gastric tube placement is not recommended as this may compromise the ability of the stomach to act as a conduit if surgical intervention is eventually pursued. Oftentimes, a multidisciplinary approach with input from medical oncology, surgery, gastroenterology, nutrition, and radiation oncology is recommended before finalizing a definitive management plan.

Surgery

There are a number of approaches for the surgical resection of ESCC and the particular method used will depend in part on surgeon experience, patient preference, and location of the tumor. In all patients without preoperative chemoradiotherapy, lymph node excision is performed with the removal of at least 20 nodes in 2 or 3 fields (mediastinal, upper abdominal, cervical) to evaluate for nodal metastases. An increase in excised nodes is associated with improved disease-specific survival.[72] Conduits (that is, tissue to connect the uninvolved proximal esophagus to the digestive tract after removal of the malignant portion) can be accomplished with the stomach, colon, or small bowel.

Ivor-Lewis esophagogastrectomy is a two-stage procedure in which a midline laparotomy is utilized to prepare the (typically gastric) conduit followed by right thoracotomy to mobilize and resect the esophagus and proceed with lymphadenectomy. Minimally invasive approaches can also be utilized. This procedure is best for tumors in the mid-lower third of the esophagus as proximal anastomoses are difficult to create via laparotomy.

McKeown (tri-incisional) esophagogastrectomy is similar to the Ivor-Lewis surgery but a third step involving a cervical incision is added to create the esophago-conduit anastomosis in the proximal esophagus. A minimally invasive approach may also be used. The McKeown Esophagogastrectomy is used in proximal tumors whereby an anastomosis cannot be created via thoracotomy or laparotomy. Given the cervical anastomosis, there is a greater risk of damage to the recurrent laryngeal nerve in addition to a higher risk of pulmonary complications.[73]

A transhiatal approach with a cervical incision for the creation of the anastomosis can be used but is limited by poor access to lymph nodes. The addition of thoracoscopy and other maneuvers can result in successful lymph node dissection. The transhiatal approach may be an option for patients with early-stage disease or those with disease amenable to endoscopic therapy but who prefer surgical management. For distal esophageal tumors, a single left thoracoabdominal approach can be used but requires a large incision (modified Ivor Lewis esophagectomy). This approach is associated with increased reflux due to the intraabdominal position of the anastomosis.

It is important to emphasize that not all surgical options are appropriate for all patients, and patient preference, surgeon/center experience, and tumor characteristics all impact the ultimate therapeutic option pursued. To that end, regardless of approach, negative circumferential margins are associated with improved overall survival, and those with positive margins have a 2 to 4 times higher odds of death within 5 years of surgery compared with those with negative margins.[74]

A cervical anastomosis may be associated with a higher rate of leaks and trauma to the recurrent laryngeal nerve compared with thoracic anastomosis, but outcomes regarding recurrence, perioperative morbidity, stricture formation, and pulmonary complications seem to be equal.[75]

Pyloromyotomy during surgery has been advocated to reduce the risk of postoperative gastric outlet obstruction (GOO), but results have been mixed. A nonrandomized large prospective study of 242 patients demonstrated no difference in GOO between patients with pyloromyotomy compared with those without. A meta-analysis of 4 studies with 533 patients demonstrated no difference in GOO rates between groups.[76,77]

Neoadjuvant therapy

Patients with good performance status and resectable disease may benefit from preoperative chemoradiotherapy. In a randomized controlled trial, patients treated with a

5-week course of carboplatin/paclitaxel demonstrated superior median survival compared with those receiving upfront surgery (49.4 months vs 24.0 months).[78] This regimen was well tolerated with less than 10% experiencing any significant side effects. Fluorouracil with oxaliplatin, irinotecan with cisplatin, and paclitaxel with fluoropyrimidine are other combinations that can be used as alternative neoadjuvant therapies. Please see the "Controversies" section within this article for greater detail regarding neoadjuvant therapies.

Metastatic and unresectable disease

The chemotherapeutic management of ESCC is complex and is reviewed in the guidelines published by the National Comprehensive Cancer Network (NCCN).[79] Preferred regimens for patients requiring definitive chemotherapy for the management of ESCC include paclitaxel with carboplatin, fluorouracil with oxaliplatin, or fluorouracil with cisplatin, combined with or without radiation therapy. All of these regimens are associated with improved survival compared with placebo.[78,80,81] A three-drug cytotoxic drug regimen (docetaxel, cisplatin, and fluorouracil) was compared with a two-drug regimen (cisplatin and fluorouracil) in a randomized study of 445 patients. The three-drug group had a significant increase in overall and 2-year survival.[82] However, this same group also had a significantly higher rate of grade 3/4 toxicities (40%–90%) compared with the two-drug group (10%–20%). Therefore, a two-drug regimen is usually preferred, but a three-drug regimen may be considered in patients with excellent health and high-performance status. Irinotecan-based therapies, typically coadministered with cisplatin or docetaxel, have also shown modest efficacy (comparable to cisplatin and fluorouracil), with manageable side effects.[83,84] Capecitabine and oxaliplatin, which may have a favorable side effect profiles when compared with cisplatin-based therapies, have also demonstrated efficacy in the management of metastatic disease with noninferior 1-year survival.[85]

Molecule targeting agents and immunotherapies

The understanding of carcinogenesis pathways has led to the identification of specific molecular targets for the management of a variety of cancers, including ESCC. Epidermal growth factor receptor (EGFR) overexpression has been identified in up to 33% of all ESCC and thus targeted therapies have been studied extensively in ESCC. One of the first studied drugs, Gefitinib, an EGFR inhibitor, showed no significant improvement in survival when compared with placebo in patients undergoing salvage therapy.[86] Several other EGFR inhibitors (cetuximab, panitumumab, and nimotuzumab), have shown efficacy with 3 to 4 months improved survival compared with cisplatin-based therapies.[87–89] HER2 status has also been evaluated as a potential therapeutic target given overexpression in ESCC. Trastuzumab, a HER2 inhibitor, has an acceptable safety profile when used in combination with traditional chemotherapy regimens.[90,91]

More recent developments in cancer therapeutics include immunotherapies to target the dysregulation of immune checkpoint inhibitors resulting in carcinogenesis. Nivolumab, a programmed cell death 1 (PD-L1) inhibitor, demonstrated prolonged survival and therapeutic efficacy in an open-label trial of 65 patients who failed first-line therapy.[92] This drug may be used after surgery with R0 margins, resulting in improved survival compared with those who received placebo.[93] Pembrolizumab, a similar PD-L1 inhibitor, has also demonstrated considerable efficacy in patients who failed first-line therapy.[94] Other immune checkpoint inhibitors that have shown promise in phase I/II trials include camrelizumab and tislelizumab.[95,96]

The Combined Positive Score (CPS) was developed to assess the prognostication of therapy success for PD-L1 inhibitors. This score is a percent of PD-L1 cells divided by viable tumor cells seen on histopathology. Pembrolizumab, as second-line therapy in patients with CPS scores greater than 10, was associated with significantly longer overall survival compared with traditional chemotherapy.[97] However, the CPS may not be a reliable predictor of response to therapy as the recent Checkmate-577 study showed no difference in survival based on PD-L1 expression whereby nivolumab was studied for use as adjuvant therapy in resected disease.[93]

Other targets of immune checkpoint inhibitors include cytotoxic T lymphocyte-associated protein 4 (CTLA-4), which is involved in the regulatory functioning of T-cells. Appropriate manipulation of this target by drugs such as ipilimumab may mediate T-cell destruction of tumor cells, and studies show promising results regarding overall survival but not progression-free, survival.[98]

Radiotherapy

Radiotherapy of ESCC seems efficacious when used as an adjunct to chemotherapy-based regimens. Treatment is usually given in a fractionated dose of 40 to 50 gray to encompass all known diseases and one nodal field beyond. Studies have demonstrated that refinements in radiation delivery, such as intensity-modulated radiotherapy, result in prolonged survival, fewer cancer-related deaths, and fewer side effects compared with traditional delivery methods.[99] Proton-beam therapy has further improved overall outcomes and safety profiles by allowing a highly targeted radiation dose with minimal effects on surrounding tissues when compared with intensity-modulated radiotherapy.[100]

For further detail on the role of radiotherapy in neoadjuvant therapy, please see the corresponding section in the "Controversies" section.

DISEASE COMPLICATIONS
Pretreatment complications

As previously discussed, patients may present with dysphagia indicating an obstructing lesion. This can result in significant malnutrition and weight loss, which can be severe enough to require enteral feedings, either in the form of nasogastric or percutaneous feeding tube placement, to optimize patient status before more definitive therapy. Sinusitis has been reported in up to 16% of patients with nasogastric tubes in an intensive care unit setting although it may be less common in other settings.,[101] Percutaneous feeding tubes may result in other complications including buried bumper syndrome, malpositioning, soft tissue infections, and tube leakage. Despite these complications, enteral feeding is generally well tolerated with serious adverse events occurring in less than 5% to 10% of patients on long-term therapy.[102] Rare cases of tumor ingrowth into surrounding tissues include the formation of esophagotracheal or esophagobronchial fistula which can result in infectious pulmonary complications.

Posttreatment complications

Endoscopic therapy for early disease (CIS, T1 tumors) is well tolerated, though significant adverse events such as strictures, bleeding, and perforation can occur. Of these, clinically significant strictures resulting in dysphagia can occur in 5% to 15% of cases.[103,104] Risk factors for stricture formation include the resection of lesions occupying greater than 75% of the esophageal circumference, longer than 3 cm, and with deep submucosal invasion.[104,105] Steroid injection at the time of resection as well as short courses of oral steroids postprocedure have been shown to reduce stricture formation.[106,107] Clinically significant bleeding requiring blood transfusion or hospital admission, and perforation occur less frequently in approximately 1% to 2% of all endoscopic resection procedures.[108,109] Although there is not a statistically significant difference in the overall complication rates of ESD and cEMR, there is a significantly higher risk of perforation with ESD.[69]

Surgical complications more frequently occur in elderly patients, as well as those with renal, hepatic, or pulmonary disease.[110] Anastomotic leaks occur in up to 25% of procedures and are more commonly seen in cases of cervical anastomoses. Frank dehiscence is exceedingly rare.[111] Patients with transthoracic/transhiatal anastomoses have leak rates of approximately 10%.[112] Anastomotic strictures can complicate approximately 30% of all esophagectomy procedures and typically can be managed with endoscopic balloon dilatation. In cases of anastomotic strictures, it is important to rule out recurrent cancer with careful inspection and targeted biopsies.[113] Aspiration may occur in 10%–15% of all esophagectomies, with cervical anastomoses further associated with higher risks of pneumonia and empyema.[114] Fistula formation to the airways is rare and may occur in less than 1% of all procedures. This complication seems to be manageable, with small case reports detailing fistula closure rates of 100% after 1.6 years.[115] Dumping syndrome with both early and late manifestations can occur in up to 20% of surgeries, although widely varying incidence rates have been reported.[116]

Previous neoadjuvant therapy is believed to play a role in conduit ischemia, but published reports have been conflicting.[117–119] Conduit ischemia is believed to impact the rate of anastomotic stricture development, which can occur in up to 40% of cases. Most of these cases can be managed with endoscopic dilation. Creation of the anastomosis with a modified Collard or hybrid staple technique is associated with lower rates of stricturing.[120,121]

Chyle leaks from traumatic injury to the thoracic duct occur in less than 10% of surgeries and are associated with significant morbidity and mortality.[122] These are typically identified by the presence of milky white drainage from chest tubes placed at the time of surgery. The management includes *nil per os* status, parenteral nutrition, and octreotide, but may require surgical intervention if no improvement occurs after several days.

In an analysis of nearly 12,000 patients from the Society for Thoracic Surgery database, overall morbidity occurred in approximately 50% of patients within 30 days of surgery, including 10% requiring reoperation, of which a quarter of these was for conduit necrosis. Other complications included sepsis (24%), myocardial infarction (33%), and acute respiratory distress syndrome (37%). Thirty-day mortality in this series was 3.3%.[123] As mentioned previously, the McKeown (tri-incisional) esophagectomy has been associated with higher morbidity and mortality, possibly mediated by the addition of cervical dissection.[73] Perioperative mortality is typically less than 10% to 15%, with likely improved outcomes in selected patients undergoing minimally invasive, robotic procedures.[73,124–126]

Chemoradiotherapy-induced strictures requiring endoscopic intervention can occur in up to 75% of all patients. In a series of patients receiving definitive management of ESCC, strictures occurred in 52% of patients receiving chemoradiotherapy, and in 76% receiving radiotherapy alone.[127] Cervical location of the primary esophageal tumor is an independent risk factor for severe stricture formation after chemoradiotherapy.[128]

CONTROVERSIES
Screening

Given the considerable morbidity and mortality associated with late-stage ESCC, which accounts for most newly diagnosed disease, screening for early-stage

ESCC or squamous dysplasia may identify candidates for minimally invasive therapies affording a chance for cure. However, given the lack of noninvasive, cost-effective screening methods, robust consensus guidelines regarding this topic are sparse.[129]

Screening high-risk populations may be warranted in endemic regions whereby the prevalence of ESCC is particularly high. In a population study from China, 4,116 volunteers from 24 villages underwent endoscopic screening examination with Lugol's solution and treatment as needed (14 communities) versus clinical follow-up by questionnaire and no endoscopic screening (10 communities). Patients in the endoscopic intervention group had a significantly lower cumulative incidence of ESCC and a significant reduction in cumulative mortality compared with the control group.[130] Other retrospective studies have demonstrated a significant cancer-survival benefit in patients living in high-risk regions undergoing endoscopic screening compared with controls, with Markov modeling suggesting this approach is cost-effective.[131–133]

Other high-risk populations that may benefit from ESCC screening include those with a history of head and neck cancer, tylosis, and history of caustic esophageal injury.[134–136] General population screening in the United States is not recommended, nor is screening for ESCC in patients with achalasia.[137]

Upper (usually sedated) endoscopy is typically used for screening but is associated with increased cost and the need for time away from work for the patient. These barriers and the need for specialized proceduralists may preclude the widespread implementation of ESCC screening. Transnasal endoscopy (TNE) uses an ultrathin endoscope inserted through the nasal cavity to allow for the visual inspection of the esophageal mucosa. This examination can be followed by a traditional upper endoscopy if suspicious lesions are found. TNE requires no sedation, is well tolerated, is not time-consuming, has good sensitivity and specificity, and can be performed at the point of care by primary care physicians.[138,139] However, TNE is not widely available limiting its applicability in the screening setting. Other potential endoscopic screening tests include high-resolution microendoscopy and endocytoscopy. However, these are not widely used, have not been studied in large or high-risk screening populations, and require a significant amount of training.

Nonendoscopic screening methods for ESCC have been advocated with the potential to increase patient uptake (given the noninvasive manner of testing), as well as reducing cost. This can be advantageous in resource-scarce regions whereby widespread endoscopic screening is not feasible but ESCC is prevalent. There is broad interest in a variety of direct sampling cell collection devices that have demonstrated efficacy in ruling out ESCC or squamous dysplasia with specificities exceeding 80% (**Fig. 6**).[140–144] Other noninvasive screening tests include analysis of exhaled volatile organic compounds,[145] as well as serum tests assessing autoantibodies,[146,147] miRNA,[148] and circulating tumor cells[149] which have all demonstrated good specificity (>90%) in preliminary trials.

Endoscopic therapy for T1b disease with deep submucosal invasion

Endoscopic management of T1a lesions and T1b lesions with invasion only into the upper half of the submucosa affords sustained long-term cancer-free survival with minimal adverse events compared with esophagectomy.[103,150] However, surgery has traditionally been recommended for patients with deep T1b disease (invasion >500 μm of submucosa) due to the increased risk of lymph node metastasis.[151,152] Some studies indicate that patients with deep T1b invasion may have reasonable survival with endoscopic therapy, which may be further improved with

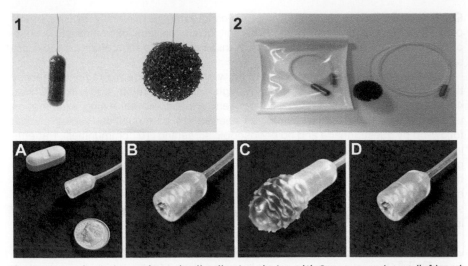

Fig. 6. Nonendoscopic esophageal cell collection devices. (1) Cytosponge: intact (left) and expanded (right; Medtronic, Minneapolis, MN). (2) EsophaCap: intact (left) and expanded (right; Capnostics, Concord, NC). (*A*) + (*B*) EsoCheck device: the device is swallowed with sips of water, inflated with 5 cm3 of air (*C*), pulled 5 cm proximal to the GEJ and then deflated into a cap (*D*) before withdrawal to avoid contamination by the squamous epithelium. (Lucid Diagnostics, New York, NY). (*From* Codipilly DC, Iyer PG. Novel Screening Tests for Barrett's Esophagus. Curr Gastroenterol Rep. 2019 Jul 25;21(9):42. https://doi.org/10. 1007/s11894-019-0710-9. PMID: 31346777; with permission.)

the addition of chemoradiotherapy.[103] For this reason, patients with otherwise low-risk disease (lack of moderate or poor differentiation, lack of lymphovascular invasion) or poor surgical candidates who have deep submucosal T1b disease may be treated with endoscopic therapy in lieu of surgery.

Neoadjuvant therapy in resectable tumors

Early trials did not demonstrate considerable improvement in cancer-related outcomes for patients receiving neoadjuvant chemotherapy followed by esophagectomy compared with those undergoing surgery alone. An initial large-scale trial with 443 patients assessing outcomes in patients receiving neoadjuvant chemotherapy with cisplatin/fluorouracil did not show cancer-related mortality benefit in the neoadjuvant group compared with the group undergoing surgery alone.[153] However, a subsequent study with 802 patients showed significant improvements in cancer-related mortality and 5-year disease-free survival in the neoadjuvant group, indicating that earlier studies may have been underpowered to detect this mortality benefit.[154] Adverse events did not differ significantly between groups in these studies.

Neoadjuvant chemoradiotherapy for resectable tumors has also been studied extensively with conflicting results regarding survival benefits y,[155,156] or rate of perioperative complications compared with surgery alone.[78] However, head-to-head comparisons of long-term outcomes between neoadjuvant chemotherapy versus neoadjuvant chemoradiotherapy show no statistically significant differences in mortality. The addition of radiotherapy to neoadjuvant treatment seems to be associated with more perioperative complications.[157] As such, neoadjuvant therapy is typically recommended for resectable patients, with no strong recommendation for or against the addition of radiotherapy to the regimen.

CLINICS CARE POINTS

- Screening for esophageal squamous carcinoma is recommended for at risk populations including those with chronic tobacco and alcohol usage, esophageal lichen planus, and tylosis.

- Screening and diagnosis should be performed with endoscopy and enhancement of the mucosa through magnification and electronic chromoendoscopy or the use of iodine to stain the mucosa.

- Treatment involves endoscopic resection of dysplastic tissue or surgical resection in combination with chemoradiotherapy for more advanced disease.

- Current chemoradiotherapy has been augmented by the use of immune checkpoint inhibitors to enhance response.

- Survivors of Stage II or greater esophageal squamous cancer should be followed for potential recurrence and also for potential complications of treatment including stricture formation, aspiration, fistula, and dumping syndrome.

FUNDING

None.

CONTRIBUTIONS

D C. Codipilly developed the initial draft of the article and subsequent revisions. K K. Wang provided essential review and feedback on the article drafts.

DISCLOSURE

D C. Codipilly: None. K K. Wang: Research funding from PCI, Interscope, Erbe, Pentax Medical Consulting: Ironwood Pharma, GIE Medical

REFERENCES

1. Sung H, Ferlay J, Siegel RL, et al. Global cancer statistics 2020: GLOBOCAN estimates of incidence and mortality worldwide for 36 cancers in 185 countries. CA: A Cancer J Clinicians 2021;71:209–49.
2. Siegel RL, Miller KD, Fuchs HE, et al. Cancer statistics, 2021. CA. Cancer J Clinicians 2021;71:7–33.
3. Arnold M, Ferlay J, van Berge Henegouwen MI, et al. Global burden of oesophageal and gastric cancer by histology and subsite in 2018. Gut 2020;69:1564.
4. Kamangar F, Nasrollahzadeh D, Safiri S, et al. The global, regional, and national burden of oesophageal cancer and its attributable risk factors in 195 countries and territories, 1990–2017: a systematic analysis for the Global Burden of Disease Study 2017. Lancet Gastroenterol Hepatol 2020;5:582–97.
5. Liang H, Fan J-H, Qiao Y-L. Epidemiology, etiology, and prevention of esophageal squamous cell carcinoma in China. Cancer Biol Med 2017;14:33–41.
6. Torre LA, Siegel RL, Ward EM, et al. Global cancer incidence and mortality rates and trends–an update. Cancer Epidemiol Biomarkers Prev 2016;25:16–27.
7. Cheng Y-F, Chen H-S, Wu S-C, et al. Esophageal squamous cell carcinoma and prognosis in Taiwan. Cancer Med 2018;7:4193–201.

8. Lu P, Gu J, Zhang N, et al. Risk factors for precancerous lesions of esophageal squamous cell carcinoma in high-risk areas of rural China: A population-based screening study. Medicine 2020;99.

9. Wang QL, Xie SH, Li WT, et al. Smoking cessation and risk of esophageal cancer by histological type: systematic review and meta-analysis. J Natl Cancer Inst 2017;109.

10. Engel LS, Chow WH, Vaughan TL, et al. Population attributable risks of esophageal and gastric cancers. J Natl Cancer Inst 2003;95:1404–13.

11. Tran GD, Sun XD, Abnet CC, et al. Prospective study of risk factors for esophageal and gastric cancers in the Linxian general population trial cohort in China. Int J Cancer 2005;113:456–63.

12. Islami F, Boffetta P, Ren J, et al. High-temperature beverages and foods and esophageal cancer risk – a systematic review. Int J Cancer J Int du Cancer 2009;125:491–524.

13. Mirvish SS. Role of N-nitroso compounds (NOC) and N-nitrosation in etiology of gastric, esophageal, nasopharyngeal and bladder cancer and contribution to cancer of known exposures to NOC. Cancer Lett 1995;93:17–48.

14. Tobey NA, Sikka D, Marten E, et al. Effect of heat stress on rabbit esophageal epithelium. Am J Physiol 1999;276:G1322–30.

15. Yu C, Tang H, Guo Y, et al. Hot tea consumption and its interactions with alcohol and tobacco use on the risk for esophageal cancer: a population-based cohort study. Ann Intern Med 2018;168:489–97.

16. Golozar A, Fagundes RB, Etemadi A, et al. Significant variation in the concentration of carcinogenic polycyclic aromatic hydrocarbons in yerba maté samples by brand, batch, and processing method. Environ Sci Technol 2012;46: 13488–93.

17. Kamangar F, Schantz MM, Abnet CC, et al. High levels of carcinogenic polycyclic aromatic hydrocarbons in mate drinks. Cancer Epidemiol Biomarkers Prev 2008;17:1262–8.

18. Islami F, Ren JS, Taylor PR, et al. Pickled vegetables and the risk of oesophageal cancer: a meta-analysis. Br J Cancer 2009;101:1641–7.

19. Liu J, Wang J, Leng Y, et al. Intake of fruit and vegetables and risk of esophageal squamous cell carcinoma: A meta-analysis of observational studies. Int J Cancer 2013;133:473–85.

20. Liu X, Wang X, Lin S, et al. Dietary patterns and oesophageal squamous cell carcinoma: a systematic review and meta-analysis. Br J Cancer 2014;110: 2785–95.

21. MacPhail AP, Simon MO, Torrance JD, et al. Changing patterns of dietary iron overload in black South Africans. Am J Clin Nutr 1979;32:1272–8.

22. Jansson C, Johansson ALV, Nyrén O, et al. Socioeconomic factors and risk of esophageal adenocarcinoma: a nationwide swedish case-control study. Cancer Epidemiol Biomarkers & Prev 2005;14:1754.

23. Talagala IA, Nawarathne M, Arambepola C. Novel risk factors for primary prevention of oesophageal carcinoma: a case-control study from Sri Lanka. BMC Cancer 2018;18:1135.

24. Ravi K, Codipilly DC, Sunjaya D, et al. Esophageal Lichen Planus Is Associated With a Significant Increase in Risk of Squamous Cell Carcinoma. Clin Gastroenterol Hepatol 2019;17:1902–3.e1.

25. Ellis A, Risk JM, Maruthappu T, et al. Tylosis with oesophageal cancer: Diagnosis, management and molecular mechanisms. Orphanet J Rare Dis 2015; 10:126.

26. Ellis A, Field JK, Field EA, et al. Tylosis associated with carcinoma of the oesophagus and oral leukoplakia in a large Liverpool family–a review of six generations. Eur J Cancer B Oral Oncol 1994;30b:102–12.

27. Farhadi M, Tahmasebi Z, Merat S, et al. Human papillomavirus in squamous cell carcinoma of esophagus in a high-risk population. World J Gastroenterol 2005; 11:1200–3.

28. Taylor PR, Abnet CC, Dawsey SM. Squamous dysplasia—the precursor lesion for esophageal squamous cell carcinoma. Cancer Epidemiol Biomarkers & Prev 2013;22:540.

29. Qiu SL, Yang GR. Precursor lesions of esophageal cancer in high-risk populations in Henan Province, China. Cancer 1988;62:551–7.

30. Dawsey SM, Lewin KJ, Wang GQ, et al. Squamous esophageal histology and subsequent risk of squamous cell carcinoma of the esophagus. A prospective follow-up study from Linxian, China. Cancer 1994;74:1686–92.

31. Wang GQ, Abnet CC, Shen Q, et al. Histological precursors of oesophageal squamous cell carcinoma: results from a 13 year prospective follow up study in a high risk population. Gut 2005;54:187–92.

32. Nagtegaal ID, Odze RD, Klimstra D, et al. The 2019 WHO classification of tumours of the digestive system. Histopathology 2020;76:182–8.

33. Hu N, Wang C, Ng D, et al. Genomic characterization of esophageal squamous cell carcinoma from a high-risk population in China. Cancer Res 2009;69: 5908–17.

34. Song Y, Li L, Ou Y, et al. Identification of genomic alterations in oesophageal squamous cell cancer. Nature 2014;509:91–5.

35. Shi ZZ, Liang JW, Zhan T, et al. Genomic alterations with impact on survival in esophageal squamous cell carcinoma identified by array comparative genomic hybridization. Genes Chromosomes Cancer 2011;50:518–26.

36. Shi ZZ, Shang L, Jiang YY, et al. Consistent and differential genetic aberrations between esophageal dysplasia and squamous cell carcinoma detected by array comparative genomic hybridization. Clin Cancer Res 2013;19:5867–78.

37. Cheng C, Zhou Y, Li H, et al. Whole-Genome Sequencing Reveals Diverse Models of Structural Variations in Esophageal Squamous Cell Carcinoma. Am J Hum Genet 2016;98:256–74.

38. Lin DC, Wang MR, Koeffler HP. Genomic and Epigenomic Aberrations in Esophageal Squamous Cell Carcinoma and Implications for Patients. Gastroenterology 2018;154:374–89.

39. Sawada G, Niida A, Uchi R, et al. Genomic landscape of esophageal squamous cell carcinoma in a japanese population. Gastroenterology 2016;150:1171–82.

40. Lima SC, Hernández-Vargas H, Simão T, et al. Identification of a DNA methylome signature of esophageal squamous cell carcinoma and potential epigenetic biomarkers. Epigenetics 2011;6:1217–27.

41. Maesawa C, Tamura G, Nishizuka S, et al. Inactivation of the CDKN2 gene by homozygous deletion and de novo methylation is associated with advanced stage esophageal squamous cell carcinoma. Cancer Res 1996;56:3875–4388.

42. Liu X, Zhang M, Ying S, et al. Genetic Alterations in Esophageal Tissues From Squamous Dysplasia to Carcinoma. Gastroenterology 2017;153:166–77.

43. Bor S, Caymaz-Bor C, Tobey NA, et al. Effect of ethanol on the structure and function of rabbit esophageal epithelium. Am J Physiology-Gastrointestinal Liver Physiol 1998;274:G819–26.

44. Brooks PJ, Theruvathu JA. DNA adducts from acetaldehyde: implications for alcohol-related carcinogenesis. Alcohol 2005;35:187–93.

45. Shi M, Ren S, Chen H, et al. Alcohol drinking inhibits NOTCH-PAX9 signaling in esophageal squamous epithelial cells. J Pathol 2021;253:384–95.

46. Enomoto N, Takase S, Yasuhara M, et al. Acetaldehyde metabolism in different aldehyde dehydrogenase-2 genotypes. Alcohol Clin Exp Res 1991;15:141–4.

47. Hecht SS. Tobacco carcinogens, their biomarkers and tobacco-induced cancer. Nat Rev Cancer 2003;3:733–44.

48. Salaspuro VJ, Hietala JM, Marvola ML, et al. Eliminating carcinogenic acetaldehyde by cysteine from saliva during smoking. Cancer Epidemiol Biomarkers & Prev 2006;15:146.

49. Miller C, Michaylira C, Nakagawa H, et al. Tobacco smoke stimulates epidermal growth factor receptor-dependent induction of cyclooxygenase-2 in primary esophageal epithelial cells, and invasion in three-dimensional organotypic culture. Cancer Res 2008;68:5402.

50. Pekarsky Y, Zanesi N, Palamarchuk A, et al. FHIT: from gene discovery to cancer treatment and prevention. Lancet Oncol 2002;3:748–54.

51. Ripley RT, Sarkaria IS, Grosser R, et al. Pretreatment dysphagia in esophageal cancer patients may eliminate the need for staging by endoscopic ultrasonography. Ann Thorac Surg 2016;101:226–30.

52. Kimura M, Ishiguro H, Tanaka T, et al. Advanced esophageal cancer with tracheobronchial fistula successfully treated by esophageal bypass surgery. Int J Surg case Rep 2015;9:115–8.

53. Sano Y, Muto M, Tajiri H, et al. Optical/digital chromoendoscopy during colonoscopy using narrow-band imaging system. Dig Endosc 2005;17:S43–8.

54. Kumagai Y, Toi M, Kawada K, et al. Angiogenesis in superficial esophageal squamous cell carcinoma: magnifying endoscopic observation and molecular analysis. Dig Endosc 2010;22:259–67.

55. Goda K, Dobashi A, Yoshimura N, et al. Narrow-band imaging magnifying endoscopy versus lugol chromoendoscopy with pink-color sign assessment in the diagnosis of superficial esophageal squamous neoplasms: a randomised noninferiority trial. Gastroenterol Res Pract 2015;2015:639462.

56. Lee CT, Chang CY, Lee YC, et al. Narrow-band imaging with magnifying endoscopy for the screening of esophageal cancer in patients with primary head and neck cancers. Endoscopy 2010;42:613–9.

57. Davila RE. Chromoendoscopy. Gastrointest Endosc Clin N Am 2009;19: 193–208.

58. Connor MJ, Sharma P. Chromoendoscopy and magnification endoscopy for diagnosing esophageal cancer and dysplasia. Thorac Surg Clin 2004;14:87–94.

59. Iacobuzio-Donahue CAME. Gastrointestinal and liver pathology 2012.

60. Jain S, Dhingra S. Pathology of esophageal cancer and Barrett's esophagus. Ann Cardiothorac Surg 2017;6:99–109.

61. DiMaio MA, Kwok S, Montgomery KD, et al. Immunohistochemical panel for distinguishing esophageal adenocarcinoma from squamous cell carcinoma: a combination of p63, cytokeratin 5/6, MUC5AC, and anterior gradient homolog 2 allows optimal subtyping. Hum Pathol 2012;43:1799–807.

62. Zhang B, Xiao Q, Yang D, et al. Spindle cell carcinoma of the esophagus: a multicenter analysis in comparison with typical squamous cell carcinoma. Medicine 2016;95:e4768.

63. Rice TW, Patil DT, Blackstone EH. 8th edition AJCC/UICC staging of cancers of the esophagus and esophagogastric junction: application to clinical practice. Ann Cardiothorac Surg 2017;6:119–30.

64. Yuequan J, Shifeng C, Bing Z. Prognostic factors and family history for survival of esophageal squamous cell carcinoma patients after surgery. Ann Thorac Surg 2010;90:908–13.
65. Cavallin F, Alfieri R, Scarpa M, et al. Nodal skip metastasis in thoracic esophageal squamous cell carcinoma: a cohort study. BMC Surg 2017;17:49.
66. Zhang X, Ly EK, Nithyanand S, et al. Learning curve for endoscopic submucosal dissection with an untutored, prevalence-based approach in the United States. Clin Gastroenterol Hepatol 2020;18:580–8.e1.
67. Yang D, Perbtani YB, Wang Y, et al. Evaluating learning curves and competence in colorectal EMR among advanced endoscopy fellows: a pilot multicenter prospective trial using cumulative sum analysis. Gastrointest Endosc 2021;93: 682–90, e4.
68. Maple JT, Abu Dayyeh BK, Chauhan SS, et al. Endoscopic submucosal dissection. Gastrointest Endosc 2015;81:1311–25.
69. Guo H-M, Zhang X-Q, Chen M, et al. Endoscopic submucosal dissection vs endoscopic mucosal resection for superficial esophageal cancer. World J Gastroenterol 2014;20:5540–7.
70. Odagiri H, Yasunaga H. Complications following endoscopic submucosal dissection for gastric, esophageal, and colorectal cancer: a review of studies based on nationwide large-scale databases. Ann translational Med 2017;5:189.
71. Ishihara R, Iishi H, Uedo N, et al. Comparison of EMR and endoscopic submucosal dissection for en bloc resection of early esophageal cancers in Japan. Gastrointest Endosc 2008;68:1066–72.
72. Greenstein AJ, Litle VR, Swanson SJ, et al. Effect of the number of lymph nodes sampled on postoperative survival of lymph node-negative esophageal cancer. Cancer 2008;112:1239–46.
73. Raymond DP, Seder CW, Wright CD, et al. Predictors of major morbidity or mortality after resection for esophageal cancer: a society of thoracic surgeons general thoracic surgery database risk adjustment model. Ann Thorac Surg 2016; 102:207–14.
74. Chan DS, Reid TD, Howell I, et al. Systematic review and meta-analysis of the influence of circumferential resection margin involvement on survival in patients with operable oesophageal cancer. Br J Surg 2013;100:456 64.
75. Biere SS, Maas KW, Cuesta MA, et al. Cervical or thoracic anastomosis after esophagectomy for cancer: a systematic review and meta-analysis. Dig Surg 2011;28:29–35.
76. Lanuti M, de Delva PE, Wright CD, et al. Post-esophagectomy gastric outlet obstruction: role of pyloromyotomy and management with endoscopic pyloric dilatation. Eur J Cardiothorac Surg 2007;31:149–53.
77. Urschel JD, Blewett CJ, Young JE, et al. Pyloric drainage (pyloroplasty) or no drainage in gastric reconstruction after esophagectomy: a meta-analysis of randomized controlled trials. Dig Surg 2002;19:160–4.
78. van Hagen P, Hulshof MCCM, van Lanschot JJB, et al. Preoperative chemoradiotherapy for esophageal or junctional cancer. N Engl J Med 2012;366: 2074–84.
79. Ajani JA, D'Amico TA, Bentrem DJ, et al. Esophageal and esophagogastric junction cancers, version 2.2019, NCCN clinical practice guidelines in oncology. J Natl Compr Canc Netw 2019;17:855–83.
80. O'Connor BM, Chadha MK, Pande A, et al. Concurrent oxaliplatin, 5-fluorouracil, and radiotherapy in the treatment of locally advanced esophageal carcinoma. Cancer J 2007;13:119–24.

81. Li Z, Zhang P, Ma Q, et al. Cisplatin-based chemoradiotherapy with 5-fluoro-uracil or pemetrexed in patients with locally advanced, unresectable esopha-geal squamous cell carcinoma: a retrospective analysis. Mol Clin Oncol 2017; 6:743–7.
82. Van Cutsem E, Moiseyenko VM, Tjulandin S, et al. Phase III study of docetaxel and cisplatin plus fluorouracil compared with cisplatin and fluorouracil as first-line therapy for advanced gastric cancer: a report of the V325 Study Group. J Clin Oncol 2006;24:4991–7.
83. Burtness B, Gibson M, Egleston B, et al. Phase II trial of docetaxel-irinotecan combination in advanced esophageal cancer. Ann Oncol 2009;20:1242–8.
84. Lordick F, von Schilling C, Bernhard H, et al. Phase II trial of irinotecan plus do-cetaxel in cisplatin-pretreated relapsed or refractory oesophageal cancer. Br J Cancer 2003;89:630–3.
85. Cunningham D, Starling N, Rao S, et al. Capecitabine and oxaliplatin for advanced esophagogastric cancer. N Engl J Med 2008;358:36–46.
86. Dutton SJ, Ferry DR, Blazeby JM, et al. Gefitinib for oesophageal cancer pro-gressing after chemotherapy (COG): a phase 3, multicentre, double-blind, pla-cebo-controlled randomised trial. Lancet Oncol 2014;15:894–904.
87. Lorenzen S, Schuster T, Porschen R, et al. Cetuximab plus cisplatin-5-fluorouracil versus cisplatin-5-fluorouracil alone in first-line metastatic squamous cell carcinoma of the esophagus: a randomized phase II study of the Arbeitsge-meinschaft Internistische Onkologie. Ann Oncol 2009;20:1667–73.
88. Moehler MH, Thuss-Patience PC, Brenner B, et al. Cisplatin/5-FU (CF)+/-panitu-mumab (P) for patients (pts) with non-resectable, advanced, or metastatic esophageal squamous cell cancer (ESCC): An open-label, randomized AIO/TTD/BDGO/EORTC phase III trial (POWER). J Clinical Oncology 2017;35:2011. https://doi.org/10.1200/JCO.2017.35.15_suppl.4011.
89. Ling Y, Chen J, Tao M, et al. A pilot study of nimotuzumab combined with cisplatin and 5-FU in patients with advanced esophageal squamous cell carci-noma. J Thorac Dis 2012;4:58–62.
90. Hardwick RH, Barham CP, Ozua P, et al. Immunohistochemical detection of p53 and c-erbB-2 in oesophageal carcinoma; no correlation with prognosis. Eur J Surg Oncol (Ejso) 1997;23:30–5.
91. Safran H, DiPetrillo T, Nadeem A, et al. Trastuzumab, paclitaxel, cisplatin, and radiation for adenocarcinoma of the esophagus: a phase I study. Cancer Invest 2004;22:670–7.
92. Kudo T, Hamamoto Y, Kato K, et al. Nivolumab treatment for oesophageal squamous-cell carcinoma: an open-label, multicentre, phase 2 trial. Lancet On-col 2017;18:631–9.
93. Kelly RJ, Ajani JA, Kuzdzal J, et al. Adjuvant nivolumab in resected esophageal or gastroesophageal junction cancer. N Engl J Med 2021;384:1191–203.
94. Kojima T, Muro K, Francois E, et al. Pembrolizumab versus chemotherapy as second-line therapy for advanced esophageal cancer: phase III KEYNOTE-181 study. J. Clinical Oncology 2019;37. https://doi.org/10.1200/JCO.2019.37.4.
95. Huang J, Xu J, Chen Y, et al. Camrelizumab versus investigator's choice of chemotherapy as second-line therapy for advanced or metastatic oesophageal squamous cell carcinoma (ESCORT): a multicentre, randomised, open-label, phase 3 study. Lancet Oncol 2020;21:832–42.
96. Xu J, Bai Y, Xu N, et al. Tislelizumab Plus chemotherapy as first-line treatment for advanced esophageal squamous cell carcinoma and gastric/gastroesophageal junction adenocarcinoma. Clin Cancer Res 2020;26:4542–50.

97. Kojima T, Shah MA, Muro K, et al. Randomized phase III KEYNOTE-181 study of pembrolizumab versus chemotherapy in advanced esophageal cancer. J Clin Oncol 2020;38:4138–48.

98. Chau I, Doki Y, Ajani JA, et al. Nivolumab (NIVO) plus ipilimumab (IPI) or NIVO plus chemotherapy (chemo) versus chemo as first-line (1L) treatment for advanced esophageal squamous cell carcinoma (ESCC): first results of the checkmate 648 study. J Clin Oncol 2021;39:LBA4001.

99. Lin SH, Wang L, Myles B, et al. Propensity score-based comparison of long-term outcomes with 3-dimensional conformal radiotherapy vs intensity-modulated radiotherapy for esophageal cancer. Int J Radiat Oncol Biol Phys 2012;84: 1078–85.

100. Lin SH, Hobbs B, Thall P, et al. Results of a phase II randomized trial of proton beam therapy vs intensity modulated radiation therapy in esophageal cancer. Int J Radiat Oncol Biol Phys 2019;105:680–1.

101. van Zanten ARH, Dixon MJ, Nipshagen MD, et al. Hospital-acquired sinusitis is a common cause of fever of unknown origin in orotracheally intubated critically ill patients. Crit Care 2005;9:R583.

102. Alivizatos V, Gavala V, Alexopoulos P, et al. Feeding tube-related complications and problems in patients receiving long-term home enteral nutrition. Indian J Palliat Care 2012;18:31–3.

103. Namikawa K, Yoshio T, Yoshimizu S, et al. Clinical outcomes of endoscopic resection of preoperatively diagnosed non-circumferential T1a-muscularis mucosae or T1b-submucosa 1 esophageal squamous cell carcinoma. Sci Rep 2021;11:6554.

104. Katada C, Muto M, Manabe T, et al. Esophageal stenosis after endoscopic mucosal resection of superficial esophageal lesions. Gastrointest Endosc 2003;57:165–9.

105. Shi Q, Ju H, Yao LQ, et al. Risk factors for postoperative stricture after endoscopic submucosal dissection for superficial esophageal carcinoma. Endoscopy 2014;46:640–4.

106. Yamaguchi N, Isomoto H, Nakayama T, et al. Usefulness of oral prednisolone in the treatment of esophageal stricture after endoscopic submucosal dissection for superficial esophageal squamous cell carcinoma. Gastrointest Endosc 2011;73:1115–21.

107. Yu JP, Liu YJ, Tao YL, et al. Prevention of esophageal stricture after endoscopic submucosal dissection: a systematic review. World J Surg 2015;39:2955–64.

108. Sato H, Inoue H, Ikeda H, et al. Clinical experience of esophageal perforation occurring with endoscopic submucosal dissection. Dis Esophagus 2014;27: 617–22.

109. Tsujii Y, Nishida T, Nishiyama O, et al. Clinical outcomes of endoscopic submucosal dissection for superficial esophageal neoplasms: a multicenter retrospective cohort study. Endoscopy 2015;47:775–83.

110. Bailey SH, Bull DA, Harpole DH, et al. Outcomes after esophagectomy: a ten-year prospective cohort. Ann Thorac Surg 2003;75:217–22 ; discussion 222.

111. Urschel JD. Esophagogastrostomy anastomotic leaks complicating esophagectomy: a review. Am J Surg 1995;169:634–40.

112. Ryan CE, Paniccia A, Meguid RA, et al. Transthoracic anastomotic leak after esophagectomy: current trends. Ann Surg Oncol 2017;24:281–90.

113. Park JY, Song H-Y, Kim JH, et al. Benign anastomotic strictures after esophagectomy: long-term effectiveness of balloon dilation and factors affecting recurrence in 155 patients. Am J Roentgenol 2012;198:1208–13.

114. Berry MF, Atkins BZ, Tong BC, et al. A comprehensive evaluation for aspiration after esophagectomy reduces the incidence of postoperative pneumonia. J Thorac Cardiovasc Surg 2010;140:1266–71.

115. Buskens CJ, Hulscher JB, Fockens P, et al. Benign tracheo-neo-esophageal fistulas after subtotal esophagectomy. Ann Thorac Surg 2001;72:221–4.

116. Boshier PR, Huddy JR, Zaninotto G, et al. Dumping syndrome after esophagectomy: a systematic review of the literature. Dis Esophagus 2016;30:1–9.

117. Koeter M, Kathiravetpillai N, Gooszen J, et al. Influence of the extent and dose of radiation on complications after neoadjuvant chemoradiation and subsequent esophagectomy with gastric tube reconstruction with a cervical anastomosis. Int J Radiat Oncol Biol Phys 2017;97:813–21.

118. Gronnier C, Tréchot B, Duhamel A, et al. Impact of neoadjuvant chemoradiotherapy on postoperative outcomes after esophageal cancer resection: results of a European multicenter study. Ann Surg 2014;260:764–71.

119. Goense L, van Rossum PS, Ruurda JP, et al. Radiation to the gastric fundus increases the risk of anastomotic leakage after esophagectomy. Ann Thorac Surg 2016;102:1798–804.

120. Beitler AL, Urschel JD. Comparison of stapled and hand-sewn esophagogastric anastomoses. Am J Surg 1998;175:337–40.

121. Ercan S, Rice TW, Murthy SC, et al. Does esophagogastric anastomotic technique influence the outcome of patients with esophageal cancer? J Thorac Cardiovasc Surg 2005;129:623–31.

122. Shah RD, Luketich JD, Schuchert MJ, et al. Postesophagectomy chylothorax: incidence, risk factors, and outcomes. Ann Thorac Surg 2012;93:897–903 ; discussion 903-904.

123. Linden PA, Towe CW, Watson TJ, et al. Mortality after esophagectomy: analysis of individual complications and their association with mortality. J Gastrointest Surg 2020;24:1948–54.

124. Steyerberg EW, Neville BA, Koppert LB, et al. Surgical mortality in patients with esophageal cancer: development and validation of a simple risk score. J Clin Oncol 2006;24:4277–84.

125. Booka E, Takeuchi H, Nishi T, et al. The impact of postoperative complications on survivals after esophagectomy for esophageal cancer. Medicine (Baltimore) 2015;94:e1369.

126. Booka E, Kikuchi H, Haneda R, et al. Short-term outcomes of robot-assisted minimally invasive esophagectomy compared with thoracoscopic or transthoracic esophagectomy. Anticancer Res 2021;41:4455–62.

127. Hamer PW, Hight SC, Ward IG, et al. Stricture rate after chemoradiotherapy and radiotherapy for oesophageal squamous cell carcinoma: a 20-year experience. ANZ J Surg 2019;89:367–71.

128. Nishibuchi I, Murakami Y, Kubo K, et al. Temporal changes and risk factors for esophageal stenosis after salvage radiotherapy in superficial esophageal cancer following non-curative endoscopic submucosal dissection. Radiother Oncol 2022;166:65–70.

129. Codipilly DC, Rubenstein JH, Leggett CL. Whether to screen, or who to screen, that is the question. Gastrointest Endosc 2021;95(2):236–8.

130. Wei WQ, Chen ZF, He YT, et al. Long-term follow-up of a community assignment, one-time endoscopic screening study of esophageal cancer in China. J Clin Oncol 2015;33:1951–7.

131. Chen Q, Yu L, Hao C, et al. Effectiveness evaluation of organized screening for esophageal cancer: a case-control study in Linzhou city, China. Sci Rep 2016;6: 35707.
132. Zheng X, Mao X, Xu K, et al. Massive endoscopic screening for esophageal and gastric cancers in a high-risk area of China. PLoS One 2015;10:e0145097.
133. Xia R, Li H, Shi J, et al. Cost-effectiveness of risk-stratified endoscopic screening for esophageal cancer in high-risk areas of China: a modeling study. Gastrointest Endosc 2021;95(2):225–35.e20.
134. Risk JM, Mills HS, Garde J, et al. The tylosis esophageal cancer (TOC) locus: more than just a familial cancer gene. Dis Esophagus 1999;12:173–6.
135. Su YY, Chen WC, Chuang HC, et al. Effect of routine esophageal screening in patients with head and neck cancer. JAMA Otolaryngol - Head Neck Surg 2013;139:350–4.
136. Mu HW, Chen CH, Yang KW, et al. The prevalence of esophageal cancer after caustic and pesticide ingestion: a nationwide cohort study. PLoS One 2020; 15:e0243922.
137. Ponds FA, Moonen A, Smout A, et al. Screening for dysplasia with Lugol chromoendoscopy in longstanding idiopathic achalasia. Am J Gastroenterol 2018; 113:855–62.
138. Huang Y-C, Lee Y-C, Tseng P-H, et al. Regular screening of esophageal cancer for 248 newly diagnosed hypopharyngeal squamous cell carcinoma by unsedated transnasal esophagogastroduodenoscopy. Oral Oncol 2016;55:55–60.
139. Arantes V, Albuquerque W, Salles JM, et al. Effectiveness of unsedated transnasal endoscopy with white-light, flexible spectral imaging color enhancement, and lugol staining for esophageal cancer screening in high-risk patients. J Clin Gastroenterol 2013;47:314–21.
140. Roth MJ, Liu SF, Dawsey SM, et al. Cytologic detection of esophageal squamous cell carcinoma and precursor lesions using balloon and sponge samplers in asymptomatic adults in Linxian, China. Cancer 1997;80:2047–59.
141. Pan QJ, Roth MJ, Guo HQ, et al. Cytologic detection of esophageal squamous cell carcinoma and its precursor lesions using balloon samplers and liquid-based cytology in asymptomatic adults in Llinxian, China. Acta Cytol 2008;52: 14–23.
142. Adams L, Roth MJ, Abnet CC, et al. Promoter methylation in cytology specimens as an early detection marker for esophageal squamous dysplasia and early esophageal squamous cell carcinoma. Cancer Prev Res 2008;1:357–61.
143. Roshandel G, Merat S, Sotoudeh M, et al. Pilot study of cytological testing for oesophageal squamous cell dysplasia in a high-risk area in Northern Iran. Br J Cancer 2014;111:2235–41.
144. Codipilly DC, Iyer PG. Novel screening tests for barrett's esophagus. Curr Gastroenterol Rep 2019;21:42.
145. Zou X, Zhou W, Lu Y, et al. Exhaled gases online measurements for esophageal cancer patients and healthy people by proton transfer reaction mass spectrometry. J Gastroenterol Hepatol 2016;31:1837–43.
146. Zhou SL, Yue WB, Fan ZM, et al. Autoantibody detection to tumor-associated antigens of P53, IMP1, P16, cyclin B1, P62, C-myc, Survivn, and Koc for the screening of high-risk subjects and early detection of esophageal squamous cell carcinoma. Dis Esophagus 2014;27:790–7.
147. Xu H-T, Miao J, Liu J-W, et al. Prognostic value of circulating tumor cells in esophageal cancer. World J Gastroenterol 2017;23:1310–8.

148. Zhang C, Wang C, Chen X, et al. Expression profile of microRNAs in serum: a fingerprint for esophageal squamous cell carcinoma. Clin Chem 2010;56: 1871–9.
149. Cao M, Yie SM, Wu SM, et al. Detection of survivin-expressing circulating cancer cells in the peripheral blood of patients with esophageal squamous cell carcinoma and its clinical significance. Clin Exp Metastasis 2009;26:751–8.
150. Lee HD, Chung H, Kwak Y, et al. Endoscopic submucosal dissection versus surgery for superficial esophageal squamous cell carcinoma: a propensity score-matched survival analysis. Clin Translational Gastroenterol 2020;11(7):e00193.
151. Qi X, Li M, Zhao S, et al. Prevalence of metastasis in T1b esophageal squamous cell carcinoma: a retrospective analysis of 258 Chinese patients. J Thorac Dis 2016;8:966–76.
152. Duan X, Shang X, Yue J, et al. A nomogram to predict lymph node metastasis risk for early esophageal squamous cell carcinoma. BMC Cancer 2021;21:431.
153. Kelsen DP, Winter KA, Gunderson LL, et al. Long-term results of RTOG trial 8911 (USA Intergroup 113): a random assignment trial comparison of chemotherapy followed by surgery compared with surgery alone for esophageal cancer. J Clin Oncol 2007;25:3719–25.
154. Allum WH, Stenning SP, Bancewicz J, et al. Long-term results of a randomized trial of surgery with or without preoperative chemotherapy in esophageal cancer. J Clin Oncol 2009;27:5062–7.
155. Burmeister BH, Smithers BM, Gebski V, et al. Surgery alone versus chemoradiotherapy followed by surgery for resectable cancer of the oesophagus: a randomised controlled phase III trial. Lancet Oncol 2005;6:659–68.
156. Bosset JF, Gignoux M, Triboulet JP, et al. Chemoradiotherapy followed by surgery compared with surgery alone in squamous-cell cancer of the esophagus. N Engl J Med 1997;337:161–7.
157. Von Döbeln G, Klevebro F, Jacobsen A, et al. Neoadjuvant chemotherapy versus neoadjuvant chemoradiotherapy for cancer of the esophagus or gastroesophageal junction: long-term results of a randomized clinical trial. Dis Esophagus 2019;32:doy078.

Management of Dysplastic Barrett's Esophagus and Early Esophageal Adenocarcinoma

Cary C. Cotton, MD, MPH[a], Swathi Eluri, MD, MPH[b],
Nicholas J. Shaheen, MD, MPH[c],*

KEYWORDS

- Endoscopic eradication therapy • Barrett's esophagus • Dysplasia
- Adenocarcinoma • Radiofrequency ablation • Cryotherapy
- Endoscopic mucosal resection

KEY POINTS

- Barrett's esophagus with low-grade dysplasia, high-grade dysplasia, or early esophageal adenocarcinoma may be treated safely and effectively with endoscopic eradication therapy.
- Endoscopic eradication therapy combines the resection of any raised neoplasia or mucosal irregularity with an ablative therapy for flat Barrett's esophagus.
- Endoscopic eradication therapy requires long-term endoscopic surveillance after successful treatment.

INTRODUCTION

Barrett's esophagus (BE) is a common premalignant condition of the esophagus associated with esophageal adenocarcinoma (EAC). BE is diagnosed by the finding of salmon-colored mucosa in the esophagus extending one or more centimeters proximal to the gastroesophageal junction (GEJ), with histologic confirmation of intestinal metaplasia.[1] While BE without dysplasia may benefit from endoscopic surveillance, therapy for the eradication of BE is appropriate in the presence of confirmed dysplasia

[a] Department of Medicine, Division of Gastroenterology and Hepatology, Center for Esophageal Diseases and Swallowing, University of North Carolina at Chapel Hill, CB#7080, 130 Mason Farm Road, Suite 4153, Chapel Hill, NC 27599-7080, USA; [b] Department of Medicine, Division of Gastroenterology and Hepatology, Center for Esophageal Diseases and Swallowing, University of North Carolina at Chapel Hill, CB#7080, 130 Mason Farm Road, Suite 4142, Chapel Hill, NC 27599-7080, USA; [c] Department of Medicine, Division of Gastroenterology and Hepatology, Center for Esophageal Diseases and Swallowing, University of North Carolina at Chapel Hill, CB#7080, 130 Mason Farm Road, Suite 4150, Chapel Hill, NC 27599-7080, USA
* Corresponding author.
E-mail address: nicholas_shaheen@med.unc.edu

Gastroenterol Clin N Am 51 (2022) 485–500
https://doi.org/10.1016/j.gtc.2022.06.004
0889-8553/22/© 2022 Elsevier Inc. All rights reserved.

or early EAC. Management of dysplastic BE and early EAC most commonly involves endoscopic eradication therapy (EET), which combines the resection of raised neoplasia[2] with the ablative treatment of the residual flat BE.[3,4] Radiofrequency ablation (RFA) is the most commonly available ablative therapy for BE,[3,4] while cryotherapy and argon plasma coagulation (APC) are also safe and effective primary treatment modalities.[5,6] Cryotherapy has been demonstrated to be effective in a meta-analysis for BE refractory to RFA.[7] Endoscopic submucosal dissection (ESD) is emerging as an endoscopic option for the treatment of patients with T1b tumors.[8] Following EET, endoscopic surveillance is recommended and is associated with a low rate of progression.[9] A growing evidence base supports decreasing the frequency of endoscopic surveillance, especially in patients with low-grade dysplasia (LGD), but as the cohort of patients who complete endoscopic eradication therapy ages, a key question remains as to when to stop surveillance.

PATIENT EVALUATION OVERVIEW

The evaluation of patients with BE requires an analysis of the clinical history, as well as the endoscopic and histologic data. A general understanding of the patient's past medical history is required, and particular attention should be paid to the presence of cardiopulmonary diseases and anticoagulation use, given the risks of endoscopy. Competing risks to the patient's mortality must be considered: the benefits of endoscopic treatment of BE and associated neoplasia is conditional on the patient surviving long enough to have developed a clinically significant cancer in the absence of endoscopic treatment. Additionally, in patients with BE with LGD, endoscopic eradication therapy is illogical in those with a short life expectancy, given that they are unlikely to benefit from a further decrease in the already-low risk of progression to EAC. As EET requires periodic endoscopic follow-up, barriers to adherence must be understood and addressed.

EET requires a diagnosis of BE with dysplasia. BE is defined by the presence of one or more centimeters of salmon-colored mucosa extending proximal to the GEJ, which is defined as the top of the gastric folds. The location of the GEJ, the length of any hiatus hernia, the maximum contiguous length of the BE segment (the Prague M length), the maximum circumferential length of the BE segment (the Prague C length), and the location of any mucosal irregularities, raised lesions, or islands of salmon-colored mucosa above the maximal contiguous length should be documented (**Fig. 1**). Current guidelines require the confirmation of any dysplasia in the BE by a second pathologist expert in gastrointestinal conditions.[1] This is especially important in the case of BE with LGD, whereby considerable inter-observer variability exists.[10] This begs the question of what qualifies a pathologist as "expert." Recent work suggests that greater than 5 years working as a subspecialty GI pathologist was protective against diagnostic errors, while working in a community-based hospital was a risk factor. Sadly, self-identification as an expert was not protective.[11]

The risk of progression to adenocarcinoma is less than 0.5% per year among patients with nondysplastic BE, and endoscopic eradication therapy is not recommended. The rationale being that the risks and costs of therapy do not justify the possible clinical benefit.[12] While associated dysplasia or neoplasia is a prerequisite to endoscopic eradication therapy, differentiation between BE with LGD, high-grade dysplasia (HGD), or intramucosal adenocarcinoma is essential to ensure appropriate triage and posttreatment surveillance intervals. To maximize accuracy for the histologic grade, the entire BE segment should be closely examined, and any mucosal irregularities should be biopsied. Random 4 quadrant biopsies should be performed within

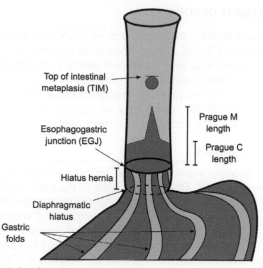

Fig. 1. Key endoscopic landmarks in the endoscopic evaluation of Barrett's esophagus.

the BE segment every 1 cm[13] Sampling any islands is indicated because it can often increase the maximum detected histologic grade.[14]

PHARMACOLOGIC TREATMENT OPTIONS

No medical therapy reliably induces reversion of BE to squamous epithelium.[15] While the management of BE with dysplasia or early EAC is predominantly endoscopic, pharmacologic treatment with high dose proton-pump inhibitors (PPIs) is used during EET to promote growth of squamous epithelium (**Table 1**).[16] The AspECT trial found a benefit of high-dose rather than low-dose PPI therapy in preventing progression of nondysplastic BE,[17] but no studies have identified an antineoplastic effect of PPIs in BE with dysplasia or early EAC. Observational studies have found protective effects of aspirin, nonsteroidal antiinflammatory drugs, and statins in BE.[15] These studies are subject to a high risk of bias due to confounding and outcome misclassification. There are no studies of these agents in populations with BE with dysplasia or early EAC.

Table 1
Standard and high-dose proton-pump inhibitor regimens

	Standard-Dose Regimen	High-Dose Regimen
Omeprazole	20 mg once daily 30 min before a meal	40 mg twice daily 30 min before meals
Pantoprazole	40 mg once daily 30 min before a meal	40 mg twice daily 30 min before meals
Lansoprazole	15 mg once daily 30 min before a meal	30 mg twice daily 30 min before meals
Esomeprazole	20 mg once daily 30 min before a meal	40 mg twice daily 30 min before meals
Rabeprazole	20 mg once daily 30 min before a meal	40 mg twice daily 30 min before meals
Dexlansoprazole	30 mg once daily 30 min before a meal	60 mg once daily 30 min before a meal

ENDOSCOPIC TREATMENT OPTIONS

Endoscopic treatments for BE with dysplasia or early EAC can be divided into ablative methods used to eradicate flat BE and methods for the endoscopic resection of raised lesions or mucosal irregularities. RFA is the most widely available ablative therapy, but cryotherapy methods, electrocoagulation, argon plasma coagulation, and wide endoscopic resection have been described. Endoscopic resection methods include endoscopic mucosal resection (EMR), which may be categorized into band-assisted and cap-assisted approaches, and endoscopic submucosal dissection.

Endoscopic Resection Methods

Before any ablative therapy, resection should be performed on any raised lesions or visible mucosal irregularities.[18] The shallow depth of the treatment of ablative modalities would only treat the surface of raised lesions and may potentially obscure deeper residual neoplasia in such lesions, making the resection of such lesions imperative before embarking on any mucosal ablation.[19] Mucosal irregularities have higher rates of neoplasia than flat areas within a Barrett's segment, and EMR before the ablation of BE increases remission of dysplasia and decreases recurrence.[20] With their low rate of lymph node metastasis, T1a intramucosal adenocarcinoma is amenable to EMR, with a meta-analysis of 70 studies reporting a 1.9% rate of lymph node metastases in BE with T1a EAC.[21]

EMR uses a hard plastic cap to capture an area of mucosa for resection with an electrosurgical snare. In the cap-assisted method, saline with or without epinephrine, or another lifting agent is injected into the submucosa. The mucosa is suctioned into the cap, the snare is deployed and constrained around the mucosa, and the lesion is resected. In band-assisted EMR, a lifting agent is not required. The mucosa is suctioned into the cap, a band is deployed, and then an electrosurgical snare is used to resect the banded mucosa (**Fig. 2**).While both cap-assisted and band ligation EMR are highly effective and resect similar-sized pieces of mucosa, band ligation EMR is significantly faster, and is, therefore, used more commonly in most centers.[22]

Endoscopic submucosal dissection (ESD) uses a lifting/dying agent along with an endoscopic electrosurgical knife to dissect the submucosa beneath a lesion. ESD allows for the resection of large lesions *en bloc* (**Fig. 3**). Whereas foci of dysplasia or T1a EAC with low-risk histologic characteristics may be resected with EMR, ESD may provide more complete resection of both T1a and T1b EAC. A retrospective cohort study of ESD in BE with early neoplasia found a rate of *en bloc* and R0 resection of 87% for HGD and T1a EAC and 49% for T1b EAC.[23] Another retrospective cohort found a 98% *en bloc* resection rate and a 58% R0 resection rate for a mix of T1a and T1b lesions.[24] A retrospective comparison found ESD had a higher rate of *en bloc* and complete resection compared with EMR, and a lower rate of recurrence.[25,26] Because ESD is more technically challenging than EMR and only necessary in highly selected lesions, expertise should be concentrated in high volume centers.

Endoscopic Ablative Methods

After the resection of any raised lesions or irregularities, the goal of endoscopic ablative therapies is the complete eradication of intestinal metaplasia (CEIM), which is defined as the absence of any visible BE with biopsies negative for intestinal metaplasia in the tubular esophagus and negative for dysplasia in the gastric cardia. RFA therapy applies radiofrequency energy by an electrode in contact with the BE segment to cause full thickness epithelial ablation while minimizing injury to the submucosa.[27] Circumferential treatment is performed using catheter-based electrodes on an

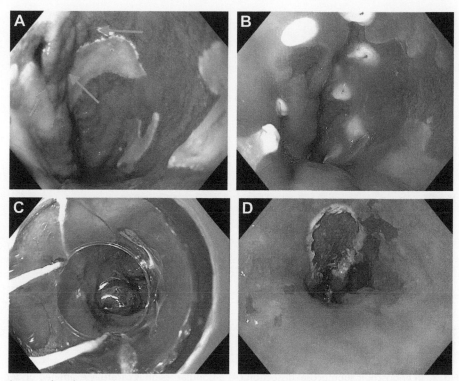

Fig. 2. In band-assisted endoscopic mucosal resection (*A*) a nodular lesion is carefully examined under white light and narrow-band imaging at the 11 o'clock position, (*B*) the perimeter is marked with a snare tip, the lesion is pulled into the endoscope cap using suction and (*C*) a band is deployed, the lesion is ensnared under the band, and (*D*) the lesion is resected en bloc by snare electrocautery. The arrows indicate the margins of a raised, dysplastic lesions before treatment. ([*A,B*] ©2022 Medtronic. All rights reserved. Used with the permission of Medtronic.)

inflatable balloon, while focal treatment is applied by an electrode either affixed to the end of the endoscope of via the working channel of the endoscope (**Fig. 4**).

Before any ablative treatment, careful inspection of the Barrett's segment is required to exclude even very slightly raised lesions, which should be first treated by a resection method. A mucolytic agent such as 1% N-acetylcysteine or saline spray is applied to the esophagus by a spray catheter advanced through the working channel of a standard gastroscope.[28] Before using a balloon catheter ablation device, a stiff guidewire is placed transorally into the stomach. While previous technology demanded that the esophageal luminal diameter be measured with sizing balloons, newer catheters (Barrx 360 Express RFA balloon catheter, Medtronic, Minneapolis, MN) are self-sizing.[26] The balloon catheter is advanced over the guidewire under endoscopic visualization and inflated. High radiofrequency energy at 10 J/centimeter^2 is applied in sequential 3-cm segments (or 4-cm segments when using the Barrx 360 Express) of the diseased esophagus with minimal overlap. The resulting coagulum is then cleaned by scraping with an endoscopy cap and spraying water in the treated segment. Then a second ablative treatment is applied in the same manner as the initial treatment.[29] Focal ablation is delivered via one of the several focal RFA devices available, which is placed in apposition to any residual islands or tongues following circumferential ablation. The focal ablation devices can also be used as primary therapy in

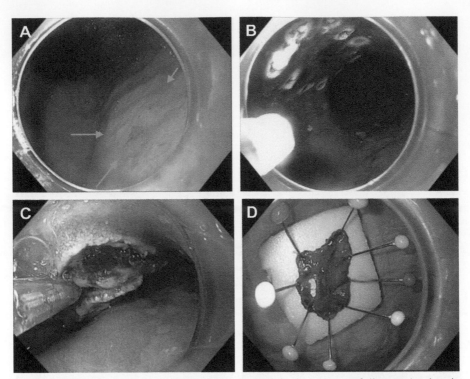

Fig. 3. In endoscopic submucosal dissection (*A*) a nodular lesion is carefully examined under white light and narrow-band imaging, (*B*) the perimeter is marked with a snare tip, the lesion is lifted by the injection of methylene blue, (*C*) the lesion is excised en bloc by submucosal dissection, and (*D*) the lesion is pinned to Styrofoam marked to indicate the spatial orientation of the specimen. The arrows indicate the margins of a raised, dysplastic lesions before treatment. (*From* Codipilly DC, Dhaliwal L, Oberoi M, et al. Comparative Outcomes of Cap Assisted Endoscopic Resection and Endoscopic Submucosal Dissection in Dysplastic Barrett's Esophagus. Clin Gastroenterol Hepatol. 2022;20(1):65-73.e1; with permission.)

cases of short-segment disease. Focal ablation is performed with 2 sequential applications of 12 J/centimeter.[2] In addition to residual islands or tongues, the GEJ is also circumferentially treated with the focal ablation catheter. Coagulum is cleaned by scraping with the distal edge of the focal catheter between treatments.

RFA results in a high rate of CEIM in LGD. In the treatment arm of the SURF Trial for BE with confirmed LGD, 88.2% achieved CEIM and 92.6% achieved eradication of dysplasia.[3] Among control patients in SURF, 26.5% progressed to HGD or EAC, while only 1.5% in the treatment arm progressed.[3] While the SURF trial was performed in a highly centralized and expert center, outcomes may vary by case volume. In the AIM-Dysplasia Trial, a smaller effect was observed on LGD, whereby 4.8% progressed in the treatment arm compared with 13.6% of the control arm.[4] Though EET is recommended as an option and is often used for LGD, uncertainty remains about its effectiveness in the North American context due to the reported lower risks of progression. A randomized controlled trial in the United States is planned. The AIM-Dysplasia Trial clearly demonstrated a benefit of RFA in BE with HGD.[4] While 19.0% in the control arm progressed to adenocarcinoma only 2.4% in the treatment arm progressed.[4]

Several modalities of cryotherapy have also been developed in the last 2 decades,[30] and are similarly safe and effective, but less widely available. Cryotherapy uses liquid

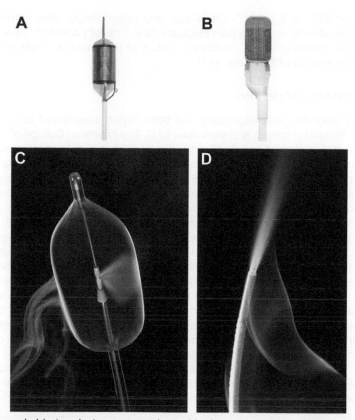

Fig. 4. Mucosal ablation devices commonly used in the management of flat Barrett's esophagus include (A) Barrx 360 Express, (B) Barrx 90, (C) C2 cryoballoon, and (D) Trufreeze liquid nitrogen spray. (*Courtesy of* (A and B) Medtronic, Minneapolis, MN; (C) Pentax, Tokyo, Japan; (D) Steris, Mentor, OH; with permission.)

nitrogen or nitrous oxide, and can be applied by spray or balloon-delivered methods. In observational studies, rates of CEIM with a variety of cryotherapy approaches range broadly from 23% to 91%, but are generally more than 60%.[31,32] Meta-analyses have been limited by high residual heterogeneity, with mean rates of CEIM ranging from 64% to 86%.[32,33] There are no comparative trials between cryotherapy and RFA, nor any comparative trials between the different cryotherapy methods. Observational comparisons between treatments are fraught, because the spectrum of disease and other confounding factors may differ between participants in treatment trials. An observational comparison using propensity-score matching to mitigate these issues found that nitrous oxide balloon cryotherapy achieved CEIM at a numerically but not statistically significant higher rate compared with RFA.[34] A cryotherapy balloon is under study that allows 3 cm hemi-circumferential treatment per application.[35]

Argon plasma coagulation (APC) uses ionized argon gas to conduct electrical current for noncontact tissue coagulation. Clinical trials of APC for the treatment of dysplastic BE have reported widely variable (57%–99%) rates of CEIM,[6,36–38] and relatively poor long-term durability (19%–38%).[37,39] Hybrid APC, an ablative method that combines a mucosal lift before APC with a single catheter, has demonstrated promising early results.[40] In 2 prospective studies, the cumulative incidence of CEIM (88%) was comparable to RFA and cryotherapy, but durability was marginally worse than RFA, at 66% at 2 years.[41] Chest pain and odynophagia were common after hybrid APC treatment, requiring pain medications in 21% of patients.[41] Fever was reported in 7%, bleeding in 4%, stricture in 4%, and there was a single esophageal perforation in a study of 154 patients.[41]

SURGICAL TREATMENT OPTIONS

Over recent decades, esophagectomy has been largely supplanted by endoscopic therapy for BE with dysplasia and superficial EAC. The American College of Gastroenterology recommends that endoscopic therapy be preferred over esophagectomy for BE with dysplasia or T1a EAC for patients with low risk features.[42] Even in high-volume centers, operative mortality of 2.5%–2.6% has been reported in esophagectomy for BE with HGD, T1a, or T1b EAC.[42,43] Serious adverse effects such as anastomotic leak, wound infection, aspiration and respiratory failure, and vocal cord paralysis are common.[42,43] In surgical series, lymph node metastasis is reported in 20%–23% in T1b lesions, although this number may be elevated due to mis-staging of T2 lesions as T1b.[44–46] A predictive model built in the National Cancer Database had moderate (C statistical 0.7)[47] discrimination between patients with and without nodal metastasis (**Tables 2** and **3**). Given the higher risk of nodal metastasis, esophagectomy with lymph node dissection may be the optimal approach to T1b lesions in good surgical candidates, especially those with poor differentiation, lymphovascular invasion, or involvement of the deep submucosa. In patients at higher risk of adverse effects from surgery, ESD offers an endoscopic alternative for the treatment of T1b lesions. Further work is ongoing to describe patients with T1b EAC who may be amenable to endoscopic management. T1b tumors of smaller size, well-differentiated histology, invasion to the superficial submucosa, and no evidence of angiolymphatic invasion may be good candidates for endoscopic management, based on low risk of lymph node involvement.

TREATMENT RESISTANCE AND COMPLICATIONS

All ablative methods have failures, and the need for second line treatment is common. Adequate control of reflux is critical to the success of any ablative method and some patients may require a surgical antireflux procedure to achieve this. The best-described salvage therapy after RFA is cryotherapy. In a meta-analysis of 8 studies, cryotherapy as salvage therapy for failed RFA showed a high rate of complete eradication of dysplasia (76%) and a smaller proportion of CEIM (46%).[7] The meta-analysis did not distinguish between balloon or spray-delivered cryotherapies, but it was

Table 2	
Points for tumor characteristics among T1a and T1b lesions in the Weksler et al. scoring system	
Tumor Characteristic	**Points**
Well differentiated	0
Moderately differentiated	2
Poorly differentiated	3
Size < 15 mm	0
Size 15–25 mm	1
Size >25 mm	2
No angiolymphatic invasion Angiolymphatic invasion	0
	2

Table 3
The proportion with lymph node metastasis among T1a and T1b lesions in the Weksler et al. scoring system

Total Points	Proportion with Lymph Node Metastasis Among T1a	Proportion with Lymph Node Metastasis Among T1b
0	0	4.3
1	0	0
2	1.9	5.7
3	2.6	13.8
4	6.5	22.0
≥5	16.1	32.4

Adapted from Weksler B, Kennedy KF, Sullivan JL. Using the National Cancer Database to create a scoring system that identifies patients with early-stage esophageal cancer at risk for nodal metastases. J Thorac Cardiovasc Surg. 2017;154(5):1787-1793; with permission.

dominated by spray-delivered methods. A subsequently published prospective study of salvage nitrous oxide balloon cryotherapy after RFA reported a similar 76% rate of complete eradication of dysplasia and a higher 72% rate of CEIM.[5]

RFA is overall safe and well tolerated. A meta-analysis of RFA with and without EMR found a rate of stricture of 5.6% (95% confidence interval [CI], 4.2%–7.4%), a rate of pain requiring medication or medical attention of 3.8% (95% CI: 1.9%–7.8%), and a rate of bleeding of 1% (95% CI: 0.8%–1.3%).[48] Two perforations occurred in 5521 United States RFA registry participants (0.04%), which is comparable to the background rate in diagnostic upper endoscopy.[49,50]

The safety of cryotherapy has been evaluated in multiple studies. A comparative study found a statistically significantly 6% increased cumulative stricture risk for cryotherapy compared with RFA (4 vs 10%).[34] Stricture rates with various cryotherapy methods have been reported from 3% to 13%, with a meta-analysis dominated by liquid nitrogen spray cryotherapy reporting a pooled rate of strictures of 7%.[5,31,32,34,51] Bleeding was not reported in most studies, but one case of delayed bleeding not requiring transfusion was reported in one study.[5] Chest pain requiring pain medication was found in 1% of treatments and chest pain was reported in 3% to 4% of patients in meta-analyses, which is less than with RFA.[31,32,48]

APC has been associated with a 3%–5% stricture rate.[6,37,38] In one study, 47% had sore throat after the procedure, 11% had difficulty swallowing, and 5% reported fever after treatment.[37] One study of 71 patients reported one perforation (1.4%) requiring esophagectomy,[6] but this was not reported in other studies of traditional APC.[36–38] In the case of hybrid APC, a prospective trial reported a 2% rate of stricture for APC following EMR, a 12% rate of chest pain, and a 4% rate of odynophagia.[52] The rate of stricture requiring dilation was reported as 3.9% in a cohort whereby most patients also underwent EMR.[41] The rate of stricture with or without dilation requirement was reported at 9.1% in a prospective study without EMR.[40]

In a pooled analysis of 15 studies, EMR of a focal lesion had an overall 0.7% stricture rate, a 1.2% rate of delayed bleeding, and a 1.2% rate of perforation.[53] In a meta-analysis of 8 studies evaluating EMR as monotherapy for the complete resection of the entire Barrett's segment, the rate of stricture formation was high at 37%, as was the rate of bleeding (8%), and perforation (2%).[54] A single-center prospective study contends that stepwise EMR, performing no more than 2 EMRs per session, reduced the stricture rates to 1%. ESD had an 11.6% rate of stricture, 1.8% rate of bleeding, and 1.5% rate of perforation in a 2018 meta-analysis of 11 studies.[55]

LONG-TERM RECOMMENDATIONS

Following endoscopic eradication of BE with dysplasia or early EAC, endoscopic surveillance is indicated to reduce the risk of recurrence and progression.[56] Recommended surveillance intervals after CEIM have been recently updated (**Table 4**).[42] Studies have found that recurrence is higher the first year after CEIM,[57] then decreases to a constant rate in the long term.[58,59] As such, the termination of surveillance should be determined by balancing the risks and benefits of surveillance endoscopy in individual patients and considering competing risks of mortality rather than at a set point in time after CEIM. Since even very late recurrence of disease has been reported, patients are never "safe" from recurrence after successful endoscopic intervention.

RECENT DEVELOPMENTS

A report from a large Dutch registry was the first to describe poor healing and poor squamous regeneration after RFA as an outcome.[60] It found that half of patients with poor healing or poor squamous regeneration at follow-up for RFA could successfully achieve CEIM with the intensification of acid suppression or longer time between treatment visits as the most successful strategies.[60]

A second multicenter randomized trial of RFA for LGD was recently reported,[61] the first reported trial to replicate the findings of the SURF trial.[3] The surveillance arm was notable for similar rates of neoplastic progression (26%) to those observed for confirmed LGD in the SURF Trial.[3] However, a high rate of regression of LGD (31%) was observed in the surveillance arm, whereas the rates of CEIM and complete remission of dysplasia were lower.[61]

An early series of 123 patients treated with the Barrx 360 Express RFA self-sizing catheter found good efficacy and safety, with lower stricture rate at a 10 J/cm^2 setting, and this has been adopted as the default energy setting for this device.[26]

A multicenter randomized clinical trial examined a nitrous oxide cryoballoon focal ablation system for the treatment of BE with dysplasia or intramucosal EAC. This study reported comparable outcomes to RFA with lower postprocedure pain.[5]

FUTURE DIRECTIONS

A fundamental challenge in the management of BE with dysplasia and early neoplasia is right-sizing the population treated by endoscopic eradication therapy in proportion to the risk of its disease. Trials demonstrating a benefit for ablative treatment of LGD included only patients with confirmed LGD, whereby the pathology was over-read by a central expert subspecialty pathologist and showed much higher rates of progression than in most community series. Future criteria for the treatment of LGD may require confirmation by 2 expert pathologists using more specific criteria such as,[62] persistent

---

Table 4
Recommended surveillance intervals of the 2020 American Gastroenterological Association Clinical Practice Update on Endoscopic Treatment of Barrett's Esophagus with Dysplasia and/or Early Cancer

Histologic Grade	Surveillance Timing
Intramucosal adenocarcinoma	At 3, 6, and 12 mo and annually thereafter.
High-grade dysplasia	At 3, 6, and 12 mo and annually thereafter.
Low-grade dysplasia	At 1 and 3 y.

LGD across examinations,[63–65] or other risk factors to identify the patients with LGD who would most benefit from endoscopic eradication.

While the literature on the endoscopic management of BE with dysplasia or early EAC has benefited from a series of randomized clinical trials,[3,4,6,22,36,37,39,56,61] none of these compare contemporary ablative therapies head-to-head. Comparing the currently available trials (featuring different patients and different methods) is fraught, and head-to-head comparative studies are needed.

Essentially no studies describe the combination of radiation or chemotherapy with endoscopic resection and mucosal ablation for early stage cancers. Neoadjuvant chemotherapy or radiation therapy could potentially down-stage lesions to an endoscopically curable stage and neoadjuvant or adjuvant therapies might mitigate the risk of concurrent lymph node metastasis. Such approaches may be particularly but not exclusively appealing for poor surgical candidates.

A core unanswered clinical question in the management of BE with dysplasia or early EAC is when to stop surveillance after successful endoscopic eradication therapy. It is not surprising, given that these patients had previously developed neoplastic BE, that they would be at risk of recurrent or progressive BE even after it is treated, and studies suggest a low but persistent rate of recurrence after 5 years. At what point does the risk of performing a surveillance endoscopy outweigh the benefits? This varies both depending on the patient's risk characteristics for undergoing an endoscopy and their risk characteristics for developing recurrent and progressive disease.

SUMMARY

In summary, endoscopic surveillance or endoscopic eradication therapy is indicated for BE with LGD, and endoscopic eradication therapy is indicated for BE with HGD or T1a EAC with low-risk histologic features. Some patients with T1b EAC may similarly benefit from endoscopic therapy. Esophagectomy with lymph node dissection is indicated for most T1b EAC and T1a EAC with high-risk histologic features. RFA and EMR remain the most widely available techniques for endoscopic eradication therapy, but the landscape of endoscopic therapies continues to evolve. Surveillance intervals after treatment are well-defined, but when to stop surveillance considering ongoing recurrence risk, decreasing life expectance, and increased adverse effect risk from endoscopy, remains an area of inquiry.

CLINICS CARE POINTS

- There is no proven benefit in the endoscopic eradication of BE without dysplasia, and endoscopic surveillance is the standard of care for these patients.

- Evaluation of a patient with BE should begin with a comprehensive clinical evaluation to judge the safety of endoscopy and competing risks to the patient, as well as the endoscopic and histologic characteristics of their disease.

- A diagnosis of BE requires at least 1 cm of salmon-colored mucosa proximal to the top of gastric folds with biopsies confirming the presence of intestinal metaplasia.

- A high-dose proton-pump inhibitor is the standard of care in the management of BE with dysplasia and early neoplasia, but other chemopreventative agents remain investigational.

- Endoscopic eradication therapy combines endoscopic resection of any raised or irregular regions, with ablative therapy for any remaining flat BE.

- Band-assisted EMR is similarly safe and effective to cap-assisted EMR but less time consuming.

- Endoscopic submucosal dissection may allow for the resection of large T1a lesions and T1b lesions in some cases, but is associated with a higher stricture and perforation rate than EMR.
- RFA is the most widely available ablative therapy. RFA is safe and effective, and is associated with self-limited postprocedure chest pain in most patients and stricture formation in about 5%.
- Hybrid APC and cryotherapy seem to offer similar effectiveness to RFA as ablative therapies. APC may have a higher rate of recurrence and cryotherapy a higher rate of stricture compared with RFA. However, cryotherapy has less postprocedure pain than RFA and APC is less costly. Head-to-head data are lacking.
- Esophagectomy is appropriate for most good surgical candidates with T1b EAC. It may also be considered in patients with T1a EAC and high risk features of poor differentiation or lymphovascular invasion, due to a higher risk of nodal metastasis.
- For patients who are refractory to RFA, cryotherapy can be used as salvage therapy with a 76% rate of complete eradication of dysplasia.
- Regular surveillance is required following the endoscopic eradication of BE with dysplasia or early EAC and should continue until an individual's risks from surveillance endoscopy outweigh the risk of recurrence and progression.

DISCLOSURE

C.C. Cotton has no conflicts of interest. S. Eluri has no conflicts of interest. N.J. Shaheen has received research funding from Medtronic, Pentax, Steris, CDx Medical, Lucid, and Interpace Diagnostics and has worked as a consultant for Boston Scientific, Cernostics, Cook Medical, Aqua, Exact Sciences, and Phathom.

REFERENCES

1. Shaheen NJ, Falk GW, Iyer PG, et al. ACG clinical guideline: diagnosis and management of barrett's esophagus. Am J Gastroenterol 2016;111:30–50 [quiz: 51].
2. Peters FP, Brakenhoff KP, Curvers WL, et al. Histologic evaluation of resection specimens obtained at 293 endoscopic resections in Barrett's esophagus. Gastrointest Endosc 2008;67:604–9.
3. Phoa KN, van Vilsteren FG, Weusten BL, et al. Radiofrequency ablation vs endoscopic surveillance for patients with Barrett esophagus and low-grade dysplasia: a randomized clinical trial. JAMA 2014;311:1209–17.
4. Shaheen NJ, Sharma P, Overholt BF, et al. Radiofrequency ablation in Barrett's esophagus with dysplasia. N Engl J Med 2009;360:2277–88.
5. Canto MI, Trindade AJ, Abrams J, et al. Multifocal cryoballoon ablation for eradication of barrett's esophagus-related neoplasia: a prospective multicenter clinical trial. Am J Gastroenterol 2020;115:1879–90.
6. Wronska E, Polkowski M, Orlowska J, et al. Argon plasma coagulation for Barrett's esophagus with low-grade dysplasia: a randomized trial with long-term follow-up on the impact of power setting and proton pump inhibitor dose. Endoscopy 2021; 53:123–32.
7. Visrodia K, Zakko L, Singh S, et al. Cryotherapy for persistent Barrett's esophagus after radiofrequency ablation: a systematic review and meta-analysis. Gastrointest Endosc 2018;87:1396–1404 e1.
8. Parikh MP, Thota PN, Raja S, et al. Outcomes of endoscopic submucosal dissection in esophageal adenocarcinoma staged T1bN0 by endoscopic ultrasound in non-surgical patients. J Gastrointest Oncol 2019;10:362–6.

9. Wolf WA, Pasricha S, Cotton C, et al. Incidence of esophageal adenocarcinoma and causes of mortality after radiofrequency ablation of barrett's esophagus. Gastroenterology 2015;149:1752–1761 e1.

10. Vennalaganti P, Kanakadandi V, Goldblum JR, et al. Discordance among pathologists in the united states and europe in diagnosis of low-grade dysplasia for patients with barrett's esophagus. Gastroenterology 2017;152:564–570 e4.

11. van der Wel MJ, Coleman HG, Bergman J, et al. Histopathologist features predictive of diagnostic concordance at expert level among a large international sample of pathologists diagnosing Barrett's dysplasia using digital pathology. Gut 2020; 69:811–22.

12. Hvid-Jensen F, Pedersen L, Drewes AM, et al. Incidence of adenocarcinoma among patients with Barrett's esophagus. N Engl J Med 2011;365:1375–83.

13. Cameron GR, Jayasekera CS, Williams R, et al. Detection and staging of esophageal cancers within Barrett's esophagus is improved by assessment in specialized Barrett's units. Gastrointest Endosc 2014;80:971–983 e1.

14. Epstein JA, Cosby H, Falk GW, et al. Columnar islands in Barrett's esophagus: Do they impact Prague C&M criteria and dysplasia grade? J Gastroenterol Hepatol 2017;32:1598–603.

15. Alkhayyat M, Kumar P, Sanaka KO, et al. Chemoprevention in Barrett's esophagus and esophageal adenocarcinoma. Therap Adv Gastroenterol 2021;14. 17562848211033730.

16. Richter JE, Penagini R, Tenca A, et al. Barrett's esophagus: proton pump inhibitors and chemoprevention II. Ann N Y Acad Sci 2011;1232:114–39.

17. Jankowski JAZ, de Caestecker J, Love SB, et al. Esomeprazole and aspirin in Barrett's oesophagus (AspECT): a randomised factorial trial. The Lancet 2018; 392:400–8.

18. Michopoulos S. Critical appraisal of guidelines for screening and surveillance of Barrett's esophagus. Ann Transl Med 2018;6:259.

19. Yang LS, Holt BA, Williams R, et al. Endoscopic features of buried Barrett's mucosa. Gastrointest Endosc 2021;94:14–21.

20. de Matos MV, da Ponte-Neto AM, de Moura DTH, et al. Treatment of high-grade dysplasia and intramucosal carcinoma using radiofrequency ablation or endoscopic mucosal resection + radiofrequency ablation: Meta-analysis and systematic review. World J Gastrointest Endosc 2019;11:239–48.

21. Dunbar KB, Spechler SJ. The risk of lymph-node metastases in patients with high-grade dysplasia or intramucosal carcinoma in Barrett's esophagus: a systematic review. Am J Gastroenterol 2012;107:850–62 [quiz: 863].

22. Pouw RE, van Vilsteren FG, Peters FP, et al. Randomized trial on endoscopic resection-cap versus multiband mucosectomy for piecemeal endoscopic resection of early Barrett's neoplasia. Gastrointest Endosc 2011;74:35–43.

23. van Munster SN, Verheij EPD, Nieuwenhuis EA, et al. Extending treatment criteria for Barrett's neoplasia: results of a nationwide cohort of 138 endoscopic submucosal dissection procedures. Endoscopy 2022;54(6):531–41.

24. Codipilly DC, Dhaliwal L, Oberoi M, et al. Comparative Outcomes of Cap Assisted Endoscopic Resection and Endoscopic Submucosal Dissection in Dysplastic Barrett's Esophagus. Clin Gastroenterol Hepatol 2022;20:65–73 e1.

25. Mejia Perez LK, Yang D, Draganov PV, et al. Endoscopic submucosal dissection vs. endoscopic mucosal resection for early Barrett's neoplasia in the West: a retrospective study. Endoscopy 2022;54(5):439–46.

26. Magee CG, Graham D, Gordon C, et al. Radiofrequency ablation for Barrett's oesophagus related neoplasia with the 360 Express catheter: initial experience

from the United Kingdom and Ireland-preliminary results. Surg Endosc 2022; 36(1):598–606.

27. Ganz RA, Utley DS, Stern RA, et al. Complete ablation of esophageal epithelium with a balloon-based bipolar electrode: a phased evaluation in the porcine and in the human esophagus. Gastrointest Endosc 2004;60:1002–10.

28. Sharma VK, Wang KK, Overholt BF, et al. Balloon-based, circumferential, endoscopic radiofrequency ablation of Barrett's esophagus: 1-year follow-up of 100 patients. Gastrointest Endosc 2007;65:185–95.

29. Pouw RE, Wirths K, Eisendrath P, et al. Efficacy of radiofrequency ablation combined with endoscopic resection for barrett's esophagus with early neoplasia. Clin Gastroenterol Hepatol 2010;8:23–9.

30. Johnston CM, Schoenfeld LP, Mysore JV, et al. Endoscopic spray cryotherapy: a new technique for mucosal ablation in the esophagus. Gastrointest Endosc 1999; 50:86–92.

31. Shaheen NJ, Greenwald BD, Peery AF, et al. Safety and efficacy of endoscopic spray cryotherapy for Barrett's esophagus with high-grade dysplasia. Gastrointest Endosc 2010;71:680–5.

32. Tariq R, Enslin S, Hayat M, et al. Efficacy of Cryotherapy as a Primary Endoscopic Ablation Modality for Dysplastic Barrett's Esophagus and Early Esophageal Neoplasia: A Systematic Review and Meta-Analysis. Cancer Control 2020;27. 1073274820976668.

33. Westerveld DR, Nguyen K, Banerjee D, et al. Safety and effectiveness of balloon cryoablation for treatment of Barrett's associated neoplasia: systematic review and meta-analysis. Endosc Int Open 2020;8:E172–8.

34. Agarwal S, Alshelleh M, Scott J, et al. Comparative outcomes of radiofrequency ablation and cryoballoon ablation in dysplastic Barrett's esophagus: a propensity score-matched cohort study. Gastrointest Endosc 2022;95(3):422–31.e2.

35. Fasullo M, Shah T, Patel M, et al. Outcomes of Radiofrequency Ablation Compared to Liquid Nitrogen Spray Cryotherapy for the Eradication of Dysplasia in Barrett's Esophagus. Dig Dis Sci 2021. https://doi.org/10.1007/s10620-021-06991-7.

36. Dulai GS, Jensen DM, Cortina G, et al. Randomized trial of argon plasma coagulation vs. multipolar electrocoagulation for ablation of Barrett's esophagus. Gastrointest Endosc 2005;61:232–40.

37. Sharma P, Wani S, Weston AP, et al. A randomised controlled trial of ablation of Barrett's oesophagus with multipolar electrocoagulation versus argon plasma coagulation in combination with acid suppression: long term results. Gut 2006; 55:1233–9.

38. Schulz H, Miehlke S, Antos D, et al. Ablation of Barrett's epithelium by endoscopic argon plasma coagulation in combination with high-dose omeprazole. Gastrointest Endosc 2000;51:659–63.

39. Sie C, Bright T, Schoeman M, et al. Argon plasma coagulation ablation versus endoscopic surveillance of Barrett's esophagus: late outcomes from two randomized trials. Endoscopy 2013;45:859–65.

40. Shimizu T, Samarasena JB, Fortinsky KJ, et al. Benefit, tolerance, and safety of hybrid argon plasma coagulation for treatment of Barrett's esophagus: US pilot study. Endosc Int Open 2021;9:E1870–6.

41. Knabe M, Beyna T, Rosch T, et al. Hybrid APC in Combination With Resection for the Endoscopic Treatment of Neoplastic Barrett's Esophagus: A Prospective, Multicenter Study. Am J Gastroenterol 2022;117:110–9.

42. Sharma P, Shaheen NJ, Katzka D, et al. AGA Clinical Practice Update on Endoscopic Treatment of Barrett's Esophagus With Dysplasia and/or Early Cancer: Expert Review. Gastroenterology 2020;158:760–9.
43. Pech O, Bollschweiler E, Manner H, et al. Comparison between endoscopic and surgical resection of mucosal esophageal adenocarcinoma in Barrett's esophagus at two high-volume centers. Ann Surg 2011;254:67–72.
44. Oetzmann von Sochaczewski C, Haist T, Pauthner M, et al. The overall metastatic rate in early esophageal adenocarcinoma: long-time follow-up of surgically treated patients. Dis Esophagus 2019;32(9):doy127.
45. Duan XF, Tang P, Shang XB, et al. The prevalence of lymph node metastasis for pathological T1 esophageal cancer: a retrospective study of 143 cases. Surg Oncol 2018;27:1–6.
46. Newton AD, Predina JD, Xia L, et al. Surgical Management of Early-Stage Esophageal Adenocarcinoma Based on Lymph Node Metastasis Risk. Ann Surg Oncol 2018;25:318–25.
47. Weksler B, Kennedy KF, Sullivan JL. Using the National Cancer Database to create a scoring system that identifies patients with early-stage esophageal cancer at risk for nodal metastases. J Thorac Cardiovasc Surg 2017;154:1787–93.
48. Qumseya BJ, Wani S, Desai M, et al. Adverse events after radiofrequency ablation in patients with barrett's esophagus: a systematic review and meta-analysis. Clin Gastroenterol Hepatol 2016;14:1086–1095 e6.
49. Quine MA, Bell GD, McCloy RF, et al. Prospective audit of upper gastrointestinal endoscopy in two regions of England: safety, staffing, and sedation methods. Gut 1995;36:462–7.
50. Silvis SE, Nebel O, Rogers G, et al. Endoscopic complications. Results of the 1974 American Society for Gastrointestinal Endoscopy Survey. JAMA 1976;235:928–30.
51. Alzoubaidi D, Hussein M, Sehgal V, et al. Cryoballoon ablation for treatment of patients with refractory esophageal neoplasia after first line endoscopic eradication therapy. Endosc Int Open 2020;8:E891–9.
52. Manner H, May A, Kouti I, et al. Efficacy and safety of Hybrid-APC for the ablation of Barrett's esophagus. Surg Endosc 2016;30:1364–70.
53. Komeda Y, Bruno M, Koch A. EMR is not inferior to ESD for early Barrett's and EGJ neoplasia: an extensive review on outcome, recurrence and complication rates. Endosc Int Open 2014;2:E58–64.
54. Tomizawa Y, Konda VJA, Coronel E, et al. Efficacy, durability, and safety of complete endoscopic mucosal resection of barrett esophagus: a systematic review and meta-analysis. J Clin Gastroenterol 2018;52:210–6.
55. Yang D, Zou F, Xiong S, et al. Endoscopic submucosal dissection for early Barrett's neoplasia: a meta-analysis. Gastrointest Endosc 2018;87:1383–93.
56. Cotton CC, Wolf WA, Overholt BF, et al. Late Recurrence of Barrett's Esophagus After Complete Eradication of Intestinal Metaplasia is Rare: Final Report From Ablation in Intestinal Metaplasia Containing Dysplasia Trial. Gastroenterology 2017;153:681–688 e2.
57. Sawas T, Iyer PG, Alsawas M, et al. Higher Rate of Barrett's Detection in the First Year After Successful Endoscopic Therapy: meta-analysis. Am J Gastroenterol 2018;113:959–71.
58. Sami SS, Ravindran A, Kahn A, et al. Timeline and location of recurrence following successful ablation in Barrett's oesophagus: an international multicentre study. Gut 2019;68:1379–85.

59. van Munster S, Nieuwenhuis E, Weusten BLAM, et al. Long-term outcomes after endoscopic treatment for Barrett's neoplasia with radiofrequency ablation ± endoscopic resection: results from the national Dutch database in a 10-year period. Gut 2022;71(2):265–76.

60. van Munster SN, Frederiks CN, Nieuwenhuis EA, et al. Incidence and outcomes of poor healing and poor squamous regeneration after radiofrequency ablation therapy for early Barrett's neoplasia. Endoscopy 2022;54(3):229–40.

61. Barret M, Pioche M, Terris B, et al. Endoscopic radiofrequency ablation or surveillance in patients with Barrett's oesophagus with confirmed low-grade dysplasia: a multicentre randomised trial. Gut 2021;70:1014–22.

62. Ten Kate FJC, Nieboer D, Ten Kate FJW, et al. Improved Progression Prediction in Barrett's Esophagus With Low-grade Dysplasia Using Specific Histologic Criteria. Am J Surg Pathol 2018;42:918–26.

63. Song KY, Henn AJ, Gravely AA, et al. Persistent confirmed low-grade dysplasia in Barrett's esophagus is a risk factor for progression to high-grade dysplasia and adenocarcinoma in a US Veterans cohort. Dis Esophagus 2020;33:doz061.

64. Kestens C, Offerhaus GJ, van Baal JW, et al. Patients With Barrett's Esophagus and Persistent Low-grade Dysplasia Have an Increased Risk for High-grade Dysplasia and Cancer. Clin Gastroenterol Hepatol 2016;14:956–962 e1.

65. Duits LC, van der Wel MJ, Cotton CC, et al. Patients with barrett's esophagus and confirmed persistent low-grade dysplasia are at increased risk for progression to neoplasia. Gastroenterology 2017;152:993–1001 e1.

Gastric Cancer
Emerging Trends in Prevention, Diagnosis, and Treatment

Dalton A. Norwood, MD[a,b,1], Eleazar E. Montalvan, MD[b,c],
Ricardo L. Dominguez, MD[b], Douglas R. Morgan, MD, MPH[a,*]

KEYWORDS

• Gastric cancer • Prevention • Diagnosis • Treatment

KEY POINTS: IMPORTANT TRENDS IN GASTRIC CANCER

- Recent guidelines for surveillance of gastric premalignant conditions (GPMCs)
  - Major paradigm shift in gastric cancer prevention
  - Surveillance endoscopy at 3 years is recommended for high-risk patients
- Advances in diagnostic technology and approaches
  - Image-enhanced endoscopy and artificial intelligence
- Dissemination of expertise in the endoscopic management of early gastric cancer
  - Endoscopic submucosal dissection is now available in US centers of excellence
- Expansion of gastric cancer targeted treatment options based on genetic biomarkers
  - Outgrowth from the National Institute of Health The Cancer Genome Atlas program
- Leverage of technology advancements

INTRODUCTION

Gastric adenocarcinoma (GC) is the third leading cause of global cancer mortality, and the leading infection-associated cancer with more than 1 million incident cases annually and nearly 800,000 deaths in 2020 (**Box 1**).[1–4]. GC was highlighted as a cancer survival "disparity" because of the breadth of 5-year survival (10%–69%), ranging from

---

[a] UAB Department of Medicine, The University of Alabama at Birmingham, Birmingham, AL 35294, USA; [b] Western Honduras Gastric Cancer Prevention Initiative, Copan Region Ministry of Health, Sala de Endoscopia, Calle 1 S, Hospital Regional de Occidente, Santa Rosa de Copán 41101, Honduras; [c] Department of Medicine, Indiana University School of Medicine, Indianapolis, IN 46202, USA
[1] Present address: 1720 2nd Avenue South BDB373, Birmingham, AL 35294, USA.
* Corresponding author. UAB Gastroenterology and Hepatology, The University of Alabama at Birmingham, BDB 373, 1808 7th Avenue South, Birmingham, AL 35233, USA
E-mail address: drmorgan@uabmc.edu

Gastroenterol Clin N Am 51 (2022) 501–518
https://doi.org/10.1016/j.gtc.2022.05.001
0889-8553/22/© 2022 Elsevier Inc. All rights reserved.

Box 1
Gastric cancer core epidemiology

Gastric cancer is an important global cancer
- Fourth leading cause of global cancer mortality
- Fifth leading cause of cancer incidence, approaching 1 million
- Incidence is expected to rise due to the growing and aging populations in the high incidence regions

Marked 5-year survival cancer disparity, range 10% to 70%
- US 5-year survival is ~30%, compared with East Asia nearly 70%, and low and low-middle income countries 10%–15%

Lead infection-associated cancer
- *Helicobacter pylori* is a WHO class I carcinogen
- The *H pylori* attributable risk is 75%–88%
- EBV coinfection drives 10% of gastric cancers

Gastric cancer represents a marked cancer disparity in the United States
- Incidence rates are nearly double in all minorities compared with Whites
- Although incidence is decreasing since WWII, it is more common than esophageal cancer

Consistent 2:1 male to female ratio in the world
- Estrogen may play a protective role by unknown mechanisms

Gastric cancer has striking geographic variability
- The high-incidence regions: Latin America, Eastern Asia, Eastern Europe
- Immigrants from high-incidence regions maintain the risk of their country of origin

Abbreviations: EBV, Epstein-Barr virus; LMICs, low and low-middle income countries; WHO, World Health Organization.

---

nearly 70% in eastern Asia to 10% to 15% in India and Latin America. In the United States, 5-year survival is 33%.[5] The principal histologic subtypes are intestinal and diffuse GC. This review focuses on distal (noncardia) gastric cancer.

Gastric cancer has remarkable geographic variability, regionally and within countries, which offers the opportunity for focused prevention programs and scientific discovery. The high-incidence regions include eastern Asia, mountainous Latin America, and areas in Eastern Europe and Russia.[2] Immigrants from high-incidence regions maintain the risk of their nation of origin.[6] Large foreign-born immigrant populations in the United States from high-incidence regions include: Mesoamerica (Southern Mexico, Central America), South America, East Asia, Eastern Europe, and Russia. The Central America four region (Honduras, El Salvador, Guatemala, Nicaragua) is the principal low and low-middle income countries region in the western hemisphere.[6–11]

In the United States, GC represents a marked cancer disparity, with nearly double the incidence rates in all non-White minorities.[12–22] Although *Helicobacter pylori* prevalence is increased in minorities, other risk factors play an important role. Additional key features of GC epidemiology in the United States include the decrease in overall incidence since World War II, and the recent increase in gastric cancer in young individuals, including young White females, which may be related to environmental factors or changes in the western microbiome.[23]

General Risk Factors

H pylori infection is the dominant risk factor for GC with an attributable risk of 75% to 88%.[24,25] *H pylori* is classified by the World Health Organization (WHO) as a class I carcinogen. *H pylori* has important virulence and oncogenic genotypes, such as CagA (cytotoxin-associated gene A) and VacA (vacuolating cytotoxin A). Additional risk factors include male sex, older age, family history of cancer, low socioeconomic status, cigarette smoking, alcohol consumption, dietary and environmental factors (eg, salt, lack of fruits and vegetables), previous gastric surgery, and pernicious anemia.[4,26–29]

BIOLOGY AND CLASSIFICATION
Gastric Carcinogenesis Pathway (Correa Cascade)

Gastric cancer is a multifactorial process, with progression through a series of histopathology stages: normal mucosa, chronic gastritis, multifocal atrophic gastritis, gastrointestinal metaplasia (GIM), dysplasia (indeterminant, low-grade, high-grade), and adenocarcinoma (**Fig. 1**).[30–39] This model fits optimally within the setting of chronic *H pylori* infection and the intestinal type GC. Progression is driven by *H pylori* virulence factors and cumulative duration of infection, host genetics and responses, and dietary and environmental factors. Atrophy, GIM, and dysplasia are considered gastric premalignant conditions (GPMCs). The accruing literature suggests that incomplete GIM (colon-like phenotype with mucin drops) has a higher risk of progression than complete GIM (small intestine–like phenotype with a brush border). Extensive GIM, involving the corpus and antrum, is also considered higher risk for progression. Although atrophy may be reversible with *H pylori* eradication, GIM and dysplasia are considered beyond the point of no return, wherein surveillance and/or endoscopic treatment is indicated in addition to *H pylori* eradication. Spasmolytic polypeptide-expressing metaplasia is a specialized form of metaplasia observed in the setting of repair, regeneration, and progression to GIM, yet its precise role in gastric carcinogenesis in humans is unclear.

Host Genetic Factors and Hereditary Gastric Cancer

Familial clustering occurs in 5% to 10% of cases and germline mutations are found in a subset of these individuals.[40–43] A proportion of the clustering is caused by *H pylori*

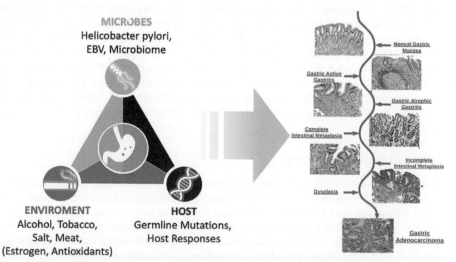

Fig. 1. Gastric cancer risk factors and pathogenesis. EBV, Epstein-Barr virus.

prevalence within families. Hereditary diffuse gastric cancer, with autosomal-dominant inheritance and *CDH1* gene mutations, represents the principal germline genetic syndrome. Surveillance and prophylactic total gastrectomy are considered for individuals with confirmed *CDH1* mutations.[44,45] Putative germline mutations (eg, in *PALB2, FBXO24, BRCA1*) in diffuse and intestinal cancers underscore ongoing investigations in the field.[44] Lastly, gastric cancer occurs more frequently in a variety of polyposis and hereditary syndromes (eg, familial adenomatous polyposis, Cowden syndrome, juvenile polyposis syndrome, Li-Fraumeni syndrome, Lynch syndrome, and Peutz-Jeghers syndrome).[40]

Histologic Classification of Gastric Cancer

Gastric cancers demonstrate significant heterogeneity in morphology and histology (discussed later). The Lauren Classification of gastric cancer histology continues to be the most commonly used system in the United States and most of the world.[46] The Lauren classification characterizes the intestinal type, diffuse type, mixed and indeterminate, or unclassifiable subtypes. Alternate classifications systems include Nakamura[47] and the WHO[48] classification. The Nakamura classification is commonly used in East Asia and is important in the setting of screening and surveillance programs for early gastric cancer (EGC). The Nakamura system discriminates between the differentiated and undifferentiated subtypes.[47,49] The WHO classification is complex, with more than 10 different subtypes, limiting its use in clinical practice. The severity of gastric atrophy and metaplasia is quantified by the Operative Link on Gastritis Assessment (OLGA) and Operative Link on Gastric Intestinal Metaplasia (OLGIM) systems, and the Correa Histopathology Score. These scoring systems are primarily used in research, although OLGA and OLGIM are used clinically in some European and South American settings.

Molecular Classification of Gastric Cancer

The molecular characterization of gastric cancer has been one of the central successes of The Cancer Genome Atlas National Institutes of Health program.[50] Four distinct molecular subtypes were categorized: chromosomal unstable (CIN), genomically stable (GS), Epstein-Barr virus–positive (EBV+), and microsatellite unstable (MSI). Supporting the Lauren classification, the CIN and GS subtypes strongly correlate with the intestinal and diffuse subtypes, respectively. The EBV and MSI subtypes each account for about 10% of cases. Limited percentages of EBV and MSI were noted in the intestinal and diffuse Lauren subtypes, and CIN and GS among the diffuse and intestinal subtypes, respectively. For cancer biology, the The Cancer Genome Atlas results are instructive (eg, defining EBV-associated GC as a distinct entity). Clinical utility in precision medicine is emerging for prognosis and targeted therapies, with *HER2* and immune checkpoint inhibitors as examples.

GASTRIC CANCER PREVENTION

General measures to reduce the risk of GC follow recommendations to reduce cancer risk in general. These measures include tobacco cessation, limited alcohol use, and dietary advice (eg, salt restriction, increased fruits and vegetables). Cumulative data from a range of studies suggest that *H pylori* eradication reduces the risk of gastric cancer, particularly in subjects with chronic gastritis and without premalignant lesions.[51,52] Population-based treatment in healthy individuals with antibiotic regimens for *H pylori* is impractical and may have adverse effects related to antibiotic resistance and the microbiome. *H pylori* treatment as a prevention measure should be individualized, with the example of patients with a family history of GC.[53]

Management of Gastric Premalignant Conditions

Recent international guidelines recommend surveillance with upper endoscopy in patients with GPMCs that are at higher risk for progression based on demographic factors and histologic diagnosis (**Table 1**).[54–56] This represents a major paradigm shift in patient management and aligns surveillance with standards for premalignant lesions of the esophagus and colon. The overall goal is to reduce the burden of gastric cancer and improve survival in regions without screening programs, such as North America and Europe. The current evidence for surveillance is modest and based on the global GC literature, and the recent recommendations are expected to generate important evidence in the coming decade. In patients with GIM, surveillance is recommended for high-risk groups (GC family history, non-White racial and ethnic groups, immigrants from high-incidence regions, autoimmune gastritis) and for those with high-risk histology (incomplete GIM, extensive GIM, severe extensive atrophy [OLGA 3–4]). For GIM or severe atrophy, the recommended interval is 3 years, but may be individualized based on the presence of other risk factors. Surveillance in 12 months is indicated for patients with low-grade dysplasia with no visible lesion. Definitive treatment (eg, endoscopic submucosal dissection [ESD]) is indicated when there is a visible lesion or high-grade dysplasia.[54–56]

Screening for GPMCs, such as intestinal metaplasia, in the general population is not recommended. Focused screening may be indicated in higher risk patients according to demographic and health factors, which include a GC family history, non-White racial and ethnic groups, immigrants from high-incidence areas, and autoimmune gastritis.

The chemoprevention of gastric cancer for patients with GPCs is not recommended, because agents and data are lacking. Observational studies suggest that regular aspirin use may reduce GC risk. Regular aspirin was associated with a significant reduction of risk of GC in women in the US Nurses Health Study.[57] Other studies in Asia and Latin America have reported the role of aspirin as protective for noncardiac GC.[58,59] There are ongoing clinical trials in high-risk populations with various agents, such as eflornithine, curcumin, and cyclooxygenase-2 inhibitors.

Table 1
Recommendations for screening and surveillance of gastric premalignant conditions

	Characteristic	Recommendation
Screening		
Average risk	Average risk	Screening not indicated
High risk	High-risk groups[a]	Individualize screening
Surveillance		
GPMC (eg, GIM)	High-risk groups[a] or histology[b]	Surveillance indicated
Low-grade dysplasia	No visible lesion	Surveillance in 6–12 mo
	Visible lesion	Definitive treatment
High-grade dysplasia	All patients	Definitive treatment

Notes: Surveillance endoscopy at 3 years should be considered for high-risk GPMCs.
[a] High-risk groups: Family history of gastric cancer, non-White racial and ethnic groups, immigrants from high-incidence regions, autoimmune gastritis.
[b] High-risk histology: Incomplete-type GIM, extensive GIM, and severe extensive atrophy (OLGA 3–4).

Helicobacter pylori Eradication

The eradication of *H pylori* is recommended for patients with GPMCs or gastric cancer, particularly EGC, to prevent progression to GC and recurrence, respectively. A recent meta-analysis of 19 studies in Japanese populations that included healthy individuals and patients with EGC showed that eradication was associated with a significant decrease in GC.[51,60] Studies are emerging for eradication in patients with GPMCs. In a recent follow-up of a 20-year Hispanic cohort high-risk population, exposure to *H pylori* therapy and *H pylori*–negative status reduced progression, as measured by the Correa score.[61] International guidelines are consistent with the recommendation for *H pylori* eradication in patients with GPMCs, including guidelines from the America Gastroenterological Association.[62]

DIAGNOSIS
Clinical Presentation

Gastric cancer is generally classified as EGC, operable GC, and advanced GC with respect to diagnosis and treatment. EGC is an invasive gastric cancer that involves the mucosa and submucosa, irrespective of the lymph node metastasis. Endoscopic resection is the treatment of choice for EGC, with a 5-year survival of greater than 90%. Operable GC is defined as resectable, locally advanced ($\geq$T2 N+) tumor. Advanced gastric cancer is inoperable locally advanced or metastatic disease.

The clinical presentation varies between individuals and may be nonspecific, ranging from mild dyspepsia to significant obstructive symptoms signaling advanced disease. The most common symptoms and signs are dyspepsia, anorexia, early satiety, weight loss, abdominal pain, and anemia. Proximal GC may present with dysphagia or regurgitation.

Endoscopic Evaluation

Esophagogastroduodenoscopy with histologic confirmation is the gold standard for gastric cancer diagnosis. The examination should include localization of any abnormality, extension and macroscopic delineation, and targeted biopsies of suspected lesions. Systematic nontargeted biopsies of the antrum, incisura, and corpus may be indicated in patients at risk for GPMCs and to define the background mucosa in those with suspected GC. Studies underscore the importance of careful inspection, which includes adequate mucosal cleansing and insufflation, systematic visual inspection, and adequate examination time. An examination time of 7 to 9 minutes has been shown to increase the detection of GMPCs and EGC, analogous to colonoscopy withdrawal time.[63–65] Visual inspection consists of at least 20 to 22 "stations," with photodocumentation of select landmarks.[66–68]

The macroscopic classification of EGC is described as type I (protruded), type II (superficial), and type III (excavated) according to the Paris Classification.[69,70] Non-EGC is classified according to the Borrmann system into four main types: type I (polypoid without ulceration and a broad base), type II (ulcerated with elevated borders and sharp margins), type III (ulcerated with diffuse infiltration at base), and type IV (diffusely infiltrative thickening of the wall) (**Fig. 2**).[71] The Borrmann type has been shown to be an independent prognostic factor.[72]

Image-Enhanced Endoscopy

Image-enhanced endoscopy, when available, in conjunction with white-light endoscopy (WLE), is indicated for EGC and operable GC, and for patients at risk for GPMCs. Gastric cancer screening programs in Eastern Asia have driven the development of

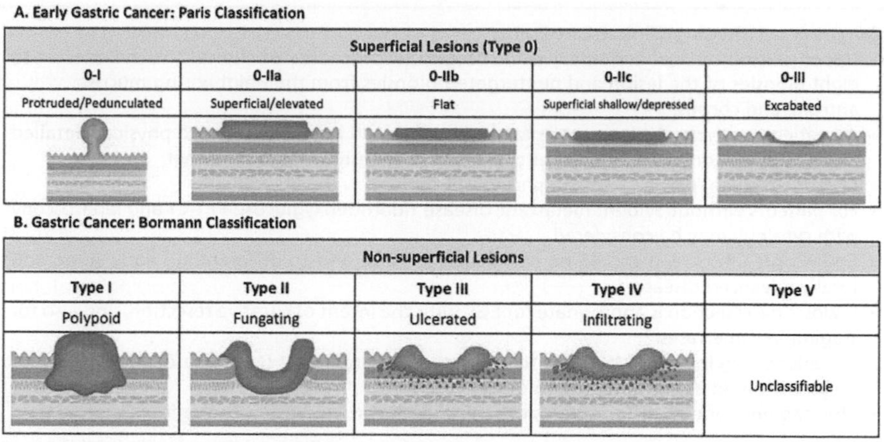

A. Early Gastric Cancer: Paris Classification

Superficial Lesions (Type 0)				
0-I	0-IIa	0-IIb	0-IIc	0-III
Protruded/Pedunculated	Superficial/elevated	Flat	Superficial shallow/depressed	Excabated

B. Gastric Cancer: Bormann Classification

Non-superficial Lesions				
Type I	Type II	Type III	Type IV	Type V
Polypoid	Fungating	Ulcerated	Infiltrating	
				Unclassifiable

Fig. 2. (A, B) Macroscopic classification of gastric cancer.

novel endoscopic imaging technologies and endoscopic resection techniques, with applications throughout the gastrointestinal tract. Image-enhanced endoscopy includes magnification (near-focus imaging and optical/digital zoom), optical technology (narrow-band imaging [NBI], autofluorescence), and chromoendoscopy (indigo carmine). In the near term, the technologies that are readily available in the United States are NBI and near-focus imaging.

NBI has demonstrated greater diagnostic accuracy over conventional WLE in several studies with sensitivity and specificity of 60% and 89%, respectively.[73–80] A substantial increase in sensitivity and specificity (95.0% and 96.8%, respectively) has been noted for the detection of small depressed gastric cancer lesions when NBI is combined with conventional WLE.[81] The criteria for a suspicious lesion are: disappearance of fine mucosal structure, microvascular dilation, and the heterogeneous shape of vessels.[82] NBI findings that are specific for GIM include marginal turbid band, light blue crest, and white opaque substance. Magnification endoscopy with the vascular surface classification system is commonly used in Eastern Asia. The vascular surface system characterizes the microvascular and microsurface patterns independently.[83,84]

Clinical Staging

Gastric cancer should be staged in accordance with standards from the American Joint Committee on Cancer, and the National Comprehensive Cancer Network. Review by a multidisciplinary tumor board is recommended to determine the treatment plan.[85,86] The staging evaluation may include: chest/abdominal/pelvic computed tomography (CT), endoscopic ultrasound, fluorodeoxyglucose-PET-CT, and laparoscopy with cytology.

Biomarkers for targeted therapies are evolving rapidly, and include MSI or dMMR in all patients, and HER2 and PD-L1 in M1 disease. High tumor mutational burden, NTRK gene fusions, and EBV status are examples of additional biomarkers that may emerge in the near term. Next-generation sequencing, when available, is appropriate for multiple determinations rather than individual assays. Lastly, circulating tumor DNA offers diagnostic and surveillance information for patient management.

Diagnosis and Staging Clinical Care Points
- Upper gastrointestinal endoscopy is the diagnostic procedure of choice. This includes six to eight biopsies of the lesion and nontargeted biopsies from the neighboring mucosa, antrum, and corpus.
- All patients with newly diagnosed gastric cancer should have a history and physical, detailed family history, complete blood count, and comprehensive metabolic panel.
- Chest/abdominal/pelvic CT for staging for all patients.
- For patients without evident metastatic disease fluorodeoxyglucose-PET-CT and laparoscopy with cytology may be considered.
- Endoscopic ultrasound should be performed for EGC and to differentiate early stage and locally advanced disease.
- Endoscopic resection is appropriate for EGC with the intent of curative resection, and also for staging in some cases.
- Genetic testing includes MSI (all patients), and HER2 and PD-L1 (M1 disease). Biomarkers for targeted therapies will continue to evolve rapidly.
- The staging work-up differentiates the three clinical stages: EGC, locoregional disease, and advanced cancer.

TREATMENT

Guidelines recommend a multidisciplinary team approach to therapeutic decisions for patients with gastric cancer.[87] GC treatment should be individualized and dependent on the consensus of the endoscopic findings, histology, and staging evaluation. We provide a brief overview of treatment approaches for EGC, locoregional operable disease, and advanced gastric cancer (**Fig. 3**). A detailed listing of targeted therapy and chemotherapeutic regimens is beyond the scope of this review.

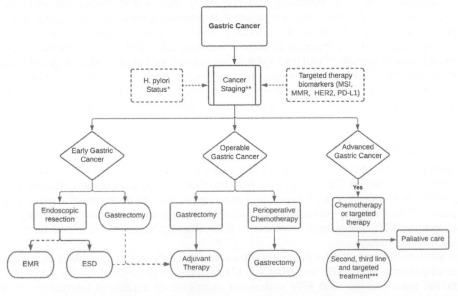

Some ESD and Gastrectomy patients might need adjuvant therapy.

Fig. 3. Gastric cancer treatment algorithm. * Individualized per patient. ** Endoscopy, Endoscopic ultrasound, abdominal/chest CT. *** See table 3.
Abbreviations: ESD, endoscopic submucosal dissection; EMR, endoscopic mucosal resection.

Helicobacter pylori Treatment

Various studies, including meta-analyses, suggest that *H pylori* eradication could reduce the development of metachronous gastric carcinoma following endoscopic resection of EGC.[88–92] Several studies have not shown a decrease in incidence of metachronous GC.[93,94] Although *H pylori* eradication is generally recommended for patients with resected EGC, the decision on treatment should be individualized and discussed with the patient.

Early Gastric Cancer

EGC involves the mucosa and submucosa, irrespective of the lymph node status (T1Nx), with 5-year survival rates greater than 90%. Endoscopic resection is the treatment of choice in patients with a criteria-based low probability of lymph node involvement. These criteria include a mucosal tumor without ulceration, size less than 20 mm in diameter, differentiated histology, and without known lymphovascular invasion.[15,95,96] Endoscopic ultrasound and CT are usually performed in the staging evaluation. Gastrectomy and adjuvant therapy are reserved for cases with a high probability of nodal involvement or a noncurative resection.

Originally developed in East Asia, there is now ample ESD experience in the United States, Europe, and Latin America in centers of excellence.[97–99] The data comparing outcomes of ESD versus endoscopic mucosal resection suggest higher rates of complete en bloc and histologic resection, curative resection, and lower risk of local recurrence with ESD. However, ESD does require more procedure time and clinical expertise.[15,95] Resections of lesions less than 1 cm may be appropriate for endoscopic mucosal resection. Some experts recommend ESD en bloc resection of high-grade dysplasia and low-grade dysplasia with mucosal irregularities to rule out an underlying EGC.[55]

Operable Gastric Cancer

For clinically staged T1 N+ and T2–T4a Nx M0 tumors, the principal treatment is surgical resection with D2 lymphadenectomy, combined with perioperative/neoadjuvant or adjuvant chemotherapy.[100,101] Notably, targeted therapies are developing rapidly and based on ongoing trials, may transition to first-line therapy (MSI/dMMR, HER2, and PD-L1 status). Curative surgery is divided into standard gastrectomy and nonstandard gastrectomy. The standard gastrectomy includes the resection of two-thirds of the stomach with D2 lymphadenectomy. Nonstandard gastrectomy includes other types of gastric resection and depends on the stage.[98] Several meta-analyses suggest equivalent or improved postoperative and long-term outcomes with laparoscopic gastrectomy versus open gastrectomy.[102]

Neoadjuvant/Perioperative Chemotherapy

Perioperative chemotherapy has become the cornerstone in the treatment of locally advanced GC. Examples of regimens include FLOT (5-fluorouracil, folinic acid, oxaliplatin, docetaxel) and ECF (epirubicin, cisplatin and infused fluorouracil). An improvement in survival from 23% to 36% is observed with the use of perioperative chemotherapy with ECF for 2 to 3 months.[103,104] The FLOT regimen demonstrated better pathologic response, higher R0 resection rates, and better survival when compared with ECF, and is the recommended standard of care for patients with locally advanced gastric cancer who can tolerate a perioperative three-drug combination regimen.[86,105,106] Chemoradiation regimens are less common in the United States, with ongoing studies.[107,108]

Advanced Gastric Cancer

Chemotherapy and targeted therapies (discussed previously) represent the standard of care in patients with metastasis or locally advanced unresectable GC.[96,109] Palliative resection or bypass surgery are commonly indicated in specific situations, such as refractory bleeding or obstruction. The only published randomized controlled trial of chemotherapy versus surgery plus chemotherapy failed to show any survival benefit.[110] The current three lines of treatment, based on response and biologic markers with their corresponding evidence, are summarized in the National Comprehensive Cancer Network Guidelines and the literature.[86,111–120]

Treatment Clinical Care Points
- Endoscopic resection is appropriate for EGC with the intent of curative resection. ESD is generally recommended. Endoscopic mucosal resection may be considered for lesions less than 1 cm.
- If the histopathology features of the EGC resection are high-risk for locoregional disease (poorly differentiated, invasion of deep submucosa, positive lateral or deep margins, lymphovascular invasion), then gastrectomy with lymphadenectomy should be considered.
- H pylori eradication is indicated, particularly in EGC patients.
- Operable gastric cancer eligible for gastrectomy with D2 lymphadenectomy includes patients with T1b-T3 Nx tumors who are medically fit.
- For operable gastric cancer T2-T3 Nx or higher, perioperative or adjuvant chemotherapy is recommended.
- For advanced gastric cancer, consideration of systemic chemotherapy and supportive care is recommended, with individualized care plans.
- Targeted therapy based on genetic markers (MSI/dMMR, HER2, PD-L1) is evolving rapidly for patients with operable and advanced disease.

GASTRIC CANCER: FUTURE TRENDS AND NEEDED RESEARCH

The gastric cancer research agenda includes a wide range of initiatives in epidemiology, prevention, diagnosis, and treatment. Gastric cancer represents an important US cancer disparity. Further research in risk factors that are specific to at-risk populations is needed, including H pylori, germline mutations, and dietary and environmental factors. The recent US and global guidelines for GPMC surveillance represents a paradigm shift and will generate important data for the first time, aligning with surveillance recommendations in the esophagus and colon. Promotion of the guidelines is important, since adoption in clinical practice is usually a lengthy process. Endoscopic technologies are changing to support new diagnostic and therapeutic approaches. Targeted therapies will continue to evolve, providing important options for patients with operable and advanced gastric cancer. Lastly, "liquid biopsy" trials are underway, and may change screening, surveillance, prognosis, and treatment monitoring paradigms in the near term.

Future Trends and the Research Agenda
- Gastric cancer represents a major US cancer disparity.
  - Intentional programs for racial and ethnic minorities are indicated.
  - Research in potential prevalent germline mutations is needed.
- Implementation of surveillance guidelines for high-risk gastric GPMCs.
  - Outcomes research with US data on GPMC surveillance programs.
- Development of novel biomarkers for gastric cancer to better define GMPC and GC risk.
  - Improved biomarkers for the risk of progression of GPMCs.

- Research in novel *H pylori* treatments beyond antibiotics.
  - Precision treatment approaches may be envisioned: who to test/treat versus not treat.
- Research in technology and quality diagnostics for GPMCs and EGC is needed.
  - Image-enhanced endoscopy, artificial intelligence (AI), and cytoendoscopy.
  - Research in quality endoscopy metrics and enhancement of training programs.
- Management of EGC will evolve in parallel with GPMC surveillance programs.
  - Outcomes data are needed for endoscopic resection (ESD) in the United States.
- Expansion of gastric cancer targeted treatment options.
- Research in "liquid biopsy" technologies have the potential to foster new paradigms.
  - Screening and GPMC surveillance, prognosis, and treatment monitoring.

FUNDING

This work was funded in part by the U.S. National Cancer Institute (NCI): P01CA028842 (DRM), R01CA190612 (DRM), PAR-15-155 (DRM), NCI CGH HSN261200800001E (DRM), P30CA068485 (DRM), K07 CA125588 (DRM).

DISCLOSURE

Cancer Prevention Pharmaceuticals and Thorne Research (NCI funded studies, with company donation of study medications) (DRM). CDx Diagnostics (Investigator initiated study, with company donation of disposables) (DRM). Freenome Inc. (Trial participation by the University) (DRM).

REFERENCES

1. de Martel C, Georges D, Bray F, et al. Global burden of cancer attributable to infections in 2018: a worldwide incidence analysis. Lancet Glob Health 2020; 8(2):e180–90.
2. GLOBOCAN I. Global cancer statistics. Available at: https://gco.iarc.fr/. Accessed January 9, 2022.
3. Coates MM, Kintu A, Gupta N, et al. Burden of non-communicable diseases from infectious causes in 2017: a modelling study. Lancet Glob Health 2020; 8(12):e1489–98.
4. Bray F, Ferlay J, Soerjomataram I, et al. Global cancer statistics 2018: GLOBOCAN estimates of incidence and mortality worldwide for 36 cancers in 185 countries. CA Cancer J Clin 2018;68(6):394–424.
5. Allemani C, Matsuda T, Di Carlo V, et al. Global surveillance of trends in cancer survival 2000-14 (CONCORD-3): analysis of individual records for 37 513 025 patients diagnosed with one of 18 cancers from 322 population-based registries in 71 countries. Lancet 2018;391(10125):1023–75.
6. Pabla BS, Shah SC, Corral JE, et al. Increased incidence and mortality of gastric cancer in immigrant populations from high to low regions of incidence: a systematic review and meta-analysis. Clin Gastroenterol Hepatol 2020;18(2): 347–359 e5.
7. Torres J, Correa P, Ferreccio C, et al. Gastric cancer incidence and mortality is associated with altitude in the mountainous regions of Pacific Latin America. Cancer Causes Control 2013;24(2):249–56.
8. Pineros M, Frech S, Frazier L, et al. Advancing reliable data for cancer control in the Central America Four Region. J Glob Oncol 2018;4:1–11.
9. Frech S, Muha CA, Stevens LM, et al. Perspectives on strengthening cancer research and control in Latin America through partnerships and diplomacy:

experience of the National Cancer Institute's Center for Global Health. J Glob Oncol 2018;4:1–11.

10. Corral JE, Delgado Hurtado JJ, Dominguez RL, et al. The descriptive epidemiology of gastric cancer in Central America and comparison with United States Hispanic populations. J Gastrointest Cancer 2015;46(1):21–8.

11. Norwood DA, Montalvan-Sanchez EE, Corral JE, et al. Western Honduras Copan Population-Based Cancer Registry: initial estimates and a model for rural Central America. JCO Glob Oncol 2021;7:1694–702.

12. Miller KD, Goding Sauer A, Ortiz AP, et al. Cancer statistics for Hispanics/Latinos, 2018. CA Cancer J Clin 2018;68(6):425–45.

13. Merchant SJ, Kim J, Choi AH, et al. A rising trend in the incidence of advanced gastric cancer in young Hispanic men. Gastric Cancer 2017;20(2):226–34.

14. Siegel RL, Fedewa SA, Miller KD, et al. Cancer statistics for Hispanics/Latinos. CA Cancer J Clin 2015;65(6):457–80.

15. Gupta S, Tao L, Murphy JD, et al. Race/ethnicity-, socioeconomic status-, and anatomic subsite-specific risks for gastric cancer. Gastroenterology 2019; 156(1):59–62 e4.

16. Klapheke AK, Carvajal-Carmona LG, Cress RD. Racial/ethnic differences in survival among gastric cancer patients in California. Cancer Causes Control 2019; 30(7):687–96.

17. Chang ET, Gomez SL, Fish K, et al. Gastric cancer incidence among Hispanics in California: patterns by time, nativity, and neighborhood characteristics. Cancer Epidemiol Biomarkers Prev 2012;21(5):709–19.

18. Morgan R, Cassidy M, DeGeus SWL, et al. Presentation and Survival of Gastric Cancer Patients at an Urban Academic Safety-Net Hospital. J Gastrointest Surg 2019;23(2):239–46.

19. Yao Q, Qi X, Cheng W, et al. A comprehensive assessment of the racial and ethnic disparities in the incidence of gastric cancer in the United States, 1992-2014. Cancer Res Treat 2019;51(2):519–29.

20. Pinheiro PS, Callahan KE, Boscoe FP, et al. Cancer site-specific disparities in New York, including the 1945-1965 birth cohort's impact on liver cancer patterns. Cancer Epidemiol Biomarkers Prev 2018;27(8):917–27.

21. Florea A, Brown HE, Harris RB, et al. Ethnic disparities in gastric cancer presentation and screening practice in the United States: analysis of 1997-2010 Surveillance, Epidemiology, and End Results-Medicare Data. Cancer Epidemiol Biomarkers Prev 2019;28(4):659–65.

22. Liu Z, Lin C, Mu L, et al. The disparities in gastrointestinal cancer incidence among Chinese populations in Shanghai compared to Chinese immigrants and indigenous non-Hispanic white populations in Los Angeles, USA. Int J Cancer 2020;146(2):329–40.

23. Anderson WF, Camargo MC, Fraumeni JF, et al. Age-specific trends in incidence of noncardia gastric cancer in US adults. JAMA 2010;303(17):1723–8.

24. Correa P, Houghton J. Carcinogenesis of *Helicobacter pylori*. Gastroenterology 2007;133(2):659–72.

25. Correa P, Piazuelo MB. The gastric precancerous cascade. J Dig Dis 2012; 13(1):2–9.

26. Arnold M, Park JY, Camargo MC, et al. Is gastric cancer becoming a rare disease? A global assessment of predicted incidence trends to 2035. Gut 2020; 69(5):823–9.

27. Morgagni P, Gardini A, Marrelli D, et al. Gastric stump carcinoma after distal subtotal gastrectomy for early gastric cancer: experience of 541 patients with long-term follow-up. Am J Surg 2015;209(6):1063–8.

28. Murphy G, Dawsey SM, Engels EA, et al. Cancer risk after pernicious anemia in the US elderly population. Clin Gastroenterol Hepatol 2015;13(13):2282–9.e1.

29. Yaghoobi M, McNabb-Baltar J, Bijarchi R, et al. What is the quantitative risk of gastric cancer in the first-degree relatives of patients? A meta-analysis. World J Gastroenterol 2017;23(13):2435–42.

30. Blaser MJ, Perez-Perez GI, Kleanthous H, et al. Infection with *Helicobacter pylori* strains possessing cagA is associated with an increased risk of developing adenocarcinoma of the stomach. Cancer Res 1995;55(10):2111–5.

31. Burucoa C, Axon A. Epidemiology of *Helicobacter pylori* infection. Helicobacter 2017;22(Suppl 1). https://doi.org/10.1111/hel.12403.

32. Correa P. Human gastric carcinogenesis: a multistep and multifactorial process: first American Cancer Society Award Lecture on cancer epidemiology and prevention. Cancer Res 1992;52(24):6735–40.

33. Correa P. *Helicobacter pylori* and gastric cancer: state of the art. Cancer Epidemiol Biomarkers Prev 1996;5(6):477–81.

34. Dixon MF, Genta RM, Yardley JH, et al. Classification and grading of gastritis. The updated Sydney System. International Workshop on the Histopathology of Gastritis, Houston 1994. Am J Surg Pathol 1996;20(10):1161–81.

35. El-Omar EM, Carrington M, Chow WH, et al. Interleukin-1 polymorphisms associated with increased risk of gastric cancer. Nature 2000;404(6776):398–402.

36. Kaurah P, MacMillan A, Boyd N, et al. Founder and recurrent CDH1 mutations in families with hereditary diffuse gastric cancer. Jama 2007;297(21):2360–72.

37. Kodaman N, Pazos A, Schneider BG, et al. Human and *Helicobacter pylori* coevolution shapes the risk of gastric disease. Proc Natl Acad Sci U S A 2014;111(4):1455–60.

38. Rugge M, Correa P, Dixon MF, et al. Gastric dysplasia: the Padova international classification. Am J Surg Pathol 2000;24(2):167–76.

39. Venerito M, Vasapolli R, Rokkas T, et al. Gastric cancer: epidemiology, prevention, and therapy. Helicobacter 2018;23(Suppl 1):e12518.

40. Van Der Post RS, Oliveira C, Guilford P, et al. Hereditary gastric cancer: what's new? Update 2013–2018. Fam Cancer 2019;18(3):363–7.

41. Huntsman DG, Carneiro F, Lewis FR, et al. Early gastric cancer in young, asymptomatic carriers of germ-line E-cadherin mutations. N Engl J Med 2001;344(25): 1904–9.

42. Oliveira C, Pinheiro H, Figueiredo J, et al. Familial gastric cancer: genetic susceptibility, pathology, and implications for management. Lancet Oncol 2015; 16(2):e60–70.

43. Worthley DL, Phillips KD, Wayte N, et al. Gastric adenocarcinoma and proximal polyposis of the stomach (GAPPS): a new autosomal dominant syndrome. Gut 2012;61(5):774–9.

44. Kupfer SS. Gaining ground in the genetics of gastric cancer. Gastroenterology 2017;152(5):926–8.

45. Tavera G, Morgan DR, Williams SM. Tipping the scale toward gastric disease: a host-pathogen genomic mismatch? Curr Genet Med Rep 2018;6(4):199–207.

46. Lauren P. The two histological main types of gastric carcinoma: diffuse and so-called intestinal-type carcinoma. An attempt at a histo-clinical classification. Acta Pathol Microbiol Scand 1965;64:31–49.

47. Nakamura K, Sugano H, Takagi K. Carcinoma of the stomach in incipient phase: its histogenesis and histological appearances. Gan 1968;59(3):251–8.

48. Nagtegaal ID, Odze RD, Klimstra D, et al. The 2019 WHO classification of tumours of the digestive system. Histopathology 2020;76(2):182–8.

49. Gotoda T, Jung HY. Endoscopic resection (endoscopic mucosal resection/endoscopic submucosal dissection) for early gastric cancer. Dig Endosc 2013;25(Suppl 1):55–63.

50. Cancer Genome Atlas Research N. Comprehensive molecular characterization of gastric adenocarcinoma. Nature 2014;513(7517):202–9.

51. Ford AC, Forman D, Hunt RH, et al. *Helicobacter pylori* eradication therapy to prevent gastric cancer in healthy asymptomatic infected individuals: systematic review and meta-analysis of randomised controlled trials. BMJ 2014;348:g3174.

52. Ford AC, Yuan Y, Forman D, et al. *Helicobacter pylori* eradication for the prevention of gastric neoplasia. Cochrane Database Syst Rev 2020;7. https://doi.org/10.1002/14651858.CD005583.pub3.

53. Choi IJ, Kook MC, Kim YI, et al. *Helicobacter pylori* therapy for the prevention of metachronous gastric cancer. N Engl J Med 2018;378(12):1085–95.

54. Chey WD, Leontiadis GI, Howden CW, et al. ACG Clinical Guideline: treatment of *Helicobacter pylori* infection. Am J Gastroenterol 2017;112(2):212–39.

55. Banks M, Graham D, Jansen M, et al. British Society of Gastroenterology guidelines on the diagnosis and management of patients at risk of gastric adenocarcinoma. Gut 2019;68(9):1545–75.

56. Pimentel-Nunes P, Libânio D, Marcos-Pinto R, et al. Management of epithelial precancerous conditions and lesions in the stomach (MAPS II): European Society of Gastrointestinal Endoscopy (ESGE), European Helicobacter and Microbiota Study Group (EHMSG), European Society of Pathology (ESP), and Sociedade Portuguesa de Endoscopia Digestiva (SPED) guideline update 2019. Endoscopy 2019;51(4):365–88.

57. Kwon S, Ma W, Drew DA, et al. Association between aspirin use and gastric adenocarcinoma: a prospective cohort study. Cancer Prev Res (Phila) 2022. https://doi.org/10.1158/1940-6207.CAPR-21-0413.

58. Wang Y, Shen C, Ge J, et al. Regular aspirin use and stomach cancer risk in China. Eur J Surg Oncol 2015;41(6):801–4.

59. Rifkin S, Estevez-Ordonez D, Dominguez RL, et al. Sa2013 aspirin is protective against gastric cancer in a high incidence region of Central America. Gastroenterology 2019;156(6). S-471-S-472.

60. Lin Y, Kawai S, Sasakabe T, et al. Effects of *Helicobacter pylori* eradication on gastric cancer incidence in the Japanese population: a systematic evidence review. Jpn J Clin Oncol 2021;51(7):1158–70.

61. Piazuelo MB, Bravo LE, Mera RM, et al. The Colombian chemoprevention trial: 20-year follow-up of a cohort of patients with gastric precancerous lesions. Gastroenterology 2021;160(4):1106–1117 e3.

62. Gupta S, Li D, El Serag HB, et al. AGA Clinical Practice Guidelines on management of gastric intestinal metaplasia. Gastroenterology 2020;158(3):693–702.

63. Teh JL, Tan JR, Lau LJ, et al. Longer examination time improves detection of gastric cancer during diagnostic upper gastrointestinal endoscopy. Clin Gastroenterol Hepatol 2015;13(3):480–487 e2.

64. Kawamura T, Wada H, Sakiyama N, et al. Examination time as a quality indicator of screening upper gastrointestinal endoscopy for asymptomatic examinees. Dig Endosc 2017;29(5):569–75.

65. Park JM, Huo SM, Lee HH, et al. Longer observation time increases proportion of neoplasms detected by esophagogastroduodenoscopy. Gastroenterology 2017;153(2):460–469 e1.

66. Yao K. The endoscopic diagnosis of early gastric cancer. Ann Gastroenterol 2013;26(1):11–22.

67. Ang TL, Khor CJ, Gotoda T. Diagnosis and endoscopic resection of early gastric cancer. Singapore Med J 2010;51(2):93–100.

68. Emura F, Gralnek I, Baron TH. Improving early detection of gastric cancer: a novel systematic alphanumeric-coded endoscopic approach. Rev Gastroenterol Peru 2013;33(1):52–8.

69. Schlemper RJ, Hirata I, Dixon MF. The macroscopic classification of early neoplasia of the digestive tract. Endoscopy 2002;34(2):163–8.

70. Participants in the Paris W. The Paris endoscopic classification of superficial neoplastic lesions: esophagus, stomach, and colon: November 30 to December 1, 2002. Gastrointest Endosc 2003;58(6):S3–43.

71. Borrmann R. Makroskopische Formen des vorgeschritteten Magenkrebses. Handbuch der speziellen pathologischen Anatomie und Histologie 1926;4:1.

72. Li C, Oh SJ, Kim S, et al. Macroscopic Borrmann type as a simple prognostic indicator in patients with advanced gastric cancer. Oncology 2009;77(3–4): 197–204.

73. Yao K. Clinical application of magnifying endoscopy with narrow-band imaging in the stomach. Clin Endosc 2015;48(6):481–90.

74. Inoue H, Fujiyoshi MRA, Toshimori A, et al. Unified magnifying endoscopic classification for esophageal, gastric and colonic lesions: a feasibility pilot study. Endosc Int Open 2021;9(9):E1306–14.

75. Kato M, Kaise M, Yonezawa J, et al. Magnifying endoscopy with narrow-band imaging achieves superior accuracy in the differential diagnosis of superficial gastric lesions identified with white-light endoscopy: a prospective study. Gastrointest Endosc 2010;72(3):523–9.

76. Miyaoka M, Yao K, Tanabe H, et al. Diagnosis of early gastric cancer using image enhanced endoscopy: a systematic approach. Translational Gastroenterol Hepatol 2020;5:50.

77. Yamada S, Doyama H, Yao K, et al. An efficient diagnostic strategy for small, depressed early gastric cancer with magnifying narrow-band imaging: a post-hoc analysis of a prospective randomized controlled trial. Gastrointest Endosc 2014;79(1):55–63.

78. Yao K, Anagnostopoulos GK, Ragunath K. Magnifying endoscopy for diagnosing and delineating early gastric cancer. Endoscopy 2009;41(5):462–7.

79. Yao K, Doyama H, Gotoda T, et al. Diagnostic performance and limitations of magnifying narrow-band imaging in screening endoscopy of early gastric cancer: a prospective multicenter feasibility study. Gastric Cancer 2014;17(4): 669–79.

80. Yoshimizu S, Yamamoto Y, Horiuchi Y, et al. Diagnostic performance of routine esophagogastroduodenoscopy using magnifying endoscope with narrow-band imaging for gastric cancer. Dig Endosc 2018;30(1):71–8.

81. Ezoe Y, Muto M, Uedo N, et al. Magnifying narrow band imaging is more accurate than conventional white-light imaging in diagnosis of gastric mucosal cancer. Gastroenterology 2011;141(6):2017–25.e3.

82. Kaise M, Kato M, Urashima M, et al. Magnifying endoscopy combined with narrow-band imaging for differential diagnosis of superficial depressed gastric lesions. Endoscopy 2009;41(04):310–5.

83. Fujiyoshi MRA, Inoue H, Fujiyoshi Y, et al. Endoscopic classifications of early gastric cancer: a literature review. Cancers 2022;14(1):100.

84. Muto M, Yao K, Kaise M, et al. Magnifying endoscopy simple diagnostic algorithm for early gastric cancer (MESDA-G). Dig Endosc 2016;28(4):379–93.

85. Amin MB, Greene FL, Edge SB, et al. The Eighth Edition AJCC Cancer Staging Manual: continuing to build a bridge from a population-based to a more "personalized" approach to cancer staging. CA Cancer J Clin 2017;67(2):93–9.

86. Smyth EC, Verheij M, Allum W, et al. Gastric cancer: ESMO Clinical Practice Guidelines for diagnosis, treatment and follow-up. Ann Oncol 2016;27(suppl 5):v38–49.

87. Ajani JA, D'Amico TA, Bentrem DJ, et al. Gastric Cancer, Version 2.2022, NCCN Clinical Practice Guidelines in Oncology. J Natl Compr Canc Netw 2022;20(2): 167–92.

88. Fukase K, Kato M, Kikuchi S, et al. Effect of eradication of *Helicobacter pylori* on incidence of metachronous gastric carcinoma after endoscopic resection of early gastric cancer: an open-label, randomised controlled trial. Lancet 2008; 372(9636):392–7.

89. Choi JM, Kim SG, Choi J, et al. Effects of *Helicobacter pylori* eradication for metachronous gastric cancer prevention: a randomized controlled trial. Gastrointest Endosc 2018;88(3):475–85.e2.

90. Shin SH, Jung DH, Kim JH, et al. *Helicobacter pylori* eradication prevents metachronous gastric neoplasms after endoscopic resection of gastric dysplasia. PLoS One 2015;10(11):e0143257.

91. Fan F, Wang Z, Li B, et al. Effects of eradicating *Helicobacter pylori* on metachronous gastric cancer prevention: a systematic review and meta-analysis. J Eval Clin Pract 2020;26(1):308–15.

92. Khan MY, Aslam A, Mihali AB, et al. Effectiveness of *Helicobacter pylori* eradication in preventing metachronous gastric cancer and preneoplastic lesions. A systematic review and meta-analysis. Eur J Gastroenterol Hepatol 2020; 32(6):686–94.

93. Choi J, Kim SG, Yoon H, et al. Eradication of *Helicobacter pylori* after endoscopic resection of gastric tumors does not reduce incidence of metachronous gastric carcinoma. Clin Gastroenterol Hepatol 2014;12(5):793–800.e1.

94. Kim SB, Lee SH, Bae SI, et al. Association between *Helicobacter pylori* status and metachronous gastric cancer after endoscopic resection. World J Gastroenterol 2016;22(44):9794–802.

95. Facciorusso A, Antonino M, Di Maso M, et al. Endoscopic submucosal dissection vs endoscopic mucosal resection for early gastric cancer: a meta-analysis. World J Gastrointest Endosc 2014;6(11):555–63.

96. Smyth EC. Chemotherapy for resectable microsatellite instability-high gastric cancer? Lancet Oncol 2020;21(2):204.

97. Draganov PV, Wang AY, Othman MO, et al. AGA Institute Clinical Practice Update: endoscopic submucosal dissection in the United States. Clin Gastroenterol Hepatol 2019;17(1):16–25.e1.

98. Japanese Gastric Cancer A. Japanese gastric cancer treatment guidelines 2018 (5th edition). Gastric Cancer 2021;24(1):1–21.

99. Chiu PW. Novel endoscopic therapeutics for early gastric cancer. Clin Gastroenterol Hepatol 2014;12(1):120–5.

100. Davis JL, Ripley RT. Postgastrectomy syndromes and nutritional considerations following gastric surgery. Surg Clin North Am 2017;97(2):277–93.

101. Hiki N, Nunobe S, Kubota T, et al. Function-preserving gastrectomy for early gastric cancer. Ann Surg Oncol 2013;20(8):2683–92.
102. Li Z, Zhao Y, Lian B, et al. Long-term oncological outcomes in laparoscopic versus open gastrectomy for advanced gastric cancer: a meta-analysis of high-quality nonrandomized studies. Am J Surg 2019;218(3):631–8.
103. Cunningham D, Allum WH, Stenning SP, et al. Perioperative chemotherapy versus surgery alone for resectable gastroesophageal cancer. N Engl J Med 2006;355(1):11–20.
104. Chua YJ, Cunningham D. The UK NCRI MAGIC trial of perioperative chemotherapy in resectable gastric cancer: implications for clinical practice. Ann Surg Oncol 2007;14(10):2687–90.
105. Al-Batran SE, Homann N, Pauligk C, et al. Perioperative chemotherapy with fluorouracil plus leucovorin, oxaliplatin, and docetaxel versus fluorouracil or capecitabine plus cisplatin and epirubicin for locally advanced, resectable gastric or gastro-oesophageal junction adenocarcinoma (FLOT4): a randomised, phase 2/3 trial. Lancet 2019;393(10184):1948–57.
106. Xiong BH, Cheng Y, Ma L, et al. An updated meta-analysis of randomized controlled trial assessing the effect of neoadjuvant chemotherapy in advanced gastric cancer. Cancer Invest 2014;32(6):272–84.
107. Anderson E, LeVee A, Kim S, et al. A comparison of clinicopathologic outcomes across neoadjuvant and adjuvant treatment modalities in resectable gastric cancer. JAMA Netw Open 2021;4(12):e2138432.
108. Thierry Andre DT, Piessen G, De La Fouchardiere C, et al. Neoadjuvant nivolumab plus ipilimumab and adjuvant nivolumab in patients (pts) with localized microsatellite instability-high (MSI)/mismatch repair deficient (dMMR) oeso-gastric adenocarcinoma (OGA): the GERCOR NEONIPIGA phase II study. Presented at: 2022 ASCO Gastrointestinal Cancers Symposium; 2022; San Francisco, CA. Session Rapid Abstract Session A: Cancers of the Esophagus and Stomach. Available at: https://meetings.asco.org/abstracts-presentations/204512?cid=DM9577&bid=137147618. Accessed March 10, 2022.
109. Murad AM, Santiago FF, Petroianu A, et al. Modified therapy with 5-fluorouracil, doxorubicin, and methotrexate in advanced gastric cancer. Cancer 1993;72(1): 37–41.
110. Fujitani K, Yang HK, Mizusawa J, et al. Gastrectomy plus chemotherapy versus chemotherapy alone for advanced gastric cancer with a single non-curable factor (REGATTA): a phase 3, randomised controlled trial. Lancet Oncol 2016; 17(3):309–18.
111. Ajani JA, D'Amico TA, Almhanna K, et al. Gastric cancer, version 3.2016, NCCN Clinical Practice Guidelines in Oncology. J Natl Compr Canc Netw 2016;14(10): 1286–312.
112. Ford HE, Marshall A, Bridgewater JA, et al. Docetaxel versus active symptom control for refractory oesophagogastric adenocarcinoma (COUGAR-02): an open-label, phase 3 randomised controlled trial. Lancet Oncol 2014;15(1): 78–86.
113. Fuchs CS, Doi T, Jang RW, et al. Safety and efficacy of pembrolizumab monotherapy in patients with previously treated advanced gastric and gastroesophageal junction cancer: phase 2 clinical KEYNOTE-059 Trial. JAMA Oncol 2018; 4(5):e180013.
114. Kang JH, Lee SI, Lim DH, et al. Salvage chemotherapy for pretreated gastric cancer: a randomized phase III trial comparing chemotherapy plus best supportive care with best supportive care alone. J Clin Oncol 2012;30(13):1513–8.

115. Kang YK, Boku N, Satoh T, et al. Nivolumab in patients with advanced gastric or gastro-oesophageal junction cancer refractory to, or intolerant of, at least two previous chemotherapy regimens (ONO-4538-12, ATTRACTION-2): a randomised, double-blind, placebo-controlled, phase 3 trial. Lancet 2017; 390(10111):2461–71.
116. Muro K, Van Cutsem E, Narita Y, et al. Pan-Asian adapted ESMO Clinical Practice Guidelines for the management of patients with metastatic gastric cancer: a JSMO-ESMO initiative endorsed by CSCO, KSMO, MOS, SSO and TOS. Ann Oncol 2019;30(1):19–33.
117. Pietrantonio F, Randon G, Di Bartolomeo M, et al. Predictive role of microsatellite instability for PD-1 blockade in patients with advanced gastric cancer: a meta-analysis of randomized clinical trials. ESMO Open 2021;6(1):100036.
118. Shitara K, Doi T, Dvorkin M, et al. Trifluridine/tipiracil versus placebo in patients with heavily pretreated metastatic gastric cancer (TAGS): a randomised, double-blind, placebo-controlled, phase 3 trial. Lancet Oncol 2018;19(11): 1437–48.
119. Thuss-Patience PC, Kretzschmar A, Bichev D, et al. Survival advantage for irinotecan versus best supportive care as second-line chemotherapy in gastric cancer: -a randomised phase III study of the Arbeitsgemeinschaft Internistische Onkologie (AIO). Eur J Cancer 2011;47(15):2306–14.
120. Wilke H, Muro K, Van Cutsem E, et al. Ramucirumab plus paclitaxel versus placebo plus paclitaxel in patients with previously treated advanced gastric or gastro-oesophageal junction adenocarcinoma (RAINBOW): a double-blind, randomised phase 3 trial. Lancet Oncol 2014;15(11):1224–35.

Endoscopic Evaluation and Management of Cholangiocarcinoma

Rohit Das, MD[a], Aatur D. Singhi, MD, PhD[b], Adam Slivka, MD, PhD[a],*

KEYWORDS

- Cholangiocarcinoma • ERCP • Next-generation sequencing

KEY POINTS

- Diagnosis of cholangiocarcinoma can be challenging due to the poor sensitivity of standard endoscopic retrograde cholangiopancreatography sampling techniques.
- Next-generation sequencing is a novel diagnostic tool that greatly improves on the accuracy of standard biliary sampling.
- Metal stents may improve the durability of biliary decompression as compared with plastic stents but add expense and do not affect prognosis.

INTRODUCTION

Cholangiocarcinoma (CCA), or cancer of the biliary tract, arises from the epithelial cells of the extrahepatic and intrahepatic bile ducts. CCA is a relatively rare condition, accounting for approximately 3% of gastrointestinal malignancies overall. In a study examining the incidence of CCA in the United States from 2001 to 2015 using the US Cancer Registry database, the calculated incidence of CCA was 1.26 cases per 100,000 people per year.[1] Although this reflects a relatively low burden of disease in high-income countries, CCA is a much more significant problem in particular parts of the world, especially in China and Thailand, where the incidence is 30- to 40-fold higher.[2] For localized disease that is amenable to resection, the 5-year survival for CCA varies between 10% and 40%, and depends on several factors, including site of disease, histologic margin status, and extent of lymph node involvement.[3] For advanced disease that is not resectable, the prognosis of CCA is poor, with a median survival of 5 to 6 months.[4]

The authors have no financial or commercial conflicts of interest to disclose.
[a] Division of Gastroenterology, Hepatology and Nutrition, UPMC Presbyterian, 200 Lothrop Street, Pittsburgh, PA 15213, USA; [b] UPMC Presbyterian, Department of Pathology, 200 Lothrop Street, Pittsburgh, PA 15213, USA
* Corresponding author. UPMC Presbyterian, 200 Lothrop Street, Mezzanine Level, C-2 Wing, Pittsburgh, PA 15213.
E-mail address: slivkaa@upmc.edu

Gastroenterol Clin N Am 51 (2022) 519–535
https://doi.org/10.1016/j.gtc.2022.06.003
0889-8553/22/© 2022 Elsevier Inc. All rights reserved.

Several risk factors for the development of CCA have been identified with strong causal association, which include primary sclerosing cholangitis (PSC),[5] cystic diseases of the liver and biliary tract such as Caroli disease and choledochal cysts,[6] chronic intrahepatic stone disease,[7] parasitic infections of the biliary tree with liver flukes,[8] certain genetic disorders including cystic fibrosis,[9] and chronic hepatitis C infection.[10] Some of these risk factors, specifically primary intrahepatic stone disease and chronic liver fluke infection, are more prevalent in Southeast Asia, accounting for the higher incidence of CCA in this region of the world.

CCA can present anywhere in the biliary tree, and a given patient's presentation depends on the site of disease. In a prospective study of 564 patients, 50% of the patients had perihilar disease, 42% had disease distal to the biliary bifurcation, and 8% had disease isolated to the intrahepatic ducts.[11] Patients with distal and perihilar disease most commonly present with painless jaundice, in the context of cross-sectional imaging evident for signs of biliary obstruction. Patients with isolated intrahepatic disease can present differently, often without jaundice, and rather with nonspecific systemic symptoms and/or cholestatic liver test abnormalities. Not uncommonly, isolated intrahepatic disease can present incidentally, diagnosed on imaging done for alternative indications.

The role of a gastroenterologist in the evaluation and management of CCA is 2-fold. Firstly, to aid in obtaining a definitive tissue diagnosis of malignancy and secondly, to palliate jaundice in patients with biliary obstruction amenable to endoscopic intervention. The former objective is especially important in patients who may have biliary stricturing disease related to benign causes, such has immunoglobulin G4–related cholangiopathy or primary sclerosing cholangitis. The latter objective is used to decrease the incidence of postprocedure infectious complications, palliate symptomatic cholestasis, and allow for the administration of full-dose systemic chemotherapy in select patients. Endoscopic retrograde cholangiopancreatography (ERCP) is the primary endoscopic procedure to achieve these goals. This article focuses on the role of ERCP in the diagnosis and management of CCA and the relative efficacy of the various endoscopic tools and techniques that have emerged over time to help us manage this disease.

THE ROLE OF IMAGING AND ENDOSCOPIC ULTRASOUND IN THE EVALUATION OF CHOLANGIOCARCINOMA

The Role of Imaging in the Evaluation of Cholangiocarcinoma

As part of the initial evaluation of CCA, cross-sectional imaging in the form of computed tomography (CT) and MRI offers valuable information that helps direct subsequent testing and management. In the absence of suspected metastatic disease, focal malignant-appearing mass lesions in the liver may represent either intrahepatic CCA or hepatocellular carcinoma (HCC). This distinction is important to make, as management differs for these 2 diseases. Typically, on CT, mass-forming intrahepatic CCA appears as a hypoattenuating lesion with associated biliary dilatation and occasionally retraction of the liver capsule. On triphasic contrast imaging, there is predominantly peripheral enhancement on both arterial and portal venous phases, in contrast to HCC that demonstrates washout of contrast on portal venous phase.[12] Importantly, a histologic subtype of intrahepatic CCA, known as combined hepatocellular-cholangiocarcinoma (HCC-CCA), may exhibit contrast enhancement patterns that overlap with HCC, making radiologic evaluation less helpful.[13]

On MRI, CCA is typically hypointense on T1-weighted images and hyperintense on T2-weighted images. On dynamic gadolinium contrast MRI, CCA usually shows peripheral enhancement on early images, with central contrast enhancement on more delayed imaging, eliciting a so-called target sign. This radiologic appearance seems to allow for better delineation between CCA and combined HCC-CCA as compared with CT scan.[14,15] MRI also offers the advantage of concurrently performing magnetic resonance cholangiopancreatography (MRCP), which can provide accurate reconstruction of the biliary tree that helps guide biliary intervention and potential operative resection (**Fig. 1**).

For extrahepatic CCA in the absence of mass-forming disease, the main role of cross-sectional imaging is to identify the site of biliary obstruction, help evaluate for other malignant processes that lead to distal biliary obstruction, and provide vascular staging for potential resectability. Although there are some data to suggest that certain MRI and CT features can help identify malignant changes of the biliary tree,[16,17] these findings are not as reliable as compared with those described for mass-forming intrahepatic CCA.

The Role of Endoscopic Ultrasound in the Evaluation of Cholangiocarcinoma

Endoscopic ultrasound (EUS) has emerged as an important tool in the diagnosis and staging of extrahepatic cholangiocarcinoma, particularly distal disease. The distal biliary tree can be very well visualized with the echoendoscope positioned in the duodenal bulb in the long position or in the second part of the duodenum with the echoendoscope usually in the short position. On EUS, extrahepatic cholangiocarcinoma typically appears as a hypoechoic lesion adjacent to or involving the biliary tree. Fine-needle aspiration (FNA) can be performed intraprocedurally to help obtain a diagnosis of malignancy. In addition, prior studies have demonstrated the utility of EUS for visualization and FNA of regional (hilar, cystic duct, common bile duct, hepatic

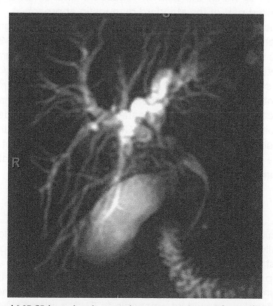

Fig. 1. Reconstructed MRCP imaging in a patient presenting with painless jaundice. Imaging is evident for marked bilateral intrahepatic biliary dilatation with a normal caliber extrahepatic duct, suspicious for proximal CCA.

artery, posterior pancreatoduodenal, and portal vein) lymphadenopathy in CCA.[18,19] In a small study of 47 patients with hilar CCA undergoing EUS evaluation, echo features and morphology of regional lymph nodes did not correlate with malignancy, with benign-appearing lymph nodes demonstrated to be malignant on EUS-FNA.[18] Subsequently, EUS characteristics of lymph nodes should not guide decisions during the procedure on what nodes to target with FNA. EUS can also provide accurate assessment of extent of portal vein involvement. Both findings of regional lymphadenopathy and portal vein involvement can help determine a given patient's eligibility for resection in distal extrahepatic disease. There are also data on EUS-FNA of regional lymph nodes in the setting of proximal extrahepatic/hilar CCA and intrahepatic CCA, suggesting a potential role of EUS in the evaluation of these patients.[19] The finding of malignant regional lymph nodes in these cases may preclude patients from further therapy and liver transplantation. Further studies are needed in this area.

In a study of 81 prospectively enrolled patients with extrahepatic CCA, EUS was found to have a sensitivity of 73% in the diagnosis of CCA. In patients with preprocedural imaging, the sensitivity of EUS was significantly superior to both dynamic contrast CT and MRI (94% vs 30% and 94% vs 42%, respectively) in the detection of tumor.[20] The sensitivity for EUS-guided diagnosis was higher for distal than proximal tumors, and this is not surprising given less accurate EUS evaluation of the proximal bile duct due to its increased distance from the duodenal lumen. EUS was also accurate in determining resectability, correctly predicting resectable tumors in 38 of 39 patients.

Importantly, there are data to indicate that FNA of proximal extrahepatic/hilar CCA, either percutaneously or via EUS, increases the risk of tumor seeding and the development of metastatic peritoneal disease.[21] For this reason, it is recommended to avoid EUS-guided FNA of hilar CCA, as the increased risk of tumor seeding could preclude curative resection or liver transplantations in select centers. For distal disease, transduodenal FNA is within the field of resection, and so EUS-guided sampling should be considered part of the standard diagnostic approach.

Intraductal ultrasound (IUS) has also been used as an adjunct diagnostic tool for the evaluation of extrahepatic CCA. These catheters are small caliber (2–3 mm), operate at a frequency of 20 MHz, and can be advanced over a guidewire through a standard duodenoscope into the biliary tree, usually via a preexisting biliary sphincterotomy. IUS findings that suggest malignancy include disruption of the normal wall layers of the bile duct, identification of a hypoechoic mass, heterogeneous/irregular wall borders, and identification of malignant-appearing peribiliary lymphadenopathy. In one study, the addition of IUS to standard ERCP diagnostic techniques increased the sensitivity diagnosing CCA from 48% to 90%.[22] Given that IUS is not widely available, unable to provide a tissue diagnosis, and associated with high interobserver variability, it is not commonly used.

Our Practice

We always obtain some form of cross-sectional imaging before endoscopic evaluation, and especially for hilar CCA, dynamic MRI with MRCP is our preferred imaging modality. For distal extrahepatic CCA, we perform EUS initially and concurrently with ERCP, to help obtain a tissue diagnosis and exclude pancreatic or ampullary neoplasms. For proximal extrahepatic CCA, we rarely consider pursuing an EUS initially even if there is a focal mass evident amenable to EUS-guided FNA. Many of our patients are considered for surgical resection, and live-donor liver transplantation is a part of our institution's management algorithm for proximal CCA.[23]

Endoscopic Retrograde Cholangiopancreatography and Diagnosis of Extrahepatic Cholangiocarcinoma

ERCP is the preferred modality for obtaining a tissue diagnosis of CCA. Standard ERCP allows for accurate delineation of extent and site of extrahepatic disease and fluoroscopically directed sampling of the biliary tree. In addition, treatment of biliary obstruction with placement of plastic or metal biliary prostheses can be performed during the same session. This section focuses on the various tools at our disposal during ERCP when evaluating suspected CCA.

Endoscopic Retrograde Cholangiopancreatography with Brushings for Cytologic Analysis

Bile duct brushings for cytologic analysis is a time-tested diagnostic tool that is commonly used for evaluation of suspected CCA during ERCP. It is technically easy to perform, carries minimal to no added risk, inexpensive, and widely available. Since the early 1990s, several studies have examined the diagnostic accuracy of bile duct brushings for diagnosis of biliary malignancy. The diagnostic accuracy has been relatively similar across multiple studies, with a sensitivity ranging between 40% and 56% and a specificity between 90% and 97%.[24–26] In the presence of concomitant inflammatory cholangiopathies, this sensitivity decreases significantly.[27] Most recently, a meta-analysis of 1123 patients with CCA was conducted examining the pooled sensitivity for various methods of endoscopic diagnosis of CCA. Among 719 patients for whom bile duct brushings were performed, the pooled sensitivity for cytologic analysis was 56%.[28] Therefore, although positive cytologic analysis accurately confirms a diagnosis of malignancy, negative cytologic analysis is fraught with a high false-negative rate, leading to repeat procedures if there remains a strong concern for malignancy.

ENDOSCOPIC RETROGRADE CHOLANGIOPANCREATOGRAPHY WITH BIOPSIES AND SINGLE-OPERATOR USE CHOLANGIOSCOPY

Histologic analysis via intraductal biopsies is another diagnostic tool commonly used during ERCP for evaluation of CCA. Although bile duct biopsies are relatively more technically challenging as compared with bile duct brushings, especially for more proximal disease, it is similarly safe, inexpensive, and widely available. Therefore, bile duct biopsies are often performed concurrently with bile duct brushings in an effort to maximize the diagnostic yield of ERCP. However, the addition of histologic analysis with bile duct biopsies unfortunately leads to only minimal improvement of diagnostic sensitivity as compared with cytologic analysis with bile duct brushings alone.[25,26,28]

Cholangioscopy has been developed over time as a means to directly visualize the bile duct for various reasons, including lithotripsy of large choledocholiths, helping to obtain guidewire access when standard fluoroscopic techniques fail, and in the case of CCA, allow for direct biliary visualization and performance of visually directed intraductal biopsies of biliary mucosal abnormalities. Single-operator use cholangioscopy (SOC) is a catheter-based system that is most commonly used and allows for a single endoscopist to control both the duodenoscope and a through-the-scope cholangioscope simultaneously. Most recent SOC platforms afford high-definition imaging that maximize detection of biliary mucosal abnormalities. The findings on cholangioscopy that suggest biliary malignancy include raised intraductal lesions, tortuous and dilated blood vessels ("tumor" vessels), mucosal friability, irregular nodularity, and mucosal ulceration (**Figs. 2** and **3**). The recently described Mendoza criteria minimizes the interobserver variability of these findings.[29] The addition of narrow-band imaging (NBI) to SOC

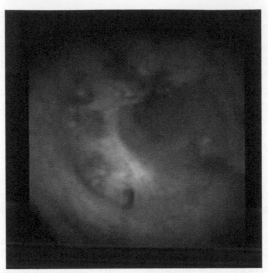

Fig. 2. Cholangioscopic image showing a papillary mass with "tumor vessels" in the left main hepatic duct. Cholangioscopy-directed biopsies confirmed an adenocarcinoma, with KRAS and TP53 mutations on next-generation sequencing.

may complement current cholangioscopy technology,[30] but more data are required, and NBI is not available on the most commonly used SOC platforms.

Since the mid-2000s when SOC first became introduced, several studies have been done examining the performance characteristics of SOC in the diagnosis of CCA. A meta-analysis was performed in 2015 summarizing the results of these studies. Across 8 different studies and 337 patients, the sensitivity for SOC visual impression

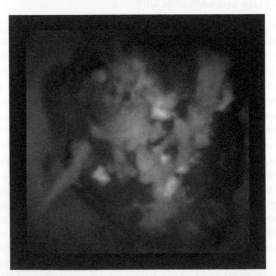

Fig. 3. Cholangioscopic image showing a friable, polypoid mass in the common hepatic duct. Cholangioscopy-directed biopsies showed intraductal papillary neoplasm of the bile duct, a diagnosis that carries a high risk for the development of CCA. The patient underwent definitive resection.

and SOC guided biopsies were 90% and 69%, respectively, whereas the opposite was the case in regard to specificity (87% and 98%, respectively).[31] These results could have several explanations, including interobserver variability of cholangioscopic findings, technique, and volume of biliary sampling. Overall, although SOC visual scoring systems are improving, the false-negative rate of SOC-guided sampling is still significant, and negative results must be interpreted with caution.

In-vivo Microscopy of Biliary Strictures

Confocal laser endomicroscopy (CLE) is a modality that has been used to obtain high-resolution imaging of gastrointestinal mucosa for various premalignant and malignant conditions, including Barrett's esophagus, colon polyps, pancreatic cysts, and so forth. CLE relies on laser technology to illuminate fluorescently highlighted tissue (using intravenous fluorescein), and subsequently capturing images reflected from the tissue that is targeted. Probe-based CLE (pCLE) has been developed to make CLE more convenient during endoscopy, as such probes can be easily passed through the working channel of endoscopes; this has allowed pCLE to have a role in evaluating CCA during ERCP.

A few studies have been performed evaluating the diagnostic utility of pCLE in CCA. Initially, the Miami classification was developed to differentiate between malignant and benign biliary strictures[32]; this was later revised to the Paris classification to include criteria for inflammatory strictures, such as those seen in PSC, and improve the specificity of pCLE.[33] In a prospective, multicenter international study, the utility of pCLE was examined in 112 patients undergoing ERCP for evaluation of biliary strictures. The combination of cholangiogram impression without pCLE and with tissue sampling yielded a sensitivity and specificity of 85% and 69%, with a diagnostic accuracy of 79%. The addition of pCLE yielded a similar sensitivity but increased specificity to 88%, and overall accuracy to 88%. This increase in accuracy was not statistically significant.

Overall, pCLE may be a promising adjunct tool when evaluating biliary strictures during ERCP. However, it is relatively expensive, and its true cost-effectiveness should be better determined. Furthermore, as with all forms of endoscopic imaging, there is a learning curve for interpretation of pCLE imaging, and consequent interobserver variability may affect its diagnostic utility.

The Role of DNA Analysis as an Adjunct to Biliary Biopsies and Brushings

As a consequence of the significant false-negative rate with standard endoscopic retrograde cholangiography (ERC) sampling, and even SOC-guided sampling, several adjunct tools focusing on detecting abnormalities associated with biliary malignancy at the molecular level have been studied in an effort to maximize the diagnostic yield of biliary biopsies and brushings; these have included looking at chromosomal structural abnormalities with various techniques, most commonly with fluorescence in situ hybridization (FISH), as well as genetic mutational analysis with next-generation sequencing (NGS).

FISH is a process by which fluorescently labeled oligonucleotide probes are used to detect chromosomal aberrations, particularly changes in chromosomal number, at loci associated with biliary malignancy. Several studies have been conducted looking at the performance characteristics of FISH in the diagnosis of CCA and how much it adds to standard sampling during ERCP. In perhaps the largest study to date, among 233 prospectively enrolled patients undergoing ERCP for evaluation of biliary strictures, an FISH probe targeting regions of chromosomes 3, 7, 9, and 17 was used. The most common abnormality found among positive diagnoses was polysomy and trisomy of chromosome 3 or 7. The sensitivity for standard cytologic analysis with bile duct brushings was approximately 20% (less than expected based on other institutions published experience, as stated earlier), and the addition of FISH increased sensitivity to approximately 60% without significantly compromising specificity.[34] Other similar studies, including one that used a different set of FISH probes optimized toward biliary malignancy, have shown similar findings.[35–37] Thus, FISH, which is expensive and operator dependent, falls short for optimizing tissue sampling of indeterminate biliary strictures.

Over the past several years, significant effort has been made to better understand the genetic landscape of biliary malignancy, from both a diagnostic and therapeutic perspective. Early studies identified alterations in several key genes that affect the pathogenesis of biliary malignancy, including *KRAS*, *TP53*, *CDKN2A*, and *SMAD4* to name a few, as well as genetic alterations that are potentially targetable for anticancer therapies.[38] As knowledge of this genetic landscape has expanded, and technology for molecular testing become more refined, the ability to perform multigene testing with NGS has transformed the evaluation and management of CCA.

Singhi and colleagues performed the largest study to date evaluating the diagnostic performance of NGS among patients with biliary strictures. This study used a targeted NGS assay, termed "BiliSeq," looking at 28 genes associated with biliary malignancy.[39] Among 220 patients (including both training and validation cohorts) with greater than 1 year of follow-up, and either pathologically proven malignancy (n = 145) or benign biliary disease as defined by clinical criteria (n = 75), the sensitivity and specificity of BiliSeq combined with pathologic evaluation of biliary brushings/biopsies was 83% and 100%, as compared with 48% and 98% with pathologic evaluation alone and 73% and 100% with BiliSeq alone. In a subset of patients with PSC (n = 37), combined BiliSeq and pathologic evaluation had nearly identical performance characteristics. Therefore, the performance of BiliSeq did not degrade in the presence of inflammatory cholangiopathies the same way standard cytology does. Finally, in 13% of cases, an actionable mutation was found that affected anticancer therapy, most commonly alterations in genes involved in the mitogen-activated protein pathway, particularly *ERBB2*.

Similar findings were reported by Dudley and colleagues who also compared the performance of NGS with FISH of bile duct brushing specimens.[40] Using a panel of 39 genes, the investigators found NGS had a sensitivity and specificity for malignancy of 74% and 98%, whereas cytopathologic evaluation had a 67% sensitivity and 98% specificity, and FISH was associated with a 55% sensitivity and 94% specificity. More importantly, the combination of cytopathologic evaluation and NGS yielded an 85% sensitivity and 96% specificity, whereas the cytopathologic evaluation plus FISH analysis achieved a 76% sensitivity and 92% specificity.

Although additional studies are needed to fully understand the utility of NGS in evaluation of CCA, based on the aforementioned data, NGS seems to confer significantly increased diagnostic accuracy as compared with other diagnostic tools and adds no technical challenge to standard ERC sampling techniques. The ability to identify actionable mutations for anticancer therapy clearly distinguishes NGS as a tool to not only aid in diagnosis but also potentially greatly improve prognosis, even among patients who are not candidates for resection. NGS assays to this point are not widely available but given the aforementioned, should be adopted as standard of care when evaluating CCA endoscopically.

Our Practice

When evaluating possible extrahepatic CCA via ERC, our standard approach is to send histologic and/or cytologic samples along with NGS on all samples, based on the strong diagnostic performance characteristics of this combined approach in our institution's experience, as detailed earlier. In patients who have negative results from this combined evaluation, we generally perform repeat sampling before considering a diagnosis and potential treatment of benign cholangiopathies. We consider performing SOC in select cases, especially in the setting of more proximal disease where standard biliary brushings and fluoroscopic biopsies can technically be more challenging. Other diagnostic tools described earlier, such as FISH and pCLE, are not part of our standard clinical practice.

Management of Cholangiocarcinoma During Endoscopic Retrograde Cholangiopancreatography

The main role of ERCP in management of CCA is to relieve biliary obstruction in patients with unresectable disease, for relief of related signs and symptoms, including jaundice and pruritis, as well as for medical optimization before systemic anticancer therapy. In patients who are candidates for definitive surgical resection, the clinical utility of preoperative biliary decompression is not completely clear. If surgery is to be delayed, preoperative biliary decompression is usually pursued to palliate symptoms and prevent chronic liver injury related to ongoing biliary obstruction. Otherwise, there are significant data to suggest that preoperative biliary decompression is not necessarily of clinical benefit and may even increase the risk of postoperative complications.[41,42]

Endoscopic Management of Distal Biliary Obstruction in Cholangiocarcinoma

In patients with extrahepatic CCA that is at least 1 to 2 cm distal to the biliary bifurcation, ERCP can usually palliate biliary obstruction effectively with a single biliary prosthesis. The question as to whether to place a plastic stent versus metal stent has been addressed in several studies, which have all looked at distal malignant biliary obstruction of various causes. In a meta-analysis of these studies from 2015, including 19 studies and nearly 2000 patients, the investigators examined plastic versus metal stents in both distal and proximal malignant biliary obstruction and subdivided their analysis based on site of disease.[43] Among patients with distal biliary obstruction, as compared with plastic stents, metal stents had significantly decreased rates of occlusion and need for reintervention, but no significant difference in short-term mortality or incidence of cholangitis. A more recent meta-analysis looking only at distal biliary obstruction showed similar findings but also suggested increased survival and decreased cholangitis with metal stents.[44] Given these data, metal stents should be favored over plastic stents in most patients with unresectable distal CCA, although plastic stents can be considered in patients with a very poor short-term prognosis to minimize expense.

When a metal stent is placed, the choice as to whether place an uncovered versus covered prosthesis is controversial. Uncovered stents are less expensive, but theoretically carry an increased risk of occlusion due to potential for in-stent tissue/tumor ingrowth. Covered stents can counteract this risk but have a higher risk of migration and theoretically an increased risk of cholecystitis if the cystic duct orifice lies within the path of the stent. A meta-analysis by Sawas and colleagues examining this question was conducted in 2018 using 11 randomized controlled trials, totaling 1272 patients.[45] Although there was an increased rate of stent ingrowth in uncovered metal stents, covered stents had a higher rate of migration, sludge/stone formation, and tumor overgrowth. Overall, there was no statistically significant difference in mortality rate or stent failure between the 2 groups. Furthermore, there was no difference in rates of adverse events, including cholangitis and cholecystitis.

Endoscopic Management of Biliary Obstruction in Proximal/Hilar Cholangiocarcinoma

Endoscopic management of biliary obstruction in patients with proximal CCA can be much more technically challenging as compared with patients with distal obstruction. On occasion, especially for angulated, severe hilar stenoses, retrograde access into obstructed biliary systems is not achievable, and percutaneous transhepatic biliary decompression may be necessary to best palliate jaundice in these patients. For this reason, ERCP for proximal CCA should be performed at centers of expertise for both advanced endoscopy and interventional radiology and decisions made in a multidisciplinary fashion.

Similar to distal obstruction, several studies have examined the comparative efficacy of plastic versus metal stents in the management of proximal, unresectable CCA. The largest randomized trial to help answer this question was published in 2012 and included 108 patients with unresectable hilar CCA. These patients already had a diagnosis, no prior biliary intervention, and received either a unilateral plastic (7-French [Fr] or 10-Fr) or an uncovered metal stent. In their intention-to-treat analysis, patients who received metal stents had a higher rate of achieving successful biliary decompression (defined as 50% decrease in total bilirubin at 4 weeks) and increased survival.[46] In the same meta-analysis by Sawas and colleagues discussed previously, in patients with proximal CCA, metal stents led to lower occlusion rates and incidence of cholangitis, and higher rates of successful drainage, but did not affect 30-day mortality or reintervention rates.[43] These data suggest that metal stents may be more beneficial than plastic stents in proximal CCA for some important clinical outcomes but not necessarily long-term survival. Importantly, uncovered stents are usually preferred in this setting, as covered stents can obstruct the contralateral tributaries of intrahepatic ducts, which can significantly increase the risk of cholangitis.

A second question to ask in the setting of proximal CCA is whether bilateral drainage offers more benefit than unilateral drainage. Several things need to be considered when approaching this issue as an endoscopist. Firstly, studies using liver volumetrics have shown that drainage of greater than 50% of the liver is required to achieve effective biliary decompression[47]; this takes into account the "quality" of the liver drained, as drainage of sectors of the liver that are atrophied, infiltrated by tumor, or affected by portal vein thrombosis does not lead to clinical benefit and likely increases the risk of infectious complications (**Fig. 4**). These factors should all be considered when deciding between unilateral versus bilateral decompression, and high-quality preprocedural imaging is paramount in guiding this decision.

Studies looking at unilateral versus bilateral stenting, either with plastic or metal stents, have been equivocal. A randomized trial in 2013 comparing plastic and metal stents in proximal CCA, with a nearly equal number of patients who underwent unilateral versus bilateral stenting, showed no difference in stent occlusion rates.[48] In their meta-analysis, Sawas and colleagues also showed no difference in clinical outcomes between unilateral versus bilateral stenting.[43] A more recent randomized trial looking at unilateral versus bilateral metal stents did show better stent patency and less need for reintervention in the bilateral stent group but no difference in survival.[49]

In some patients, ERCP fails to address biliary obstruction; this could be due to a wide variety of reasons, including failed biliary cannulation, surgically altered anatomy, or inability to access desired obstructed segments retrograde. Percutaneous transhepatic biliary drain placement is the most commonly used management alternative in this setting. However, EUS-guided biliary drainage (EUS-BD) is an emerging endoscopic alternative whereby decompression can be achieved in a transduodenal (for

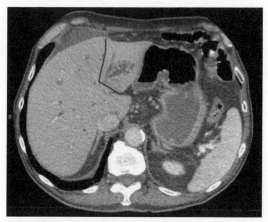

Fig. 4. Contrast-enhanced CT imaging in a patient with hilar CCA. The patient has left-sided biliary dilatation, but the left lobe is atrophic. In such a scenario, left-sided biliary intervention may not be of clinical benefit.

distal obstruction) or transgastric (for proximal obstruction, targeting left intrahepatic ducts) fashion. EUS-BD has been shown to be effective, but associated with significant morbidity, and should only be performed at centers of expertise.[50]

Novel intraductal ablative techniques have also been studied in the setting of unresectable proximal CCA. Photodynamic therapy (PDT) is an ablative technique that destroys tumor tissue through the interaction of locally applied light and an intravenously administered photosensitizing agent that is preferentially absorbed by neoplastic tissue. Modalities to apply PDT within the biliary tree have been developed, and its utility in management of CCA has been examined in several studies. A meta-analysis of these studies does suggest that the addition of PDT to standard endoscopic management improves survival.[51] The largest randomized trial (39 patients) actually prematurely halted their study due to the increased benefit of PDT immediately seen in their population, with a median survival of 493 days in the PDT group versus 98 days in the group receiving standard of care.[52] PDT is expensive, often not covered by insurance, and requires patients to avoid sunlight for prolonged periods of time.

Radiofrequency ablation (RFA) is another ablative technique that is becoming a more popular alternative to PDT, which uses heat energy to induce tissue necrosis. RFA probes that can be advanced through the working channel of a duodenoscope have been developed, and consequently, the utility of RFA in management of unresectable extrahepatic CCA has been examined. The largest randomized trial consisted of 96 patients and compared 8.5-Fr stent placement with and without RFA. The study did show significantly improved stent patency and overall mean survival in the RFA group, without an increase in adverse events.[53] Importantly, patients with more complex stenoses (Bismuth III or IV) were excluded from this study, questioning whether RFA would have shown any benefit if a metal stent was used. Overall, for both PDT and RFA, more data are needed to determine their true cost-effectiveness, as they are relatively expensive technologies and not widely available.

Our Practice

For patients presenting with suspected biliary obstruction from distal CCA, we usually place a covered metal or plastic stent at initial ERCP while awaiting the results of

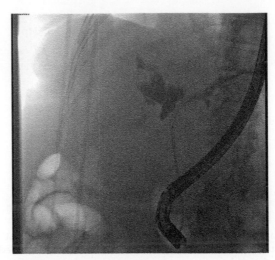

Fig. 5. Cholangiogram image of a patient with hilar CCA, showing bilateral biliary dilatation. A guidewire and balloon are in place in the left intrahepatic duct. Access into the dilated right intrahepatic system is later achieved.

sampling and plan of management. Once a diagnosis of CCA has been confirmed and a patient is deemed unresectable, in patients who started with a plastic stent, we place uncovered stents due to the added expense of covered metal stents and lack of data supporting their use over their uncovered counterparts.

In the case of more proximal disease, we use MRCP and dynamic cross-sectional imaging to help determine which liver sectors are worth draining and the utility of unilateral versus bilateral decompression. As in distal disease, we place plastics stents at index ERCP while awaiting the results of biliary sampling and plan of management (**Figs. 5** and **6**). We generally exchange to plastic stents during subsequent ERCPs

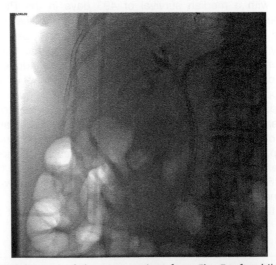

Fig. 6. Cholangiogram image of the same patient from **Fig. 5**, after bilateral 10-Fr plastic stent placement into the systems that were accessed and opacified.

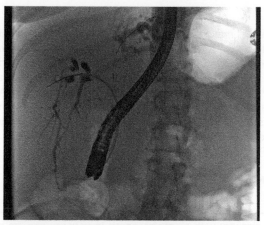

Fig. 7. Cholangiogram image of a patient with hilar CCA, showing bilateral biliary dilatation and access into both opacified systems. This patient had recurrent cholangitis with bilateral plastic stents, and this procedure was performed with the intent of exchanging to bilateral uncovered metal stents.

mainly because of their reduced expense and longer survival in these patients as compared with patients with pancreatic cancer with obstructive jaundice. Subsequent uncovered metal stent—related complications can be challenging to manage endoscopically and is another important consideration.

The use of uncovered metal versus plastic stents in patients in whom bilateral stenting is being contemplated is determined on a case-by-case basis, considering access to anatomic segments and prognosis. Guidewire access without contrast injection, and subsequent anterograde contrast injection, is useful to fulfill the "drain what you fill" axiom and minimize infectious complications (**Figs. 7** and **8**). Preprocedural and postprocedural antibiotics are used for all cases of proximal CCA. Adjunct endoscopic modalities, such as RFA and PDT, are not part of our standard practice, but we have been using RFA in selected patients with increasing frequency.

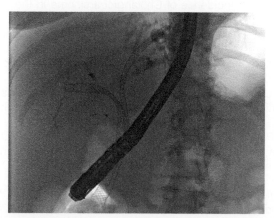

Fig. 8. Cholangiogram image of the same patient from **Fig. 7**, after successful placement of bilateral uncovered metal stents.

SUMMARY

Among gastrointestinal malignancies, CCA is a relatively rare condition, which, in the absence of resection, has a poor prognosis. Obtaining a tissue diagnosis of malignancy can be challenging in CCA due to the poor sensitivity of standard ERCP sampling techniques. More novel diagnostic tools, particularly DNA analysis of biliary tissue with NGS, has greatly improved our ability to diagnose CCA and differentiate between benign and malignant biliary disease. ERCP with placement of plastic or metal biliary stents remains the mainstay of managing biliary obstruction related to CCA, although evolving intra-ductal ablative platforms may significantly improve the capability of ERCP to palliate this disease.

CLINICS CARE POINTS

- CCA is a rare malignancy with a poor prognosis in patients who are not candidates for definitive resection. Strong risk factors for CCA include primary sclerosing cholangitis, cystic diseases of the biliary tree, and chronic intrahepatic stone disease, among others.

- Dynamic contrasted cross-sectional imaging is a key part of the evaluation in CCA, especially in patients with intrahepatic disease, where differentiation from other hepatic lesions/malignancies is imperative.

- For extrahepatic CCA, standard sampling techniques have a high specificity but are fraught by poor sensitivity that often leads to repeat procedural evaluation. DNA analysis of biliary tissue with NGS significantly improves on the sensitivity of ERCP sampling, without sacrificing specificity nor adding technical complexity to ERCP.

- In endoscopic management of CCA, metal stents may offer more durability and less need for reintervention as compared with plastic stents in both distal and proximal extrahepatic CCA but do not necessarily affect long-term outcome. Whether to pursue unilateral or bilateral drainage should be determined on a case-by-case basis, using preprocedural imaging as a guide.

REFERENCES

1. Patel N, Benipal B. Incidence of Cholangiocarcinoma in the USA from 2001 to 2015: A US Cancer Statistics Analysis of 50 States. Cureus 2019;11(1):e3962.
2. Ouyang G, Liu Q, Wu Y, et al. The global, regional, and national burden of gallbladder and biliary tract cancer and its attributable risk factors in 195 countries and territories, 1990 to 2017: A systematic analysis for the Global Burden of Disease Study 2017. Cancer 2021;127(13):2238–50.
3. Murakami Y, Uemura K, Sudo T, et al. Prognostic factors after surgical resection for intrahepatic, hilar, and distal cholangiocarcinoma. Ann Surg Oncol 2011; 18(3):651–8.
4. Lamarca A, Palmer DH, Wasan HS, et al. Second-line FOLFOX chemotherapy versus active symptom control for advanced biliary tract cancer (ABC-06): a phase 3, open-label, randomised, controlled trial. Lancet Oncol 2021;22(5): 690–701.
5. Burak K, Angulo P, Pasha TM, et al. Incidence and risk factors for cholangiocarcinoma in primary sclerosing cholangitis. Am J Gastroenterol 2004;99(3):523–6.
6. He XD, Wang L, Liu W, et al. The risk of carcinogenesis in congenital choledochal cyst patients: an analysis of 214 cases. Ann Hepatol 2014;13(6):819–26.

7. Lee CC, Wu CY, Chen GH. What is the impact of coexistence of hepatolithiasis on cholangiocarcinoma? J Gastroenterol Hepatol 2002;17(9):1015–20.

8. Watanapa P, Watanapa WB. Liver fluke-associated cholangiocarcinoma. Br J Surg 2002;89(8):962–70.

9. Yamada A, Komaki Y, Komaki F, et al. Risk of gastrointestinal cancers in patients with cystic fibrosis: a systematic review and meta-analysis. Lancet Oncol 2018; 19(6):758–67.

10. Mahale P, Torres HA, Kramer JR, et al. Hepatitis C virus infection and the risk of cancer among elderly US adults: A registry-based case-control study. Cancer 2017;123(7):1202–11.

11. DeOliveira ML, Cunningham SC, Cameron JL, et al. Cholangiocarcinoma: thirty-one-year experience with 564 patients at a single institution. Ann Surg 2007; 245(5):755–62.

12. Iavarone M, Piscaglia F, Vavassori S, et al. Contrast enhanced CT-scan to diagnose intrahepatic cholangiocarcinoma in patients with cirrhosis. J Hepatol 2013;58(6):1188–93.

13. Fowler KJ, Sheybani A, Parker RA 3rd, et al. Combined hepatocellular and cholangiocarcinoma (biphenotypic) tumors: imaging features and diagnostic accuracy of contrast-enhanced CT and MRI. AJR Am J Roentgenol 2013;201(2): 332–9.

14. Hwang J, Kim YK, Park MJ, et al. Differentiating combined hepatocellular and cholangiocarcinoma from mass-forming intrahepatic cholangiocarcinoma using gadoxetic acid-enhanced MRI. J Magn Reson Imaging 2012;36(4):881–9.

15. Manfredi R, Barbaro B, Masselli G, et al. Magnetic resonance imaging of cholangiocarcinoma. Semin Liver Dis 2004;24(2):155–64.

16. Choi SH, Han JK, Lee JM, et al. Differentiating malignant from benign common bile duct stricture with multiphasic helical CT. Radiology 2005;236(1):178–83.

17. Cui XY, Chen HW, Cai S, et al. Diffusion-weighted MR imaging for detection of extrahepatic cholangiocarcinoma. Eur J Radiol 2012;81(11):2961–5.

18. Gleeson FC, Rajan E, Levy MJ, et al. EUS-guided FNA of regional lymph nodes in patients with unresectable hilar cholangiocarcinoma. Gastrointest Endosc 2008; 67(3):438–43.

19. Malikowski T, Levy MJ, Gleeson FC, et al. Endoscopic Ultrasound/Fine Needle Aspiration Is Effective for Lymph Node Staging in Patients With Cholangiocarcinoma. Hepatology 2020;72(3):940–8.

20. Mohamadnejad M, DeWitt JM, Sherman S, et al. Role of EUS for preoperative evaluation of cholangiocarcinoma: a large single-center experience. Gastrointest Endosc 2011;73(1):71–8.

21. Heimbach JK, Sanchez W, Rosen CB, et al. Trans-peritoneal fine needle aspiration biopsy of hilar cholangiocarcinoma is associated with disease dissemination. HPB (Oxford) 2011;13(5):356–60.

22. Farrell RJ, Agarwal B, Brandwein SL, et al. Intraductal US is a useful adjunct to ERCP for distinguishing malignant from benign biliary strictures. Gastrointest Endosc 2002;56(5):681–7.

23. Olthoff KM, Smith AR, Abecassis M, et al. Defining long-term outcomes with living donor liver transplantation in North America. Ann Surg 2015;262(3):465–75.

24. Glasbrenner B, Ardan M, Boeck W, et al. Prospective evaluation of brush cytology of biliary strictures during endoscopic retrograde cholangiopancreatography. Endoscopy 1999;31(9):712–7.

25. Ponchon T, Gagnon P, Berger F, et al. Value of endobiliary brush cytology and biopsies for the diagnosis of malignant bile duct stenosis: results of a prospective study. Gastrointest Endosc 1995;42(6):565–72.

26. Weber A, von Weyhern C, Fend F, et al. Endoscopic transpapillary brush cytology and forceps biopsy in patients with hilar cholangiocarcinoma. World J Gastroenterol 2008;14(7):1097–101.

27. Trikudanathan G, Navaneethan U, Njei B, et al. Diagnostic yield of bile duct brushings for cholangiocarcinoma in primary sclerosing cholangitis: a systematic review and meta-analysis. Gastrointest Endosc 2014;79(5):783–9.

28. Yoon SB, Moon SH, Ko SW, et al. Brush Cytology, Forceps Biopsy, or Endoscopic Ultrasound-Guided Sampling for Diagnosis of Bile Duct Cancer: A Meta-Analysis. Dig Dis Sci 2022;67(7):3284–97.

29. Kahaleh M, Gaidhane M, Shahid HM, et al. Digital single-operator cholangioscopy interobserver study using a new classification: the Mendoza Classification (with video). Gastrointest Endosc 2022;95(2):319–26.

30. Mounzer R, Austin GL, Wani S, et al. Per-oral video cholangiopancreatoscopy with narrow-band imaging for the evaluation of indeterminate pancreaticobiliary disease. Gastrointest Endosc 2017;85(3):509–17.

31. Sun X, Zhou Z, Tian J, et al. Is single-operator peroral cholangioscopy a useful tool for the diagnosis of indeterminate biliary lesion? A systematic review and meta-analysis. Gastrointest Endosc 2015;82(1):79–87.

32. Meining A, Chen YK, Pleskow D, et al. Direct visualization of indeterminate pancreaticobiliary strictures with probe-based confocal laser endomicroscopy: a multicenter experience. Gastrointest Endosc 2011;74(5):961–8.

33. Caillol F, Filoche B, Gaidhane M, et al. Refined probe-based confocal laser endomicroscopy classification for biliary strictures: the Paris Classification. Dig Dis Sci 2013;58(6):1784–9.

34. Moreno Luna LE, Kipp B, Halling KC, et al. Advanced cytologic techniques for the detection of malignant pancreatobiliary strictures. Gastroenterology 2006;131(4):1064–72.

35. Barr Fritcher EG, Voss JS, Brankley SM, et al. An Optimized Set of Fluorescence In Situ Hybridization Probes for Detection of Pancreatobiliary Tract Cancer in Cytology Brush Samples. Gastroenterology 2015;149(7):1813–1824 e1811.

36. Levy MJ, Baron TH, Clayton AC, et al. Prospective evaluation of advanced molecular markers and imaging techniques in patients with indeterminate bile duct strictures. Am J Gastroenterol 2008;103(5):1263–73.

37. Liew ZH, Loh TJ, Lim TKH, et al. Role of fluorescence in situ hybridization in diagnosing cholangiocarcinoma in indeterminate biliary strictures. J Gastroenterol Hepatol 2018;33(1):315–9.

38. Lowery MA, Ptashkin R, Jordan E, et al. Comprehensive Molecular Profiling of Intrahepatic and Extrahepatic Cholangiocarcinomas: Potential Targets for Intervention. Clin Cancer Res 2018;24(17):4154–61.

39. Singhi AD, Nikiforova MN, Chennat J, et al. Integrating next-generation sequencing to endoscopic retrograde cholangiopancreatography (ERCP)-obtained biliary specimens improves the detection and management of patients with malignant bile duct strictures. Gut 2020;69(1):52–61.

40. Dudley JC, Zheng Z, McDonald T, et al. Next-Generation Sequencing and Fluorescence in Situ Hybridization Have Comparable Performance Characteristics in the Analysis of Pancreaticobiliary Brushings for Malignancy. J Mol Diagn 2016;18(1):124–30.

41. Liu F, Li Y, Wei Y, et al. Preoperative biliary drainage before resection for hilar cholangiocarcinoma: whether or not? A systematic review. Dig Dis Sci 2011; 56(3):663–72.
42. Pisters PW, Hudec WA, Hess KR, et al. Effect of preoperative biliary decompression on pancreaticoduodenectomy-associated morbidity in 300 consecutive patients. Ann Surg 2001;234(1):47–55.
43. Sawas T, Al Halabi S, Parsi MA, et al. Self-expandable metal stents versus plastic stents for malignant biliary obstruction: a meta-analysis. Gastrointest Endosc 2015;82(2):256–267 e257.
44. Moole H, Jaeger A, Cashman M, et al. Are self-expandable metal stents superior to plastic stents in palliating malignant distal biliary strictures? A meta-analysis and systematic review. Med J Armed Forces India 2017;73(1):42–8.
45. Tringali A, Hassan C, Rota M, et al. Covered vs. uncovered self-expandable metal stents for malignant distal biliary strictures: a systematic review and meta-analysis. Endoscopy 2018;50(6):631–41.
46. Sangchan A, Kongkasame W, Pugkhem A, et al. Efficacy of metal and plastic stents in unresectable complex hilar cholangiocarcinoma: a randomized controlled trial. Gastrointest Endosc 2012;76(1):93–9.
47. Vienne A, Hobeika E, Gouya H, et al. Prediction of drainage effectiveness during endoscopic stenting of malignant hilar strictures: the role of liver volume assessment. Gastrointest Endosc 2010;72(4):728–35.
48. Mukai T, Yasuda I, Nakashima M, et al. Metallic stents are more efficacious than plastic stents in unresectable malignant hilar biliary strictures: a randomized controlled trial. J Hepatobiliary Pancreat Sci 2013;20(2):214–22.
49. Lee TH, Kim TH, Moon JH, et al. Bilateral versus unilateral placement of metal stents for inoperable high-grade malignant hilar biliary strictures: a multicenter, prospective, randomized study (with video). Gastrointest Endosc 2017;86(5): 817–27.
50. Wang K, Zhu J, Xing L, et al. Assessment of efficacy and safety of EUS-guided biliary drainage: a systematic review. Gastrointest Endosc 2016;83(6):1218–27.
51. Lu Y, Liu L, Wu JC, et al. Efficacy and safety of photodynamic therapy for unresectable cholangiocarcinoma: A meta-analysis. Clin Res Hepatol Gastroenterol 2015;39(6):718–24.
52. Ortner ME, Caca K, Berr F, et al. Successful photodynamic therapy for nonresectable cholangiocarcinoma: a randomized prospective study. Gastroenterology 2003;125(5):1355–63.
53. Yang J, Wang J, Zhou H, et al. Efficacy and safety of endoscopic radiofrequency ablation for unresectable extrahepatic cholangiocarcinoma: a randomized trial. Endoscopy 2018;50(8):751–60.

Pancreatic Cystic Neoplasms

Sahin Coban, MD[a],*, Omer Basar, MD[b], William R. Brugge, MD[c]

KEYWORDS

- Pancreatic cysts • Neoplasms • Diagnostic modalities • Treatment

KEY POINTS

- Pancreatic cystic neoplasms continue to be a diagnostic and management dilemma to clinicians and may require a multidisciplinary approach.
- Differentiating premalignant and malignant cysts from nonmalignant ones remains challenging.
- Emerging diagnostic tools, including the needle biopsy with microforceps and needle-based confocal laser endomicroscopy, are of exciting potential along with cyst fluid analysis.
- Minimally invasive surgical approaches and newly developed endoscopic ultrasound-guided ablation techniques are promising as treatment options.

INTRODUCTION

A cystic lesion of the pancreas can be caused by various conditions, including cystic neoplasm, a non-neoplastic cyst, or a solid tumor with cystic degeneration. Histologically, non-neoplastic pancreatic cysts are mainly categorized as nonepithelial and epithelial cysts. Nonepithelial cysts include pancreatic pseudocysts (the most common) and infection-related cysts. Epithelial cysts include retention cysts (the most common), mucinous nonneoplastic cysts, squamoid cysts, lymphoepithelial cysts, enterogenous cysts, endometrial cysts, and para-ampullary duodenal wall cysts.[1,2]

Pancreatic cystic neoplasms (PCN), they are a heterogeneous group of pancreatic cysts mainly categorized as mucinous cystic lesions and nonmucinous cystic lesions, according to the epithelial lining of the cyst. Mucinous cystic lesions include intraductal papillary mucinous neoplasms (IPMNs) and mucinous cystic neoplasms (MCNs). Both these lesions produce mucin. Therefore, they are called either mucinous neoplasms or mucin-producing neoplasms and have similar cyst fluid features that can transform into pancreatic adenocarcinoma. Nonmucinous neoplastic cystic lesions consist of serous cystic neoplasms (SCNs) and other rare cystic lesions, including

[a] Department of Gastroenterology, Mount Auburn Hospital, 330 Mt Auburn St, Cambridge, MA 02138, USA; [b] Department of Gastroenterology, The University of Missouri, Columbia, MO 65211, USA; [c] Department of Gastroenterology, Harvard Medical School, Mount Auburn Hospital, 330 Mt Auburn St, Cambridge, MA 02138, USA
* Corresponding author. 330 Mt Auburn St, Cambridge, MA 02138, USA
E-mail addresses: sahin.coban@mah.org; scoban72@yahoo.com

Gastroenterol Clin N Am 51 (2022) 537–559
https://doi.org/10.1016/j.gtc.2022.06.008
0889-8553/22/© 2022 Elsevier Inc. All rights reserved.

solid pseudopapillary neoplasms (SPNs) and cystic pancreatic neuroendocrine tumors (cPNETs).[3] These cystic neoplasms have various clinical, pathological, and radiological features and are mainly detected incidentally (**Table 1**).

Increasing awareness and widespread use of high-quality cross-sectional imaging and the trend for healthy individuals to undergo preventive health check-ups (including imaging) have increased PCN detection. PCN prevalence varies among studies, depending on the type of imaging used. Whereas abdominal ultrasonography only detected PCN in 0.21% of participants,[4] they are identified in up to 20% of MRI[5] and 3% of computed tomography (CT) scans. Indeed, MRI with cholangiopancreatography (MRCP) revealed PCN in up to 49.1% of scanned individuals.[6] Similarly, in autopsy studies, PCNs are detected in up to 50% of patients[4,7]

The presence of PCN strongly correlates with increasing age, but there is no difference between genders.[6] Additionally, diabetes mellitus and chronic pancreatitis are risk factors associated with the development of IPMNs.[8,9]

The identification of a pancreatic cyst causes anxiety in both patients and physicians due to its malignant potential. Thus, further medical evaluation usually is needed for more clarification of the cysts' nature. The risk of malignancy of incidental pancreatic cysts varies among studies. A retrospective study of Veterans Administration patients with pancreatic cysts reported a hazard ratio of 19.64 for developing pancreatic cancer.[10] A Japanese study demonstrated that patients with pancreatic cysts have an observed incidence of pancreatic cancer 22.5 times higher than that of the expected mortality from pancreatic cancer in the general population (95% CI, 11.0–45.3).[11] However, another study of incidental pancreatic cysts stated a lower risk of malignancy for pancreatic cancer with a hazard ratio of 3.0.[12] The 2015 American Gastroenterological Association (AGA) technical review of incidental asymptomatic neoplastic pancreatic cysts estimated an incident risk of malignancy at 0.24% per year with a prevalent malignant risk of 0.25% at the time the cyst is detected.[13] These data justify the anxiety of patients and physicians that no matter how asymptomatic a pancreatic cyst is at initial presentation, either it can be malignant at the time of diagnosis or it has the potential of turning into cancer.

More than two-thirds of PCN are diagnosed incidentally and are more frequently diagnosed at smaller sizes in the last decades. The most common pathological diagnosis has been IPMN, which has malignant potential in resected PCN series.[14,15] Therefore, differentiation between PCN subtypes is crucial since their malignancy potential varies. Whereas SCNs are mostly benign and do not need surveillance, other types of cystic lesions such as main duct IPMN (MD-IPMN), side-branch IPMN (SB-IPMN), MCN, SPN, and cPNET, are considered premalignant and require either a curable treatment or surveillance.[16,17] The risk of advanced neoplasia (high-grade dysplasia [HGD] or invasive cancer) in IPMN is increased predominantly by main duct involvement, reported in up to 100%, of resected specimens.[8,17–19] Additionally, individuals with IPMN are at increased risk of developing conventional pancreatic ductal adenocarcinoma.[20] Advanced neoplasia has also been reported in up to 39% of patients in resected MCN,[21,22] up to 30% of those in resected side-branch IPMN specimens,[23,24] up to 15% of those with resected SPN,[25] and 10% of those with resected cPNET.[26]

Clinical Presentation

Most PCNs are detected incidentally during the imaging workup for an unrelated medical situation. Namely, they are mostly asymptomatic in terms of typical pancreatic symptoms such as jaundice, pancreatitis, or new-onset diabetes mellitus. However,

Table 1
General features of cystic neoplasms of the pancreas

Features	MD/IPMN	SB/IPMN	MCN	SCN	SPN	cPNET
Median age at diagnosis	5th to 7th decade	5th to 7th decade	5th to 7th decade	5th to 7th decade	2nd to 3rd decade	5th to 6th decade
Gender distribution	M = F	M = F	F	F	F	M = F
Localization	Head	Entire pancreas	Body and tail	Entire pancreas	Body and tail	Entire pancreas
Morphology	Unilocular, dilated MPD	Multilocular, septated, normal MPD	Unilocular	Microcystic	Mixed solid and cystic	Associated mass
Communication with the MPD	Yes	No	No	No	No	No
Solitary/Multifocal	Solitary or multifocal	Solitary or multifocal	Solitary	Solitary	Solitary	Solitary
Clinical presentation	Pancreatitis, jaundice, exocrine insufficiency, malignancy-related	Pancreatitis, jaundice, malignancy-related	Abdominal pain, malignancy-related	Abdominal pain, mass effect	Abdominal pain, mass effect	Abdominal pain, mass effect
Typical imaging features	Dilated MPD or dilated MPD with dilated side branches	Dilated side branches	Unilocular, macrocystic	Microcystic (honeycomb appearance)	Solid and cystic mass	Solid and cystic mass, hypervascularity
Risk of malignancy	High	High	High	Low	Low	Low
Fluid analysis	High CEA, high amylase, high viscosity	High CEA, high amylase, high viscosity	High CEA, variable amylase, low viscosity	Low CEA, low amylase/lipase, low viscosity	Low CEA, low amylase/lipase, low viscosity	Low CEA, low amylase/lipase, low viscosity
Common molecular markers in cyst fluid	KRAS, GNAS	KRAS, GNAS	KRAS	vHL	Variable	Variable

Abbreviations: MD/IPMN, main duct/intraductal papillary mucinous neoplasm; SB/IPMN, side-branch/intraductal papillary mucinous neoplasm; MCN, mucinous cystic neoplasm; SCN, serous cystic neoplasm; SPN, solid-pseudopapillary neoplasm; cPNET, cystic pancreatic neuroendocrine tumor.

MCNs can be symptomatic in up to 10% of cases.[27] If they are large, symptoms can be caused by the mass effect of these neoplasms.

In most cases, patients with IPMN are asymptomatic. Nonetheless, both MD-IPMNs and SB-IPMNs can cause mild and often recurrent flares of acute pancreatitis due to transient mucinous ductal obstruction in 7%–34.6% of cases.[28,29] Progressive inflammatory changes and development of atrophy and fibrosis in the pancreas, secondary to main pancreatic duct (MPD) obstruction, can also result in permanent structural damage, leading to endocrine and exocrine pancreatic insufficiency. In addition, if there is obstructive jaundice in a patient with IPMN, it indicates that the lesion is in the pancreatic head and may suggest the features of high-risk malignant lesions, including mass size of >3 cm, enhancing solid component, and MPD size of ≥10 mm.[30]

cPNETs are most often detected as an incidental finding on imaging. A vast majority of cPNETs are nonfunctioning, whereas active neuroendocrine tumors hypersecrete single or multiple hormones and can present with symptoms such as tachycardia, flushing, or lightheadedness.[31] Patients with ductal adenocarcinoma with a cystic component—despite its rarity—can present with abdominal pain or discomfort, weight loss, jaundice, or recurrent pancreatitis.[32]

Intraductal Papillary Mucinous Neoplasms

IPMNs may occur at any age; however, the mean age at diagnosis is 65 years, and it is seen equally in both sexes. However, IPMNs can arise from the main duct or side branches only, or a combination of both, known as mixed IPMN (**Fig. 1**). They are characteristically lined with intraductal papillary mucin-producing neoplastic epithelium and have different levels of malignancy potential.

MD-IPMN has the highest malignant potential and is characterized by diffuse or segmental dilatation of the MPD due to a mucus-producing cystic tumor within the duct. The most common IPMN is the side-branch IPMN. Most SB-IPMNs do not progress to pancreatic cancer.[33] Multifocal SB-IPMNs can occur in up to 40% of cases but there is no evidence that the risk of malignant transformation is higher in these cysts.[34] SB-IPMNs are classically thin-walled cysts without calcification, and there is usually a connection between the cyst and the MPD.

Although the localization of cysts is not helpful in the differentiation of PCNs, being multifocal and communicating with the MPD is suggestive of SB-IPMNs. Alternatively, most MCNs are solitary. Both main-duct and side-branch IPMNs may lead to acute pancreatitis, caused by occlusion of the pancreatic duct orifice by thick mucin. In addition, patients may present with abdominal pain, malaise, jaundice, or weight loss. However, most patients with IPMNs are free of symptoms and diagnosed incidentally.

High-risk features of malignant IPMNs include having an enhancing nodule or a solid component, MPD dilation of >1 cm, jaundice, and cytology with advanced neoplasia (HGD or cancer), which are associated with a lower 5-year survival rate compared to those who do not have these high-risk features.[35]

Histologically, IPMNs are classified into four subtypes: gastric foveolar (predominant in SB-IPMNs), intestinal (predominant in MD-IPMNs), pancreaticobiliary, and oncocytic. According to histological studies, this categorization is highly efficient in predicting the biological behavior of IPMNs. The gastric foveolar subtype is more commonly found in SB-IPMN and mixed type IPMN, and exhibits the best prognosis. In contrast, the intestinal subtype tends to occur in MD-IPMNs and exhibits a worse prognosis.[36]

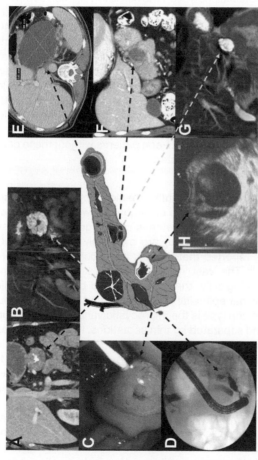

Fig. 1. An illustration of PCNs along with various examples of imaging. (*A*) Axial view of CT scan of a 6 cm multicystic serous cystic adenoma (with central (calcification). (*B*) Axial view of MRI of a 6 cm multicystic serous cystic adenoma (same patient). (*C*) Endoscopic view of the ampulla of Vater with leaking mucus indicative of an MD-IPMN (fish-mouth appearance). (*D*) ERCP view of an MD-IPMN (same patient). (*E*) Axial view of CT scan of a large pseudocyst with debris. (*F*) Axial view of CT scan of an MCN. (*G*) Axial view of MRI of an MCN (same patient). (*H*) EUS view of a serous SPN.

Mucinous Cystic Neoplasms

MCNs occur almost entirely in middle-age women. They are characterized by the presence of ovarian-like stroma, explaining why they occur predominantly in women. The term "mother cysts" is generally applied to them. The pathognomonic ovarian-like stroma, which surrounds the cyst's inner epithelial layer, helps to differentiate MCNs from IPMNs.

On imaging, MCNs can be seen as unilocular cysts located in the body or tail of the pancreas in over 97% of cases (see **Fig. 1**E, F).[37] Unlike SB-IPMNs, there is typically no communication with the MPD which is of normal caliber.

MCNs have malignant potential; however, the risk is lower when compared to IPMNs. Risk factors for malignancy include size >6 cm, enhancing nodule, thick irregular wall, and peripheral calcifications, which are found in approximately 25% of MCNs.[13]

A review of 90 resected MCNs reported that only 10% of the lesions contained advanced neoplasia.[21] In this study and in a review covering 344 MCNs, there were no cases of advanced neoplasia in MCNs of <3 cm in diameter.[21,38] Therefore, there is a conflict regarding whether MCNs should be surgically resected or followed by imaging. There is an agreement on immediate resection of MCNs, in patients with symptoms (such as pancreatitis), and in patients with concerning endoscopic ultrasound (EUS) features such as solid component or positive cytology for HGD or adenocarcinoma. However, there is still a conflict between patients without these concerning features and MCNs less than 3 cm in diameter.

Serous cystic neoplasms

SCNs are nonmucinous, predominantly benign cystic neoplasms (serous cystadenomas-SCAs). SCAs occur more commonly in women (75%), who are typically in their 60s. They are therefore sometimes called "grandmother cysts."[39] Malignant cases (serous cystadenocarcinoma) are extremely rare. A recent multicenter study of over 2500 SCAs reported that the risk of serous cystadenocarcinoma was extremely low at 0.1%.[40] The vast majority of SCAs are asymptomatic, mostly detected incidentally. Histologically, the cysts are lined by a single, uniform layer of glycogen-containing cuboidal epithelial cells with round nuclei and abundant clear cytoplasm. The more common type is the microcystic variant, in which numerous multiple cysts are grouped and separated by thin septations. It makes the classic imaging features of a honeycomb or sponge-like appearance. A central scar is also a characteristic imaging feature caused by calcifications but is present in less than 30% of SCAs (see **Fig. 1**A, B). Calcification occurs at the center of SCNs, whereas it is peripheral in MCNs. The oligo- or macrocystic variant is the less common type and is difficult to differentiate from an SB-IPMN or MCN.

SCNs are slow-growing cysts. Although related symptoms are rare, SCAs can cause symptoms due to their size. The prognosis of SCNs is excellent and given their benign nature, they should be followed by surveillance imaging; however, most asymptomatic SCAs do not require surveillance. Surgical resection is not recommended unless there is uncertainty about malignancy, rapid growth, or significant symptoms. The intervals of surveillance imaging remain unclear.

Solid Pseudopapillary Neoplasms

Solid SPNs are rare heterogeneous lesions, predominant in women, with a 10:1 female-to-male ratio. They are most frequently present in women in their 20s but have a wide age range with cases described in children and adults over 50. They can occur in any part of the pancreas and have malignant potential. Histologically, they are characterized by pseudopapillary and cystic spaces containing hemorrhage and cholesterol clefts in myxoid stroma alternating with solid tissue. Therefore, these lesions appear cystic and solid (see **Fig. 1**H). A systematic review of 484 studies including 2744 patients with SPN showed that the most common presentations were abdominal pain (63%) or asymptomatic incidental finding (38%). Smaller tumors tend to be solid, whereas larger ones have a mixed solid and cystic appearance. Typically, SPNs are benign or low-grade malignant tumors. Advanced neoplasia (HGD or invasive carcinoma) is found in approximately 10% of SPNs. In contrast to pancreatic adenocarcinoma, outcomes of patients with PCNs are excellent with a 5-year disease-free survival of over 98%.[41]

Cystic Pancreatic Neuroendocrine Tumors

cPNETs are rare variants of pancreatic neuroendocrine tumors that are usually nonfunctioning and often diagnosed incidentally. Morphologically, they can be solid, cystic, or mixed with a variable malignant potential. They can occur sporadically or in individuals with multiple endocrine neoplasia type 1, Von Hippel Lindau (VHL) syndrome, and neurofibromatosis type 1. Sexes are equally affected with peak presentation in the 60s. Incidence increases with age. Imaging reveals a well-circumscribed multi- or unilocular cyst surrounded by a thick fibrous capsule. EUS-guided fine needle aspiration (FNA) is often required to reach an accurate diagnosis. Surgical resection is the optimal treatment modality for clinically active cPNETs; however, asymptomatic cPNETs of <1 cm are managed with surveillance. Patients with resected cPNETs have an excellent prognosis.[42,43]

Diagnostic Approaches to PCNs

Cystic lesions of the pancreas are more commonly diagnosed because of the widespread use of cross-sectional imaging. Incidentally detected pancreatic cystic lesions are challenging to physicians, and typically require a multidisciplinary approach. The most crucial concern is differentiating neoplastic lesions from non-neoplastic ones. The distinction between the different subtypes is also important since the management of PCNs varies according to their subtype.

Assessment of a patient with an incidental pancreatic cyst should begin with a detailed history including any description of acute or chronic pancreatitis, and a family history of pancreatic cancer or hereditary cancer syndromes. For newly diagnosed PCNs, imaging may include a pancreatic protocol CT or gadolinium-enhanced MRI with MRCP.[16,17,44] EUS is kept as a next step if there are suspicious features of concern for PCNs such as nodules, dilatation of the pancreatic duct, or a thickened enhancing wall. In addition, EUS can be used to obtain cyst fluid for cytology and biochemical analysis to get a more precise diagnosis.

MRI with MRCP is usually preferred over CT as a surveillance modality for several reasons. Firstly, MRI/MRCP is more sensitive than CT in detecting communication between a lesion and the MPD. In addition, MRI/MRCP is an excellent imaging modality for outlining the gross appearance of PCNs including the presence of enhancing mural nodules, any solid component within a cystic lesion, or internal septations.[45] Secondly, MRI does not expose patients to the ionizing radiation of CT scanning with its increased risk for malignancy.[46] If MRI cannot be performed, a pancreatic protocol CT with contrast-enhanced images should be obtained. The imaging findings will help define the next steps in management and these may include EUS for further diagnostic assessment, surgical resection, or the initiation of a surveillance program.[47]

On imaging, PCNs can be identified by some of their unique features. MD-IPMN can be recognized by marked dilation of the MPD. In some cases, a bulging ampulla with leaking thick mucin from the orifice can be observed during endoscopic examination (fish-mouth appearance), which is practically pathognomonic for MD-IPMN (see

Fig. 1C). SB-IPMN can be predicted by the dilation of side branches of the MPD, or a "grape-shaped" cystic lesion that communicates with the MPD. Mixed-type IPMN may show features of both types of IPMNs. However, IPMNs appear in the head of the pancreas in up to 70% of the patients, but 20% occur in the body or tail. Alternatively, 5%–10% of IPMNs are multifocal.

MCNs usually arise from the body or tail of the pancreas, mainly being unilocular or septated macrocystic lesions.[48–50]

Morphologically, SCN can appear in microcystic, macrocystic (or oligocystic), or mixed microcystic and macrocystic. A central calcification or scar can occur in SCN (see **Fig. 1**A, B). Macrocystic or oligocystic SCNs are composed of more extensive and fewer cysts that can be unilocular; however, this variant is not common. Distinguishing a macrocystic SCN from an MCN or SB-IPMN can be difficult because of the similarity in shape. Also, differentiating a solid SCN can be difficult from an SPN or cPNET, which are most commonly identified as a mixed appearance lesion with cystic and solid components, but they can also appear as a cystic mass or a calcified cystic mass in the pancreas.[51,52]

In recent years, secretin-enhanced MRCP has been developed to improve the visualization of a connection between a pancreatic cyst and the pancreatic duct.[53] Secretin is a polypeptide hormone that stimulates the release of pancreatic juice from acinar cells into the pancreatic ducts, leading to enlargement and visibility of the MPD.[54] Several studies have shown that secretin-enhanced MRCP provides better visualization of the MPD than conventional MRCP.[53,55,56]

Endoscopic Ultrasound

EUS is an important diagnostic modality in the evaluation of pancreatic cystic lesions as MRI, MRCP, and CT have less than 50% accuracy for differentiating PCNs.[47] Following radiologic imaging, a pancreatic cyst should be evaluated by EUS if the cyst is indeterminate, has high-risk features, or when the results are likely to alter management. EUS imaging provides visualization of borders, wall thickness, septations, masses, mural nodules, and papillary projections and demonstrates communication with the MPD. However, EUS alone also has limitations similar to CT and MRI. Brugge and colleagues[57,58] reported that EUS imaging alone showed only 51% diagnostic accuracy for differentiating mucinous from nonmucinous cysts. However, the addition of FNA, which allows for cytological, biochemical, and DNA analysis, can further help in diagnosis and differentiation.[57,59]

Societal guidelines published in recent years provide guidance as to when EUS evaluation is indicated in the management of PCNs (**Box 1**). It is reasonable to perform EUS-FNA in a PCN with clinical and imaging features that are indeterminate, or in the setting of worrisome features. However, EUS-FNA may not always be feasible in PCNs if they are small in size or because of their location. Generally, EUS can be recommended in patients with worrisome features such as cyst of $\geq$30 mm, thickened/enhanced cyst wall, MPD between 5 mm and 9 mm, nonenhancing mural nodule, and abrupt change in MPD caliber with atrophy.

Currently, contrast-enhanced EUS seems the most accurate diagnostic modality for differentiating mural nodules from mucin clots or debris, producing a low false-negative rate compared to other imaging modalities.[60–62] Contrast-enhanced harmonic EUS is a unique imaging technique in which particular intravenous contrast agents are used to highlight microvasculature differences between normal and abnormal tissue. Contrast-enhanced EUS can identify vascularity by detecting signals from microbubbles in vessels produced by intravenously administered contrast agents. In addition, contrast-enhanced EUS seems to help diagnose not only mural

Box 1	
Indications of EUS in diagnosing PCN	
2015 AGA guideline[44]	At least two of the following worrisome features: • Cyst size $\not\geq$ 30 mm • Dilated MPD • Presence of a solid component (mural nodule)
2017 IAP guideline[17]	If any of the following present: • Cyst size ≥30 mm • Growth rate ≥5 mm/2 years • MPD dilatation between 5 and 9 mm • Acute pancreatitis due to cyst • Enhancing mural nodule (<5 mm) • Increased levels of serum CA19–9 • Abrupt change in caliber of MPD with distal pancreatic atrophy • Thickened/enhancing cyst walls • Lymphadenopathy
2018 ACG guideline[47]	If any of the following present: • IPMN or MCN $\not\geq$ 30 mm • MPD $\not\geq$ 5 mm • Change in MPD caliber with marked atrophy • Increase in cyst size of $\not\geq$ 3 mm/year during surveillance • Jaundice due to cyst • Acute pancreatitis due to cyst • Presence of solid component (mural nodule)
2018 European guideline[16]	• Clinical or radiological worrisome features for malignancy—EUS can be alternated or performed in conjunction with MRI during surveillance

Abbreviations: ACG, American College of Gastroenterology; AGA, American Gastroenterological Association; CA19-9, cancer antigen 19-9; European, European Study Group on Cystic Tumors of the Pancreas; EUS, endoscopic ultrasound; FNA, fine needle aspiration; IAP, International Association of Pancreatology; IPMN, intraductal papillary mucinous neoplasm; MPD, main pancreatic duct; PCN, pancreatic cystic neoplasm.

nodules but also differentiate nodules with advanced neoplasia from nodules with low-grade dysplasia (LGD).[63] Recently, Marchegiani and colleagues[64] published a meta-analysis including 70 studies with 2297 resected IPMNs and reported a positive predictive value of 62% for the presence of advanced neoplasia in the histology of an enhancing mural nodule on contrast-enhanced EUS.

Cyst Fluid Analysis

Researchers have focused on searching for the ideal cyst fluid markers to distinguish mucinous from nonmucinous cysts and to predict the malignant progression of cysts. EUS-FNA provides for cytopathological examination, identification of cyst fluid, biochemical analyses, and analysis of molecular biomarkers.[65] EUS-FNA is a safe procedure with a low risk of complications estimated to be 2%–3%, including abdominal pain, infection, intracystic bleeding, and pancreatitis.[16,66] In malignant lesions, needle tract seeding is extremely rare through EUS-FNA; thus, the risk of peritoneal metastases is not increased, and it can be ignored.[67]

The cyst fluid is viscous in mucin-producing neoplasms but nonviscous in SCNs. Macroscopically, the string sign is the most informative indicator in differentiating between mucinous and nonmucinous PCNs as mucinous PCNs typically contain highly viscous cyst fluid.[68] For the string sign, a drop of aspirated cyst fluid is placed between the thumb and index finger and stretched. A string length measuring at least 3.5–10 mm indicates a mucinous PCN, with a pooled sensitivity of 58% and specificity of 95%.[69] The string sign has limitations due to the subjective nature of the interpretation of the test.

Cyst fluid obtained during EUS-FNA is often acellular. Therefore, cytopathological examination typically has a low diagnostic yield with less than 50% sensitivity for mucinous lesions. However, if positive, it is helpful for a specific diagnosis.[44] In a meta-analysis of cytopathological cyst fluid analyses, Thornton and colleagues[70] reported a sensitivity of 54% and specificity of 93% for differentiating between mucinous and nonmucinous PCNs. Cyst fluid cytology is highly specific for malignancy with at best 60% sensitivity for malignant lesions.[44] Further, cyst fluid cytology appears more useful for the diagnosis of SPEN and cPNETs with 70%–89% and 70%–81% accuracy, respectively.[71,72]

For mucinous or malignant cysts, a 29% improvement in diagnostic yield has been reported with cyst wall cytology using a technique of puncturing the wall of the cyst and repeatedly passing the needle back and forth through the collapsed cyst wall.[73] Phan and colleagues[74] looked at 47 patients who underwent EUS-FNB (core biopsy) of the cyst wall following complete aspiration of the cyst. This study revealed a higher diagnostic yield with EUS-FNB compared to cyst fluid cytology. Therefore, cyst wall cytology might be preferred over cyst fluid alone in the diagnosis of PCNs.

Recently, through-the-needle forceps have been introduced for EUS-guided tissue acquisition. These microforceps have an outer diameter of < 1 mm and can be advanced through a standard 19-gauge EUS needle to obtain samples of the cyst wall and/or mural nodules for histological evaluation (**Fig. 2**). In a multicenter study

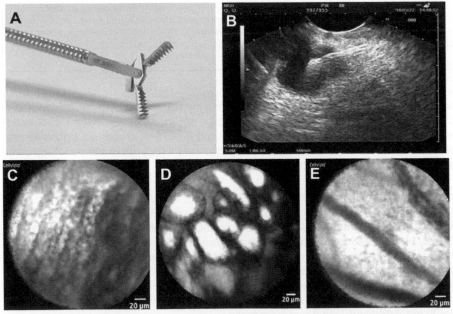

Fig. 2. New diagnostic approaches in PCNs. (*A*) A microbiopsy forceps wide open outside of a cyst. (*B*) EUS view showing a microbiopsy forceps used for tissue acquisition. (*C*) Confocal endomicroscopy view showing superficial network in an SCA. (*D*) Confocal endomicroscopy view showing papillary structures in an IPMN. (*E*) Confocal endomicroscopy view showing epithelial borders in an MCN.

of 42 patients, Basar and colleagues[75] reported that microforceps were significantly superior to cytology alone for providing a specific cyst diagnosis. Recently, a systematic review of 9 studies with 463 patients undergoing EUS with microbiopsy forceps reported a 68.6% diagnostic accuracy and a 10% complication rate, with intracystic hemorrhage and mild acute pancreatitis reported more frequently.[76] Currently, further studies are needed to increase the experience with this sampling technique.

The quantification of tumor marker carcinoembryonic antigen (CEA) levels, which is a glycoprotein found in the embryonic endodermal epithelium, is the most helpful biomarker for differentiating between mucinous and nonmucinous PCN in biochemical analyses of pancreatic cystic fluid.[65] Whereas mucinous cysts are lined by endoderm-derived columnar epithelial cells secreting CEA, nonmucinous cysts are lined by simple cuboidal epithelium, containing little or no CEA. However, CEA levels of >192 ng/mL in cyst fluid favor a diagnosis of a mucinous cyst rather than that of an SCN. CEA levels of <5 ng/mL are suggestive of an SCN.[16,17,58,65] The presence of mucin on cytology or a positive string sign with a high cyst fluid CEA level is nearly diagnostic for a mucin-producing neoplasm.[69]

Another biomarker used in the evaluation of PCNs is the cyst fluid amylase level, which is usually high in IPMNs and low in MCNs and SCNs. Although not specific, high levels of amylase in cyst fluid strongly suggest a connection between the cyst and the pancreatic ductal system (IPMN and pseudocysts).[77,78] Pancreatic cyst fluid glucose levels have also been studied as a potential biomarker for differentiating mucinous from nonmucinous PCNs. Two studies have reported that cyst fluid glucose levels have similar diagnostic accuracy when compared to cyst fluid CEA, amylase, and cytological tests, with the added advantage that is rapid, inexpensive, and require minimal cyst fluid.[79,80] Again, further confirmatory evidence is needed in large, prospective, multicenter trials.

DNA testing of pancreatic cyst fluid is also helpful to differentiate mucinous cysts from nonmucinous ones. It also seems to help distinguish between mucinous pancreatic lesions sub-types (IPMN vs. MCN) and between premalignant lesions and advanced neoplasia.[81–83] Investigating mutated genes in cyst fluid (released into pancreatic cyst fluid after cell death), also has a high potential in differentiating mucinous cyst subtypes. The presence of cystic fluid KRAS and GNAS mutations is highly sensitive for IPMN and specific for mucinous PCNs.[82]

KRAS mutations are frequently seen in MCN, and the prevalence of these mutations is reported to be correlated with the severity of dysplasia. Singhi and colleagues[82] reported that KRAS mutations were detected in 13% of patients with LGD MCN and 100% in those with HGD MCN.

However, GNAS mutations are not detected in MCN; however, when present, it could be useful to differentiate IPMN from MCN. VHL mutations or deletions are associated with SCN.[84,85] SMAD4, CDKN2A, TP53, PIK3CA, and PTEN mutations or deletions are also related to advanced neoplasia in PCNs.[83,86] Singhi and colleagues[82] demonstrated in their prospective study that the combination of KRAS or GNAS mutations and alterations in TP53, PIK3CA, or PTEN had an 89% sensitivity and 100% specificity for advanced pancreatic neoplasia. Nonetheless, further studies are still needed to integrate DNA-based molecular testing in pancreatic cyst fluid into current management guidelines.

Other Diagnostic Modalities

Newly developed tools during EUS that may improve the diagnosis of pancreatic cysts have been introduced in recent years, including needle-based confocal laser endomicroscopy (nCLE) and microforceps.[87] Confocal laser endomicroscopy is a novel imaging method providing in vivo histologic imaging. EUS-nCLE using a confocal probe through a 19-gauge FNA needle provides real-time visualization of the microscopic cellular features of the cyst wall (see **Fig. 2**). EUS-nCLE imaging is obtained after the intravenous injection of fluorescein. Visualizing a superficial vascular network pattern has over 90% sensitivity and 100% specificity for the diagnosis of SCA. Sensitivity for mucinous cysts ranges from 59% to 100%, with finger-like papilla noted in IPMN and epithelial bands are seen in MCN.[88]

Both nCLE and microbiopsy forceps are exciting tools capable of improving the diagnosis of PCNs; however, further studies are necessary to understand their safety profile and find the optimal place for these tools along with currently available cyst fluid biomarkers.

Treatment

Surgery

Surgery should be considered when the cyst is malignant, has a high risk for malignancy, or when symptomatic. Surgical resection is recommended for symptomatic SCAs.[16] In contrast, surgical resection should be considered for all MCN patients. Similarly, surgical resection is suggested for MD-IPMN and mixed-type IPMNs due to their higher malignant risk.[17,89] As per guidelines, surgical resection indications for MCNs and IPMNs are shown in **Table 2**. SPNs are considered for surgical resection due to their malignancy potential, favorable post-resection outcomes, and presence mainly in young women.[16,41]

A recent meta-analysis comparing the Fukuoka and AGA guidelines reported that they both had similarly modest sensitivity (67% and 59%, respectively) and specificity (64% and 77%, respectively) for identifying HGD and invasive cancer [61].

The AGA technical review covering asymptomatic cysts determined the following as the most significant risk factors for malignancy in incidental pancreatic cysts: solid component [odds ratio (OR) 7.7], cyst size of >3 cm (OR 3), and dilated MPD (OR 2.4).[13] Studies have reported that the size of MPD correlates with varying malignant potential. A study of 563 radiologically diagnosed and resected branch duct IPMNs (BD-IPMNs) revealed that 18% of cysts of >3 cm had advanced neoplasia. In contrast, no malignancy was detected in cysts of <2 cm, and no HGD was noted in lesions of <1 cm.[90] Larger cysts seem to be associated with the development of high-risk features, including nodules and MPD dilation.[91]

EUS-guided ablation modalities

Current guidelines for managing MCNs and IPMNs recommend either long-term surveillance, which is expensive or nontherapeutic or surgical resection which is associated with high morbidity. Moreover, surgery may not be an option for patients with significant comorbidities. Therefore, EUS-guided cyst ablation was developed to destroy the neoplastic epithelial lining of cysts in patients who decline surgery or are not operative candidates. Cyst ablation can be performed by injecting ethanol or antitumor agents such as paclitaxel; or by radiofrequency ablation (RFA). Pancreatic cysts can be resolved by EUS-guided ablation in 33% to 79% of cases and improve quality of life by avoiding surgery.[92] A propensity score matching analysis comparing a EUS-guided ethanol ablation (EUS-EA) group (n = 118) and a group without an endoscopic intervention (or natural course of disease group, n = 428) revealed that the EUS-EA group had a significantly lower rate of surgical resection when compared to the control group (4.8% vs. 26.2%) with a mean follow up of over 6 years.[93] Ideal cyst features for EUS-guided ablation include unilocular cysts or oligolocular cysts with fewer than 3–7 locules (to ensure each locule is injected properly), cyst size 2–6 cm, and no open communication with the MPD.[92]

Table 2
Indications for surgical resection of PCN by different guidelines

	Cytology	Imaging
2015 AGA guideline[44]	Positive for malignancy	• Both a solid component and dilated PD (MPD $\not\geqq$ 5 mm
2017 IAP guideline[17]	Suspicious or positive for malignancy	• Obstructive jaundice with PCN in head of pancreas • Enhanced mural nodule $\not\geqq$ 5 mm • MPD $\not\geqq$ 10 mm • MD-IPMN
2018 ACG guideline[47]	Positive for advanced neoplasia (HGD or malignancy)	• Mural nodule • Concerning features on EUS • All MD-IPMNs
2018 European guideline[16]	Suspicious or positive for advanced neoplasia	Absolute indications: • Solid component • Obstructive jaundice in head of the pancreas (PCN related) • Enhancing mural nodule >5 mm • MPD $\not\geqq$ 10 mm • Symptoms due to PCN Relative indications: • PCN growth rate $\not\geqq$ 5 mm/year • Elevated CA-19-9 level (>37 U/mL) • MPD 5–9.9 mm • PCN size $\not\geqq$ 40 mm • New-onset diabetes mellitus • Acute pancreatitis (due to IPMN) • Enhancing mural nodule <5 mm

Abbreviations: ACG, American College of Gastroenterology; AGA, American Gastroenterological Association; CA19-9, cancer antigen 19-9; European, European Study Group on Cystic Tumors of the Pancreas; EUS, endoscopic ultrasound; FNA, fine needle aspiration; HGD, high-grade dysplasia; IAP, International Association of Pancreatology; IPMN, intraductal papillary mucinous neoplasm; MPD, main pancreatic duct; PCN, pancreatic cystic neoplasm.

Response to ablation is described by volume reduction in the cyst. Complete response is defined as at least 95% reduction in volume, partial response as 75% to 95%, and nonresponse as 0% to 74%.[94]

Paclitaxel, a quite viscous and hydrophobic chemotherapeutic agent, is theoretically capable of remaining in the cyst for a long time to exert its apoptotic effects along the epithelial lining. A prospective study of 164 patients investigated the effect of cyst ablation with alcohol and paclitaxel combined and reported complete resolution, partial resolution, and persistent cyst rates in 72%, 20%, and 8% of patients, respectively. Only 1.7% cyst recurrence was detected during the 6-year follow-up period in the 114 patients who had complete cyst resolution after this combination therapy.[93] Cyst size of <35 mm and absence of septa were predictors of complete response.[95,96] Moreover, it has been demonstrated that in 72% of the cysts where the ethanol–paclitaxel combination was applied, baseline DNA mutations were eliminated in the post-ablation cyst fluid.[97]

The ethanol–paclitaxel combination therapy has replaced ethanol alone for cyst ablation because of increased efficacy and decreased complications such as pancreatitis, attributed to the ethanol.[98] Therefore, other ablation regimens without ethanol have been investigated. In a randomized trial of paclitaxel and gemcitabine with and without ethanol, comparable complete ablation rates with no adverse effects were observed in the ethanol-free group.[99] Recently, in a long-term analysis of 36 patients, Lester and colleagues[100] showed that complete cyst resolution in mucinous pancreatic cysts after EUS-guided chemoablation with paclitaxel and gemcitabine is long-lasting, with 87% of complete responders at 12 months having maintained resolution at their latest follow up. The application of EUS-guided cyst ablation will be more common with the development of new delivery agents, improved techniques, and standardized definitions of clinical success in future studies.

Radiofrequency ablation

RFA is a safe and effective technique to treat cystic lesions. RFA induces direct cell death via coagulative necrosis and hyperthermic energy. Currently, only a 19-gauge EUS-guided RFA needle is available, and only a few studies have investigated the role of EUS-RFA in treating PCNs.[101,102]

In a prospective study, Barthet and colleagues[101] treated 16 BD-IPMNs and 1 MCN using EUS-guided RFA. Complete resolution at 6 and 12 months was shown in 47% and 64.7% of the 17 PCNs, respectively. This delayed response can be due to the immunostimulatory effects of RFA. At the end of the 42 months of follow up, the authors reported that there was still a significant response in 66.6% of the 15 patients

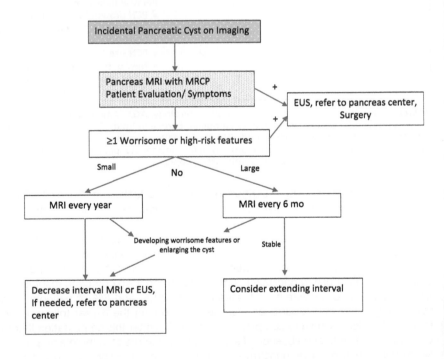

EUS: Endoscopic ultrasonography

MRI: Magnetic resonance imaging

MRCP: Magnetic resonance cholangiopancreatography

Fig. 3. Approach to an incidental pancreatic cyst. EUS, Endoscopic ultrasound; MRCP, Magnetic resonance cholangiopancreatography.

with no mural nodules.[102] However, larger- and longer-term studies are required to assess the efficacy and safety of EUS-RFA in PCNs.

Surveillance

Although newer diagnostic techniques have been developed, the management of PCNs is still very challenging, and a constant source of debate among experts due to the malignant potential of these cysts. A practical algorithm can be suggested as a framework for approaching these lesions (**Fig. 3**). However, it is vital to decide whether the patient needs further evaluation before proceeding with this management algorithm. Is the cyst an asymptomatic or a benign lesion that needs no follow up? Or if required, is the patient eligible for surgery? Several scoring indexes, including the Charlson Comorbidity Index and the Adult Comorbidity Evaluation 27, have been used to help with clinical decisions. High scores on the Charlson Comorbidity Index (>7) are associated with shorter survival and a higher risk of dying from non-IPMN-related causes.[103,104] In another study that used the Adult Comorbidity Evaluation 27 scoring system, 793 patients with IPMNs were assessed. The study showed that patients with higher scores were more likely to die from non-IPMN-related causes.[105] These scoring systems, therefore, can help clinical decision-making, especially if significant comorbidities are present.

The AGA 2015 guideline recommends stopping surveillance after 5 years of stability in cysts' condition; however, long-term studies of pancreatic cysts reveal that this guideline may place some patients at risk. A retrospective study, in which 108 patients with SB-IPMN $\leq$ 1.5 cm were followed for more than 5 years, found there was a low rate of malignant progression of 0.9%.[106] Another study following 144 BD-IPMNs without worrisome or high-risk features for a median of 84 months revealed that in 18%, worrisome or high-risk features developed beyond 5 years of follow up.[107] In line with those, in a cohort of 1036 BD-IPMNs without worrisome features, after a median of 62 months, worrisome features and pancreatic cancer were observed in 4% and 1% of cysts, respectively.[108] Given these studies, surveillance should not be stopped in all patients after 5 years. Further long-term studies

Table 3
Recommendations of the guidelines based on the PCN size detected incidentally (if no high-risk or worrisome features)

Guidelines	PCN sizes	Recommendations
2015 AGA guideline[44]	1–4 cm	MRI in 1 year
2017 IAP guideline[17]	1–2 cm	MRI or CT in 1 year
	2–3 cm	EUS in 3–6 months
	>3 cm	Alternating MRI with EUS in 3–6 months, strongly consider surgery in young and fit patients
2018 ACG guideline[47]	1–2 cm	MRI in 1 year
	2–3 cm	MRI or EUS in 6–12 months
	>3 cm	MRI or EUS every 6–12 months (and refer to the multidisciplinary task)
2018 European guideline[16]	1–4 cm	MRI or EUS in 6 months (together with serum CA-19–9 level and clinical evaluation)

Abbreviations: ACG, American College of Gastroenterology; AGA, American Gastroenterological Association; CA19-9, cancer antigen 19-9; European, European Study Group on Cystic Tumors of the Pancreas; EUS, endoscopic ultrasound; IAP, International Association of Pancreatology; PCN, pancreatic cystic neoplasm.

are required to determine a subgroup of patients in whom follow up can be safely discontinued.

SUMMARY

PCNs continue to be a diagnostic and management challenge to clinicians and may require a multidisciplinary approach, including gastroenterology, radiology, surgery, and pathology. Currently, early detection of high-risk lesions enables potentially curative surgical resection. Furthermore, early detection of lesions without worrisome features can lead to appropriate surveillance. However, differentiating premalignant and malignant cysts from nonmalignant ones remains a difficult task. Emerging diagnostic tools, such as the needle biopsy with microforceps and nCLE, are of exciting potential along with cyst fluid analysis. Although there is no single algorithm for PCN management because of the lack of high-quality evidence, current guidelines provide recommendations for the management of these lesions based on cumulative data (**Table 3**). Ongoing prospective studies with a larger number of patients will be helpful to modify these recommendations and future guidelines. Clinicians should discuss the management of these patients with a multidisciplinary team with expertise in the diagnosis and surgical treatment of PCNs, especially in the setting of indeterminate cysts or worrisome high-risk features. Minimally invasive surgical approaches and newly developed EUS-guided ablation techniques are promising, but their effectiveness needs further validation in more extensive studies.

CLINICS CARE POINTS

- Endoscopic ultrasound remains the main diagnostic modality for further assessing PCNs since imaging modalities have less than 50% accuracy for differentiating PCNs. Currently, contrast-enhanced EUS seems the most accurate diagnostic modality for differentiating mucinous and nonmucinous PCNs, producing a very low false-negative rate compared to other imaging modalities.
- EUS-FNA helps differentiate mucinous from nonmucinous cysts when imaging is indeterminate. However, EUS-FNA may not always be feasible if a pancreatic cyst is small in size or because of its location.
- The guidelines are helpful on whom to select for EUS and EUS-FNA based on the presence of specific risk features.
- EUS–FNA provides cyst fluid analysis including cytopathological examination, identification of cyst fluid, biochemical analyses, and analysis of molecular biomarkers. Cyst fluid analysis has been the ideal method for distinguishing a mucinous cyst from the nonmucinous one and predicting the malignant progression of a cyst.
- Emerging additional diagnostic tools, including through the needle biopsy with microforceps and needle-based confocal laser endomicroscopy, are of exciting potential along with cyst fluid analysis.
- Minimally invasive surgical approaches and newly developed EUS-guided ablation techniques are promising in the treatment of PCNs.

DISCLOSURE

The authors have nothing to disclose.

ACKNOWLEDGMENTS

The authors give special thanks to Mehmet Emre Coban for preparing the illustration and figures.

REFERENCES

1. Goh BK, Tan YM, Chung YF, et al. Non-neoplastic cystic and cystic-like lesions of the pancreas: may mimic pancreatic cystic neoplasms. ANZ J Surg 2006; 76(5):325–31.
2. Del Chiaro M, Verbeke C, Salvia R, et al. European experts consensus statement on cystic tumours of the pancreas. Dig Liver Dis 2013;45(9):703–11.
3. Brugge WR, Lauwers GY, Sahani D, et al. Cystic neoplasms of the pancreas. N Engl J Med 2004;351(12):1218–26.
4. Ikeda M, Sato T, Morozumi A, et al. Morphologic changes in the pancreas detected by screening ultrasonography in a mass survey, with special reference to main duct dilatation, cyst formation, and calcification. Pancreas 1994;9(4): 508–12.
5. de Oliveira PB, Puchnick A, Szejnfeld J, et al. Prevalence of incidental pancreatic cysts on 3 tesla magnetic resonance. PLoS One 2015;10(3):e0121317.
6. Kromrey ML, Bulow R, Hubner J, et al. Prospective study on the incidence, prevalence and 5-year pancreatic-related mortality of pancreatic cysts in a population-based study. Gut 2018;67(1):138–45.
7. Kimura W, Nagai H, Kuroda A, et al. Analysis of small cystic lesions of the pancreas. Int J Pancreatol 1995;18(3):197–206.
8. Salvia R, Fernandez-del Castillo C, Bassi C, et al. Main-duct intraductal papillary mucinous neoplasms of the pancreas: clinical predictors of malignancy and long-term survival following resection. Ann Surg 2004;239(5):678–85 [discussion: 85-7].
9. Ridtitid W, DeWitt JM, Schmidt CM, et al. Management of branch-duct intraductal papillary mucinous neoplasms: a large single-center study to assess predictors of malignancy and long-term outcomes. Gastrointest Endosc 2016;84(3): 436–45.
10. Munigala S, Gelrud A, Agarwal B. Risk of pancreatic cancer in patients with pancreatic cyst. Gastrointest Endosc 2016;84(1):81–6.
11. Tada M, Kawabe T, Arizumi M, et al. Pancreatic cancer in patients with pancreatic cystic lesions: a prospective study in 197 patients. Clin Gastroenterol Hepatol 2006;4(10):1265–70.
12. Chernyak V, Flusberg M, Haramati LB, et al. Incidental pancreatic cystic lesions: is there a relationship with the development of pancreatic adenocarcinoma and all-cause mortality? Radiology 2015;274(1):161–9.
13. Scheiman JM, Hwang JH, Moayyedi P. American gastroenterological association technical review on the diagnosis and management of asymptomatic neoplastic pancreatic cysts. Gastroenterology 2015;148(4):824–848 e22.
14. Valsangkar NP, Morales-Oyarvide V, Thayer SP, et al. 851 resected cystic tumors of the pancreas: a 33-year experience at the Massachusetts General Hospital. Surgery 2012;152(3 Suppl 1):S4–12.
15. Gaujoux S, Coriat R. [Cystic lesion of the pancreas. The epidemic in yet not under control!]. Presse Med 2019;48(7–8 Pt 1):749–51.
16. European Study Group on Cystic Tumours of the P. European evidence-based guidelines on pancreatic cystic neoplasms. Gut 2018;67(5):789–804.
17. Tanaka M, Fernandez-Del Castillo C, Kamisawa T, et al. Revisions of international consensus Fukuoka guidelines for the management of IPMN of the pancreas. Pancreatology 2017;17(5):738–53.
18. Lee SY, Lee KT, Lee JK, et al. Long-term follow up results of intraductal papillary mucinous tumors of pancreas. J Gastroenterol Hepatol 2005;20(9):1379–84.

19. Salvia R, Burelli A, Perri G, et al. State-of-the-art surgical treatment of IPMNs. Langenbecks Arch Surg 2021;406(8):2633–42.
20. Felsenstein M, Noe M, Masica DL, et al. IPMNs with co-occurring invasive cancers: neighbours but not always relatives. Gut 2018;67(9):1652–62.
21. Park JW, Jang JY, Kang MJ, et al. Mucinous cystic neoplasm of the pancreas: is surgical resection recommended for all surgically fit patients? Pancreatology 2014;14(2):131–6.
22. Zamboni G, Scarpa A, Bogina G, et al. Mucinous cystic tumors of the pancreas: clinicopathological features, prognosis, and relationship to other mucinous cystic tumors. Am J Surg Pathol 1999;23(4):410–22.
23. Kanno A, Satoh K, Hirota M, et al. Prediction of invasive carcinoma in branch type intraductal papillary mucinous neoplasms of the pancreas. J Gastroenterol 2010;45(9):952–9.
24. Rodriguez JR, Salvia R, Crippa S, et al. Branch-duct intraductal papillary mucinous neoplasms: observations in 145 patients who underwent resection. Gastroenterology 2007;133(1):72–9 [quiz: 309-10].
25. Lee SE, Jang JY, Hwang DW, et al. Clinical features and outcome of solid pseudopapillary neoplasm: differences between adults and children. Arch Surg 2008;143(12):1218–21.
26. Koh YX, Chok AY, Zheng HL, et al. A systematic review and meta-analysis of the clinicopathologic characteristics of cystic versus solid pancreatic neuroendocrine neoplasms. Surgery 2014;156(1):83–96 e2.
27. Crippa S, Salvia R, Warshaw AL, et al. Mucinous cystic neoplasm of the pancreas is not an aggressive entity: lessons from 163 resected patients. Ann Surg 2008;247(4):571–9.
28. Jang JW, Kim MH, Jeong SU, et al. Clinical characteristics of intraductal papillary mucinous neoplasm manifesting as acute pancreatitis or acute recurrent pancreatitis. J Gastroenterol Hepatol 2013;28(4):731–8.
29. Ringold DA, Shroff P, Sikka SK, et al. Pancreatitis is frequent among patients with side-branch intraductal papillary mucinous neoplasia diagnosed by EUS. Gastrointest Endosc 2009;70(3):488–94.
30. Ozaki K, Ikeno H, Kaizaki Y, et al. Pearls and pitfalls of imaging features of pancreatic cystic lesions: a case-based approach with imaging-pathologic correlation. Jpn J Radiol 2021;39(2):118–42.
31. Goh BK, Ooi LL, Tan YM, et al. Clinico-pathological features of cystic pancreatic endocrine neoplasms and a comparison with their solid counterparts. Eur J Surg Oncol 2006;32(5):553–6.
32. Sheehan MK, Beck K, Pickleman J, et al. Spectrum of cystic neoplasms of the pancreas and their surgical management. Arch Surg 2003;138(6):657–60 [discussion: 60-2].
33. Stark A, Donahue TR, Reber HA, et al. Pancreatic cyst disease: a review. JAMA 2016;315(17):1882–93.
34. Gardner TB, Glass LM, Smith KD, et al. Pancreatic cyst prevalence and the risk of mucin-producing adenocarcinoma in US adults. Am J Gastroenterol 2013; 108(10):1546–50.
35. Capurso G, Crippa S, Vanella G, et al. Factors associated with the risk of progression of low-risk branch-duct intraductal papillary mucinous neoplasms. JAMA Netw Open 2020;3(11):e2022933.
36. Yamada S, Fujii T, Shimoyama Y, et al. Clinical implication of morphological subtypes in management of intraductal papillary mucinous neoplasm. Ann Surg Oncol 2014;21(7):2444–52.

37. Scott J, Martin I, Redhead D, et al. Mucinous cystic neoplasms of the pancreas: imaging features and diagnostic difficulties. Clin Radiol 2000;55(3):187–92.
38. Goh BK, Tan YM, Chung YF, et al. A review of mucinous cystic neoplasms of the pancreas defined by ovarian-type stroma: clinicopathological features of 344 patients. World J Surg 2006;30(12):2236–45.
39. Sakorafas GH, Smyrniotis V, Reid-Lombardo KM, et al. Primary pancreatic cystic neoplasms revisited. Part I: serous cystic neoplasms. Surg Oncol 2011;20(2): e84–92.
40. Jais B, Rebours V, Malleo G, et al. Serous cystic neoplasm of the pancreas: a multinational study of 2622 patients under the auspices of the International Association of Pancreatology and European Pancreatic Club (European Study Group on Cystic Tumors of the Pancreas). Gut 2016;65(2):305–12.
41. Law JK, Ahmed A, Singh VK, et al. A systematic review of solid-pseudopapillary neoplasms: are these rare lesions? Pancreas 2014;43(3):331–7.
42. Kunz PL, Reidy-Lagunes D, Anthony LB, et al. Consensus guidelines for the management and treatment of neuroendocrine tumors. Pancreas 2013;42(4): 557–77.
43. Gaujoux S, Tang L, Klimstra D, et al. The outcome of resected cystic pancreatic endocrine neoplasms: a case-matched analysis. Surgery 2012;151(4):518–25.
44. Vege SS, Ziring B, Jain R, et al. Clinical Guidelines C, American Gastroenterology A. American gastroenterological association institute guideline on the diagnosis and management of asymptomatic neoplastic pancreatic cysts. Gastroenterology 2015;148(4):819–22 [quize: 12-3].
45. Waters JA, Schmidt CM, Pinchot JW, et al. CT vs MRCP: optimal classification of IPMN type and extent. J Gastrointest Surg 2008;12(1):101–9.
46. Sodickson A, Baeyens PF, Andriole KP, et al. Recurrent CT, cumulative radiation exposure, and associated radiation-induced cancer risks from CT of adults. Radiology 2009;251(1):175–84.
47. Elta GH, Enestvedt BK, Sauer BG, et al. ACG clinical guideline: diagnosis and management of pancreatic cysts. Am J Gastroenterol 2018;113(4):464–79.
48. Sugiyama M, Atomi Y. Intraductal papillary mucinous tumors of the pancreas: imaging studies and treatment strategies. Ann Surg 1998;228(5):685–91.
49. Postlewait LM, Ethun CG, McInnis MR, et al. Association of preoperative risk factors with malignancy in pancreatic mucinous cystic neoplasms: a multicenter study. JAMA Surg 2017;152(1):19–25.
50. Keane MG, Shamali A, Nilsson LN, et al. Risk of malignancy in resected pancreatic mucinous cystic neoplasms. Br J Surg 2018;105(4):439–46.
51. Papavramidis T, Papavramidis S. Solid pseudopapillary tumors of the pancreas: review of 718 patients reported in English literature. J Am Coll Surg 2005;200(6): 965–72.
52. Lewis RB, Lattin GE Jr, Paal E. Pancreatic endocrine tumors: radiologic-clinicopathologic correlation. Radiographics 2010;30(6):1445–64.
53. Rastegar N, Matteoni-Athayde LG, Eng J, et al. Incremental value of secretin-enhanced magnetic resonance cholangiopancreatography in detecting ductal communication in a population with high prevalence of small pancreatic cysts. Eur J Radiol 2015;84(4):575–80.
54. Chey WY, Chang TM. Secretin, 100 years later. J Gastroenterol 2003;38(11): 1025–35.
55. Akisik MF, Sandrasegaran K, Aisen AA, et al. Dynamic secretin-enhanced MR cholangiopancreatography. Radiographics 2006;26(3):665–77.

56. Tirkes T, Sandrasegaran K, Sanyal R, et al. Secretin-enhanced MR cholangio-pancreatography: spectrum of findings. Radiographics 2013;33(7):1889–906.

57. Brugge WR. Evaluation of pancreatic cystic lesions with EUS. Gastrointest Endosc 2004;59(6):698–707.

58. Brugge WR, Lewandrowski K, Lee-Lewandrowski E, et al. Diagnosis of pancreatic cystic neoplasms: a report of the cooperative pancreatic cyst study. Gastroenterology 2004;126(5):1330–6.

59. Brugge WR. Pancreatic fine needle aspiration: to do or not to do? JOP 2004; 5(4):282–8.

60. Yamashita Y, Ueda K, Itonaga M, et al. Usefulness of contrast-enhanced endoscopic sonography for discriminating mural nodules from mucous clots in intraductal papillary mucinous neoplasms: a single-center prospective study. J Ultrasound Med 2013;32(1):61–8.

61. Yamamoto N, Kato H, Tomoda T, et al. Contrast-enhanced harmonic endoscopic ultrasonography with time-intensity curve analysis for intraductal papillary mucinous neoplasms of the pancreas. Endoscopy 2016;48(1):26–34.

62. Fusaroli P, Serrani M, De Giorgio R, et al. Contrast harmonic-endoscopic ultrasound is useful to identify neoplastic features of pancreatic cysts (with videos). Pancreas 2016;45(2):265–8.

63. Kamata K, Kitano M. Endoscopic diagnosis of cystic lesions of the pancreas. Dig Endosc 2019;31(1):5–15.

64. Marchegiani G, Andrianello S, Borin A, et al. Systematic review, meta-analysis, and a high-volume center experience supporting the new role of mural nodules proposed by the updated 2017 international guidelines on IPMN of the pancreas. Surgery 2018;163(6):1272–9.

65. Dumonceau JM, Deprez PH, Jenssen C, et al. Indications, results, and clinical impact of endoscopic ultrasound (EUS)-guided sampling in gastroenterology: European Society of Gastrointestinal Endoscopy (ESGE) Clinical Guideline - Updated January 2017. Endoscopy 2017;49(7):695–714.

66. Tanaka M, Fernandez-del Castillo C, Adsay V, et al. International consensus guidelines 2012 for the management of IPMN and MCN of the pancreas. Pancreatology 2012;12(3):183–97.

67. Yoon WJ, Daglilar ES, Fernandez-del Castillo C, et al. Peritoneal seeding in intraductal papillary mucinous neoplasm of the pancreas patients who underwent endoscopic ultrasound-guided fine-needle aspiration: the PIPE Study. Endoscopy 2014;46(5):382–7.

68. Leung KK, Ross WA, Evans D, et al. Pancreatic cystic neoplasm: the role of cyst morphology, cyst fluid analysis, and expectant management. Ann Surg Oncol 2009;16(10):2818–24.

69. Bick BL, Enders FT, Levy MJ, et al. The string sign for diagnosis of mucinous pancreatic cysts. Endoscopy 2015;47(7):626–31.

70. Thornton GD, McPhail MJ, Nayagam S, et al. Endoscopic ultrasound guided fine needle aspiration for the diagnosis of pancreatic cystic neoplasms: a meta-analysis. Pancreatology 2013;13(1):48–57.

71. Karsenti D, Caillol F, Chaput U, et al. Safety of endoscopic ultrasound-guided fine-needle aspiration for pancreatic solid pseudopapillary neoplasm before surgical resection: a european multicenter registry-based study on 149 patients. Pancreas 2020;49(1):34–8.

72. Ridtitid W, Halawi H, DeWitt JM, et al. Cystic pancreatic neuroendocrine tumors: outcomes of preoperative endosonography-guided fine needle aspiration, and recurrence during long-term follow-up. Endoscopy 2015;47(7):617–25.

73. Hong SK, Loren DE, Rogart JN, et al. Targeted cyst wall puncture and aspiration during EUS-FNA increases the diagnostic yield of premalignant and malignant pancreatic cysts. Gastrointest Endosc 2012;75(4):775–82.

74. Phan J, Dawson D, Sedarat A, et al. Clinical Utility of Obtaining Endoscopic Ultrasound-Guided Fine-Needle Biopsies for Histologic Analyses of Pancreatic Cystic Lesions. Gastroenterology 2020;158(3):475–477 e1.

75. Basar O, Yuksel O, Yang DJ, et al. Feasibility and safety of microforceps biopsy in the diagnosis of pancreatic cysts. Gastrointest Endosc 2018;88(1):79–86.

76. Balaban VD, Cazacu IM, Pinte L, et al. EUS-through-the-needle microbiopsy forceps in pancreatic cystic lesions: a systematic review. Endosc Ultrasound 2021; 10(1):19–24.

77. Al-Rashdan A, Schmidt CM, Al-Haddad M, et al. Fluid analysis prior to surgical resection of suspected mucinous pancreatic cysts. A single centre experience. J Gastrointest Oncol 2011;2(4):208–14.

78. van der Waaij LA, van Dullemen HM, Porte RJ. Cyst fluid analysis in the differential diagnosis of pancreatic cystic lesions: a pooled analysis. Gastrointest Endosc 2005;62(3):383–9.

79. Carr RA, Yip-Schneider MT, Simpson RE, et al. Pancreatic cyst fluid glucose: rapid, inexpensive, and accurate diagnosis of mucinous pancreatic cysts. Surgery 2018;163(3):600–5.

80. Zikos T, Pham K, Bowen R, et al. Cyst fluid glucose is rapidly feasible and accurate in diagnosing mucinous pancreatic cysts. Am J Gastroenterol 2015; 110(6):909–14.

81. Wu J, Jiao Y, Dal Molin M, et al. Whole-exome sequencing of neoplastic cysts of the pancreas reveals recurrent mutations in components of ubiquitin-dependent pathways. Proc Natl Acad Sci U S A 2011;108(52):21188–93.

82. Singhi AD, McGrath K, Brand RE, et al. Preoperative next-generation sequencing of pancreatic cyst fluid is highly accurate in cyst classification and detection of advanced neoplasia. Gut 2018;67(12):2131–41.

83. Singhi AD, Wood LD. Early detection of pancreatic cancer using DNA-based molecular approaches. Nat Rev Gastroenterol Hepatol 2021;18(7):457–68.

84. Nikiforova MN, Khalid A, Fasanella KE, et al. Integration of KRAS testing in the diagnosis of pancreatic cystic lesions: a clinical experience of 618 pancreatic cysts. Mod Pathol 2013;26(11):1478–87.

85. Singhi AD, Nikiforova MN, Fasanella KE, et al. Preoperative GNAS and KRAS testing in the diagnosis of pancreatic mucinous cysts. Clin Cancer Res 2014; 20(16):4381–9.

86. Yu J, Sadakari Y, Shindo K, et al. Digital next-generation sequencing identifies low-abundance mutations in pancreatic juice samples collected from the duodenum of patients with pancreatic cancer and intraductal papillary mucinous neoplasms. Gut 2017;66(9):1677–87.

87. Coban S, Basar O, Brugge WR. Future directions for endoscopic ultrasound: where are we heading? Gastrointest Endosc Clin N Am 2017;27(4):759–72.

88. Coban S, Brugge W. EUS-guided confocal laser endomicroscopy: can we use thick and wide for diagnosis of early cancer? Gastrointest Endosc 2020;91(3): 564–7.

89. Anonsen K, Sahakyan MA, Kleive D, et al. Trends in management and outcome of cystic pancreatic lesions - analysis of 322 cases undergoing surgical resection. Scand J Gastroenterol 2019;54(8):1051–7.

90. Sahora K, Mino-Kenudson M, Brugge W, et al. Branch duct intraductal papillary mucinous neoplasms: does cyst size change the tip of the scale? A critical

analysis of the revised international consensus guidelines in a large single-institutional series. Ann Surg 2013;258(3):466–75.

91. Han Y, Lee H, Kang JS, et al. Progression of pancreatic branch duct intraductal papillary mucinous neoplasm associates with cyst size. Gastroenterology 2018; 154(3):576–84.

92. Canakis A, Law R, Baron T. An updated review on ablative treatment of pancreatic cystic lesions. Gastrointest Endosc 2020;91(3):520–6.

93. Choi JH, Lee SH, Choi YH, et al. Clinical outcomes of endoscopic ultrasound-guided ethanol ablation for pancreatic cystic lesions compared with the natural course: a propensity score matching analysis. Therap Adv Gastroenterol 2018; 11:1–13.

94. Teoh AY, Seo DW, Brugge W, et al. Position statement on EUS-guided ablation of pancreatic cystic neoplasms from an international expert panel. Endosc Int Open 2019;7(9):E1064–77.

95. Choi JH, Seo DW, Song TJ, et al. Long-term outcomes after endoscopic ultrasound-guided ablation of pancreatic cysts. Endoscopy 2017;49(9):866–73.

96. Oh HC, Seo DW, Song TJ, et al. Endoscopic ultrasonography-guided ethanol lavage with paclitaxel injection treats patients with pancreatic cysts. Gastroenterology 2011;140(1):172–9.

97. DeWitt JM, Al-Haddad M, Sherman S, et al. Alterations in cyst fluid genetics following endoscopic ultrasound-guided pancreatic cyst ablation with ethanol and paclitaxel. Endoscopy 2014;46(6):457–64.

98. Attila T, Adsay V, Faigel DO. The efficacy and safety of endoscopic ultrasound-guided ablation of pancreatic cysts with alcohol and paclitaxel: a systematic review. Eur J Gastroenterol Hepatol 2019;31(1):1–9.

99. Moyer MT, Sharzehi S, Mathew A, et al. The Safety and Efficacy of an Alcohol-Free Pancreatic Cyst Ablation Protocol. Gastroenterology 2017;153(5): 1295–303.

100. Lester C, Walsh L, Hartz KM, et al. The durability of EUS-Guided chemoablation of mucinous pancreatic cysts: a long-term follow-up of the CHARM trial. Clin Gastroenterol Hepatol 2022;20(2):e326–9.

101. Barthet M, Giovannini M, Lesavre N, et al. Endoscopic ultrasound-guided radiofrequency ablation for pancreatic neuroendocrine tumors and pancreatic cystic neoplasms: a prospective multicenter study. Endoscopy 2019;51(9):836–42.

102. Barthet M, Giovannini M, Gasmi M, et al. Long-term outcome after EUS-guided radiofrequency ablation: Prospective results in pancreatic neuroendocrine tumors and pancreatic cystic neoplasms. Endosc Int Open 2021;9(8):E1178–85.

103. Sahora K, Ferrone CR, Brugge WR, et al. Effects of comorbidities on outcomes of patients with intraductal papillary mucinous neoplasms. Clin Gastroenterol Hepatol 2015;13(10):1816–23.

104. Kwok K, Chang J, Duan L, et al. Competing risks for mortality in patients with asymptomatic pancreatic cystic neoplasms: implications for clinical management. Am J Gastroenterol 2017;112(8):1330–6.

105. Kawakubo K, Tada M, Isayama H, et al. Risk for mortality from causes other than pancreatic cancer in patients with intraductal papillary mucinous neoplasm of the pancreas. Pancreas 2013;42(4):687–91.

106. Pergolini I, Sahora K, Ferrone CR, et al. Long-term risk of pancreatic malignancy in patients with branch duct intraductal papillary mucinous neoplasm in a referral center. Gastroenterology 2017;153(5):1284–12894 e1.

107. Crippa S, Pezzilli R, Bissolati M, et al. Active surveillance beyond 5 years is required for presumed branch-duct intraductal papillary mucinous neoplasms

undergoing non-operative management. Am J Gastroenterol 2017;112(7): 1153–61.

108. Marchegiani G, Andrianello S, Pollini T, et al. "Trivial" cysts redefine the risk of cancer in presumed branch-duct intraductal papillary mucinous neoplasms of the pancreas: a potential target for follow-up discontinuation? Am J Gastroenterol 2019;114(10):1678–84.

Familial Pancreatic Cancer

Helena Saba, MD[a], Michael Goggins, MD[a,b,c,d],*

KEYWORDS

- Pancreatic cancer • Familial • Hereditary • Pancreas surveillance • Screening

KEY POINTS

- First-degree relatives of individuals with familial pancreatic cancer and individuals with a deleterious germline mutation in one of the pancreatic cancer susceptibility genes are at significantly increased risk of developing pancreatic cancer and can potentially benefit from surveillance.
- Surveillance focuses on the early detection of pancreatic ductal adenocarcinoma and its high-grade precursor lesions using endoscopic ultrasound examination and/or magnetic resonance imaging/magnetic resonance cholangiopancreatography.
- Patients undergoing pancreas surveillance are more likely to be diagnosed with low-stage resectable pancreatic cancers and to achieve long-term survival.
- Novel strategies are needed to better stratify pancreatic cancer risk. Emerging tests are currently being evaluated, which could eventually improve the detection of high-grade precancerous lesions and early-stage invasive pancreatic cancer.

INTRODUCTION

Pancreatic ductal adenocarcinoma (PDAC) is the deadliest of all major cancer types with most patients having advanced disease at diagnosis. Recent data from the National Cancer Institute's (NCI) Surveillance, Epidemiology, and End Results (SEER) registry reveal a 5-year survival rate of 3% for patients with metastatic pancreatic cancer, increasing to 14.4% for those with regional (node-positive) disease and 41.6% for those with localized disease confined to the pancreas.[1] Pancreatic cancer survival rates have increased significantly in the past decade, and the current 5-year

The authors have no disclosures to report.
[a] Departments of Pathology, Johns Hopkins Medical Institutions, CRB2 351, 1550 Orleans Street, Baltimore, MD 21231, USA; [b] Departments of Medicine, Johns Hopkins Medical Institutions, CRB2 351, 1550 Orleans Street, Baltimore, MD 21231, USA; [c] Departments of Oncology, Johns Hopkins Medical Institutions, CRB2 351, 1550 Orleans Street, Baltimore, MD 21231, USA; [d] Bloomberg School of Public Health, The Sol Goldman Pancreatic Cancer Research Center, Johns Hopkins Medical Institutions, CRB2 351, 1550 Orleans Street, Baltimore, MD 21231, USA
* Corresponding author. The Sol Goldman Pancreatic Cancer Research Center, Johns Hopkins Medical Institutions, CRB2 351, 1550 Orleans Street, Baltimore, MD 21231.
E-mail address: mgoggins@jhmi.edu

survival is 11%. Experts predict that by 2030 PDAC will be the second-leading cause of cancer death in the United States.[2]

Progress is needed, not only in the treatment of this disease but also in the diagnosis and pancreatic risk assessment that would enable more individuals to pursue early detection. Despite the high mortality associated with pancreatic cancer, screening the general population for PDAC is not recommended.[3] The average lifetime risk of developing PDAC is low (1.6%, 1 in 64), and more importantly, the age-specific incidence in the general population is low (approximately 1/1000 to 1/10,000, depending on age). As a result, even the best screening tests would generate hundreds to thousands of false positives for every true positive test.[4] However, individuals with an estimated 5% or a higher lifetime risk of developing PDAC are now encouraged to undergo surveillance, as per the International Cancer of the Pancreas Screening (CAPS) Consortium recommendations.[5] The so-called high-risk individuals (HRIs) carry either a deleterious germline mutation in one of the pancreatic cancer susceptibility genes and/or have a strong family history of PDAC, with at least one first-degree and one second-degree relative affected with PDAC.[5]

In this review, we elaborate on the inherited predisposition to familial pancreatic cancer (FPC) and focus on the role of surveillance for individuals at high risk of pancreatic cancer.

INHERITED PREDISPOSITION

Pancreatic cancer has a significant inherited predisposition.[6–8] It is well-known that having a family history of PDAC increases the risk of developing the disease. The entity of FPC refers to kindred with at least a pair of first-degree relatives with pancreatic cancer, a definition that helps quantify risk. Both the number of family members affected, and their degree relation to one another can be used to estimate this risk. For example, Klein and colleagues[6] found that having two first-degree relatives with pancreatic cancer equates to an elevated PDAC risk ratio of 6.4-fold over average risk, corresponding to a lifetime risk of 8% to 12%. The magnitude of the risk is also associated with the age-at-PDAC of the relatives, with higher risk observed among relatives diagnosed at younger than 50 years.[9] Further studies are needed to better define these risk estimates, including how inherited susceptibility gene variants modify the risk in families. The definition of FPC was created before the availability of widespread gene testing. Nowadays, individuals at increased risk are typically grouped according to whether they have a familial-only risk or if they have a known pancreatic cancer susceptibility gene variant.[3,10]

Despite the value of obtaining a detailed cancer family history, relying on a family history of pancreatic or other cancers to identify potential gene mutation carriers will miss most mutation carriers, and most affected individuals do not come from kindred with a recognizable inherited cancer syndrome.[8] When multigene panel testing is applied to unselected patients with PDAC, close to 10% are found to have a high-penetrance pathogenic variant in one of the known pancreatic cancer susceptibility genes,[11–13] including BRCA2 (breast cancer 2), ATM (ataxia telangiectasia mutated), BRCA1 (breast cancer 1), Lynch syndrome-associated genes, CDKN2A (cyclin dependent kinase inhibitor 2A) (responsible for Familial Atypical Mole and Multiple Melanoma)[7] or STK11 (serine threonine kinase 11) (responsible for Peutz–Jeghers syndrome), among others (**Table 1**).

The significant potential of lowering cancer mortality by identifying close relatives of PDAC cases who have deleterious susceptibility gene variants has led the National Comprehensive Cancer Network[14,15] and the American Society of Clinical Oncology[16] to develop guidelines recommending germline gene testing to all patients diagnosed

Table 1
Pancreatic cancer susceptibility genes

Gene Name	Average Lifetime Risk for PDAC	Increased Relative Risk of Developing PDAC	Associated Inherited Syndromes	Other Cancers/Clinical Manifestations	Mechanism of Action
BRCA2	5–10%[13,17]	~4–6x[13]	Hereditary breast and ovarian cancer	Breast, ovarian, prostate, gastric cancers[17]	Homologous repair
BRCA1	3%[13,17]	~2.5x[13]		Breast, ovarian, prostate, colorectal, gallbladder cancers[17]	
ATM	9.5%[18]	~6x[13]	Ataxia telangiectasia	Breast, prostate cancers	DNA repair
CDK2NA	17%[19,20]	~12–20x[13]	Familial atypical mole and multiple melanoma syndrome	Melanoma	Cell cycle regulation
MLH1	4%[21]	~7x[13]	Lynch syndrome	Colorectal, gynecologic, urothelial, brain cancers intestinal, gastric	Mismatch repair
MSH2		~7x[13]			
MSH6		Unknown			
PALB2	2–3%[22]	~6x[13]	None	Breast cancer	Homologous repair
TP53	Unknown	~7x[13]	Li–Fraumeni syndrome	Most human cancers	DNA repair
PRSS1	7–40%[23,24]	~10x[13]	Hereditary pancreatitis	Recurrent acute pancreatitis	Trypsin activation
STK11	11–36%[25,26]	~30x[13]	Peutz–Jeghers syndrome	Breast, GIT, gynecologic, lung cancers	AMPK signaling
CPA1	~0.5%	~3x	Hereditary pancreatitis	None	Acinar-cell ER stress
CPB1		~9x[27]	Subclinical pancreatitis		

Abbreviations: AMPK, adenosine monophosphate-activated protein kinase; CPA1, carboxypeptidase A1; CPB1, carboxypeptidase B1; ER, endoplasmic reticulum; GIT, Gastrointestinal tract; MLH1, mutL homolog 1; MSH2, mutS homolog 2; MSH6, mutS homolog 6; PALB2, partner and localizer of BRCA2; PRSS1, serine protease 1; TP53, tumor protein p53.

with PDAC regardless of their age at diagnosis or family history, and if appropriate, their first-degree relatives.

For most of these pancreatic cancer susceptibility genes, deleterious variants predispose to other cancers as well.[8] Hereditary recurrent acute pancreatitis, mostly due to deleterious variants in *PRSS1* is a rare but important mechanism of pancreatic cancer susceptibility.[8]

In most populations, deleterious susceptibility gene variants are most commonly identified in *BRCA2* and *ATM* among unselected PDAC cases, with a prevalence of approximately 2%.[11,13] Founder mutations are an important contributor in certain populations such as the common *BRCA2* founder mutation in individuals of Ashkenazi Jewish descent[28] and the *CDK2NA* founder mutation in the Dutch.[19]

The average lifetime risk of PDAC is highest among patients with Peutz–Jeghers syndrome (11% to 36%[25,26]) and those who have a germline pathogenic variant in *CDKN2A* (17%).[19,20] The risk of pancreatic cancer is also high for *PRSS1* mutation carriers with earlier studies estimating a lifetime risk of approximately 40%. However, a more recent study estimated a much lower risk of about 7%.[23,24]

The lifetime risk for *BRCA2* and *ATM* mutation carriers is estimated to be approximately 10%. For *ATM* mutation carriers, this risk has been estimated to be about 1.0% by age 50 years, increasing to 6.3% by 70 years of age, and to 9.5% by 80 years.[18] Among *BRCA2* mutation carriers, estimates of the relative risk[17] and the odds ratio (OR)[13] are similar (approximately 6-fold overall in most studies). In contrast, the lifetime risk among *BRCA1* mutations carriers is approximately 3%, below the 5% risk threshold that risk experts have used as a guideline when considering who should be screened for pancreatic cancer in the absence of a family history.

The PDAC risk among carriers with Lynch syndrome-associated germline mutations (in *MLH1*, *MSH2*, PMS2, and *MSH6*) is also estimated to be near the 5% threshold for surveillance,[21] and the PDAC risk among *PALB2* germline mutation carriers is thought to be similar to *BRCA2*, though limited data are available (see **Table 1**).

Recent efforts to identify additional FPC susceptibility genes have identified several genes with variants that are thought to contribute to pancreatic cancer risk by inducing pancreatic acinar cell endoplasmic reticulum stress, a mechanism known to contribute to some forms of hereditary pancreatitis.[27] The case-control studies[27,29] have found evidence that rare variants in *CPA1* and *CPB1* (functionally classified as endoplasmic reticulum [ER] stress-inducing variants genes) are more common in patients with PDAC than in non-cancer controls (OR for *CPA1*: 3.65 [95% CI, 1.58–8.39] and OR for *CPB1*: 9.51 [95% CI, 3.46–26.15]).[27] A recent genome-wide association study identified a common deletion variant in *CTRB2* (chymotrypsinogen B2) as ER-stress inducing (OR for PDAC 1.36).[30] Of note, acute pancreatitis is usually not a feature of PDAC cases associated with ER stress variants.

The aforementioned risk values are subject to variation depending on the germline variant itself as well as additional inherited and environmental factors.[8] For example, smoking is a major nongenetic factor that independently contributes to the increased risk of PDAC with OR, 3.7 (95% CI, 1.8–7.6).[6,7] Smoking is also associated with a substantially lower average age-at-diagnosis in familial PDAC kindred. In individuals with hereditary pancreatitis, smoking lowers the age of onset by approximately 20 years.[31] Overall, pathogenic variants in the known germline pancreatic susceptibility genes known to date explain only a minor portion (less than 20%) of the familial clustering of pancreatic cancer.[8]

Polygenic risk scores (the risk of developing a disease based on the total number of changes related to the disease) are being developed for several cancer types in an effort to refine risk estimates.[32] Although polygenic risk scores can refine risk and have promise for common diseases, their clinical value for less common diseases such as pancreatic cancer is currently limited, even when combined with other risk factors (family history, smoking, obesity, and so forth).[33] One study has used polygenic risk scores to estimate PDAC risk among patients with new-onset diabetes.[34]

PANCREATIC CANCER SURVEILLANCE

For over two decades, the potential of early detection to reduce pancreatic cancer mortality has formed the basis of pancreas surveillance studies. In recent years, the accumulated evidence of these studies finds that pancreatic surveillance of HRIs can downstage tumors with significantly improved outcomes among those diagnosed with pancreatic cancer. Candidates for pancreatic surveillance should have a detailed discussion about the potential benefits and risks of surveillance and the need for long-term compliance. A patient-tailored approach should consider an individual's family history, germline mutation status, most recent imaging findings, and genetic and environmental factors.

Goals of Surveillance

In 2020, the International CAPS Consortium issued its modified recommendations with regard to pancreatic surveillance, updating the CAPS consensus statements from 2013.[35] Consensus regarding the main goal of pancreatic surveillance did not change: reducing pancreatic cancer-related deaths by the detection and treatment of Stage I PDAC and precursor lesions with high-grade dysplasia.[5,36] The clearest evidence to date that pancreatic surveillance can improve long-term outcomes is reported in a study of 354 HRIs enrolled in the CAPS program, where long-term survival was common among patients who maintained surveillance compared with those whose surveillance lapsed.[37]

Whom to Screen and When

The selection of individuals eligible for pancreatic surveillance currently relies on three key criteria: family history, germline mutation status, and age (**Table 2**). These criteria allow clinicians to best assess pancreatic cancer risk.[5]

 Current recommendations of the International CAPS Consortium regarding family history (when there is no known susceptibility gene mutation) state that individuals are eligible for surveillance if they have at least two affected blood relatives with PDAC on the same side of the family, of whom at least one is an affected first-degree relative, who in turn has an affected first-degree relative.[5] The recommendations regarding age-to-commence surveillance are based on the age-at-diagnosis of pancreatic cancer in HRIs. Most pancreatic cancers in individuals with a family history of PDAC are diagnosed after age 55, and on average have a later age-at-diagnosis than those with a known pancreatic cancer susceptibility variant.[11,37] The consensus at the last International CAPS Consortium was to initiate surveillance at age 50 years or later for this group, although 22.1% of the experts considered 55 years as the adequate age to begin. This was consistent with the latest American Gastroenterological Association (AGA) clinical practice update recommendations[36] and the American College of Gastroenterology (ACG) guidelines.[38]

 The recommendations for surveillance of those with susceptibility gene variants are specific for each gene.[5,36,38] Given their high lifetime risk of pancreatic cancer, carriers of mutations in STK11 (Peutz–Jeghers syndrome) and CDKN2A (Familial Atypical Multiple Mole Melanoma, only mutations that inactivate p16) are advised to participate in pancreatic surveillance, regardless of their family history.[5] Initiating surveillance for

Table 2
Summary of the pancreatic cancer surveillance recommendations in high-risk individual by organization

	International CAPS Consortium[5] (2020)	AGA[36] (2020)	ACG[38] (2015)
Who?	• All patients with Peutz–Jeghers syndrome • All patients with hereditary pancreatitis • All carriers of a germline CDKN2A mutation • Carriers of a germline BRCA2, PALB2, ATM, MLH1, MSH2, or MSH6 gene mutation with at least one affected FDR or SDR • Individuals from familial pancreatic cancer kindred, defined as at least two affected FDRs who are an FDR to at least one with pancreatic cancer. • Carriers of a germline BRCA1 gene mutation with at least one affected FDR[a]		• Carriers of a germline BRCA2, PALB2, ATM, MLH1, MSH2, or MSH6 gene mutation with at least one affected FDR or SDR • Carriers of a germline BRCA1 gene mutation with at least one affected FDR or SDR
When?	• Age to begin surveillance depends on patient's gene mutation status and family history • There is no consensus on the age to end surveillance • Start surveillance at age 40 y for all individuals with Peutz–Jeghers syndrome • Start surveillance at age 40 y for all carriers of a germline CDKN2A mutation and individuals with hereditary pancreatitis • Start surveillance at age 45 or 50 y or 10 y younger than youngest affected blood relative for all carriers of a germline BRCA2, BRCA1, PALB2, ATM, MLH1, MSH2, or MSH6 mutation • Start surveillance at age 50 or 55 y[a] or 10 y younger than youngest affected blood relative for FPC kindred (without a known germline mutation)	• Start surveillance at age 35 y for all individuals with Peutz–Jeghers syndrome • Start surveillance at age 50 y, or 10 y younger than the earliest age of PC in the family for all carriers of a germline CDKN2A mutation • Start surveillance at age 50 y, or 10 y younger than the earliest age of PC in the family for all carriers of a germline BRCA2, BRCA1, PALB2, ATM, MLH1, MSH2, or MSH6 mutation and for individuals with FPC kindred (without a known germline mutation)	
How?	• MRI/MRCP and EUS at baseline • Alternate MRI/MRCP and EUS (no consensus if and how to alternate) during follow-up • Serum CA19–9 and CT only for concerning findings • Surveillance annually if no or only non-concerning abnormalities • Surveillance every 3 or 6 mo if concerning abnormalities for which immediate surgery is not indicated • Surgery if positive FNA and/or high suspicion of malignancy on imaging	• Not considered	

FDR, first-degree relative; SDR, second-degree relative; FPC, Familial Pancreatic Cancer; MRI, magnetic resonance imaging; MRCP, magnetic resonance cholangio-pancreatography; EUS, endoscopic ultrasound; FNA, fine-needle aspiration; CT, computed tomography; PC, pancreatic cancer.
[a] Consensus was not reached.

CDKN2A mutation carriers is recommended at age 40 years and at age 30 to 40 years for patients with Peutz–Jeghers syndrome,[5] with the ACG suggesting 35 years as a suitable age.[38] For patients with hereditary pancreatitis, owing to disease-causing variants in *PRSS1*, *CPA1*, and *CTRC*,[5] surveillance is recommended after age 40 years, or 20 years after the first pancreatitis attack, irrespective of gene status.[5,31,36,38]

Discriminating changes of pancreatitis from the presence of pancreatic neoplasia using current imaging tests is challenging, and for this reason, pancreas surveillance of those with a history of recurrent acute pancreatitis should be undertaken at centers of excellence.[36] For *ATM*, *BRCA2*, *PALB2*, and Lynch syndrome mutation carriers, most guidelines recommend surveillance if individuals have at least one affected first-degree blood relative with pancreatic cancer.[5,36] Consensus as to the pancreatic cancer family history criteria for *BRCA1* mutation carriers (who have a low average lifetime risk of developing PDAC) was not reached among CAPS experts, although most still encourage surveillance in this group.[5]

Among mutation carriers, a family history of pancreatic cancer modifies risk, but the extent to which it does is not well-defined. In the early years of pancreas surveillance, before much evidence and experience had been accumulated, it was considered important to limit eligibility to the highest risk individuals. In recent years, groups have begun investigating the yield of surveillance among mutation carriers without a family history of PDAC. Katona and colleagues[39] examined this question among *BRCA1*, *BRCA2*, *ATM*, and *PALB2* mutation carriers. The sample size was too small to adequately address this question, but two individuals (3%) developed PDAC, a similar detection rate to that reported in other studies among high-risk groups with a family history of PDAC (yielding an estimate that 111 to 135 patients will need to be screened to identify one with a PDAC or a high-grade precursor lesion).[40,41]

Some studies have reported a low diagnostic yield among individuals under surveillance with familial-only risk. For example, the Dutch FPC Surveillance Study Group reported on 366 HRIs (including 201 mutation-negative FPC kindred and 165 PDAC susceptibility gene mutation carriers) and revealed a cumulative PDAC incidence of 9.3% in the mutation carriers group, as opposed to 0% in the FPC kindred one ($P < 0.001$).[42] These findings led Overbeek and colleagues[42] to question the value of surveillance in those with meeting only familial risk criteria. However, this conclusion is likely premature as this has not been the experience in the CAPS program, although not all familial risk patients undergo gene testing. Indeed, most of the risk estimates in FPC kindred were based on genetically untested families.[6,43] However, the low number of PDAC cases and the relatively young age of their cohort (whose risk of PDAC will increase with time) were limitations of their study. Abe and colleagues[44] demonstrated through a study involving 464 HRIs that the risk of neoplastic progression is higher among patients with a known deleterious germline mutation than in those with a familial risk alone [hazard ratio (HR), 2.85; 95% CI, 1.0 to 8.18; $P < 0.05$]. Abe and colleagues[44] showed the risk of developing PDAC among individuals with familial risk alone is still significant and recommended surveillance in this group. The latest AGA Clinical Practice Update recommended as their third best practice advice that genetic testing should be offered to FPC kindred who meet the criteria for surveillance.[36]

Pancreas Surveillance Tests

Endoscopic ultrasound (EUS) and magnetic resonance imaging (MRI)/magnetic retrograde cholangiopancreatography (MRCP) are currently the most widely used modalities for pancreatic surveillance. Pancreatic protocol computed tomography

(CT) has been shown to be useful in characterizing solid lesions after they were found on surveillance imaging,[7] but CT is not generally used as a first-line test because of the radiation dose and intravenous contrast requirement. Furthermore, EUS and MRI/MRCP have the advantage of being superior at detecting very small pancreatic cysts.[5,45] Developments in CT, such as the use of artificial intelligence methods to improve the detection of subtle lesions, could change that recommendation in the future.[46]

Several studies have attempted to compare the diagnostic yield of these imaging technologies. For example, Canto and colleagues [47]compared EUS, MRI/MRCP, and CT and found that the detection of subcentimeter pancreatic cysts was superior with EUS and MRI/MRCP. Some studies have compared overall diagnostic yield that includes cysts and solid lesions. A meta-analysis of 2,122 HRIs who underwent imaging found no significant difference between EUS and MRI in their ability to detect high-grade dysplasia, T1N0M0 PDAC, or cysts.[40] This study and prior studies[40,48,49] found that EUS can detect subtle focal parenchymal abnormalities which might result from pancreatic intraepithelial neoplasia (PanIN), although their clinical significance in the setting of surveillance has yet to be defined.

The detection of PanIN remains a major challenge of pancreatic surveillance. Most PDACs are thought to originate from PanIN, whether the individual has a family history, inherited susceptibility gene mutation, or a sporadic form of cancer. As subcentimeter pancreatic cysts with imaging characteristics of intraductal papillary mucinous neoplasms (IPMNs) are commonly observed in patients undergoing surveillance, it would be easy to conclude (incorrectly) that PDACs that emerge in those with a familial/inherited risk often go through an IPMN-like pathway. However, PDACs that do arise in the background of pancreatic cysts, often do so away from preexisting, non-worrisome pancreatic cysts, and have independent genetics.[50] Indeed, even among patients with large sporadic IPMNs, it is common to find that the pancreatic cancer is genetically distinct from the IPMN and presumed to have arisen from PanIN.[51] Concomitant high-grade PanINs originating in areas of the pancreas distinct from pancreatic cysts are often found in subjects with resected sporadic low-grade IPMNs. Among HRIs, the presence of pancreatic cysts is associated with a modest increased relative risk of developing PDAC compared with those without such cysts.[37]

Developments in imaging may one day allow for the detection of PanIN within the intact pancreas, but this remains a challenge. Some investigators are looking at pancreatic juice collected from the duodenum at the time of EUS (pancreatic juice profiling) using digital next-generation sequencing. Such profiling can reveal the molecular alterations within the pancreas, but they are not sufficient to localize PanIN.[52] Other approaches using molecular imaging such as those targeting the integrin $\alpha_v\beta6$-binding peptide which has been used to image pancreatic cancer[53] could have utility for detecting large PanIN.

The most important question regarding the diagnostic yield of imaging tests in the setting of pancreatic surveillance is the accuracy for detecting small (1 cm or less) pancreatic cancers. Many factors contribute to diagnostic performance including clinician/radiologist expertise, imaging technique used, and the variable imaging characteristics of small tumors. The low incidence of PDAC even in high-risk cohorts has made it a difficult question to answer definitively. A multicenter blinded prospective study by Harinck and colleagues,[45] comparing the efficacy of MRI and EUS in HRIs revealed that EUS was particularly sensitive for the detection of solid lesions less than 20 mm, with two PDACs (including a Stage I PDAC) detected by EUS but not by MRI.

Outcomes of Surveillance

Few studies of pancreatic surveillance among HRIs have reported sufficient numbers of patients diagnosed with PDAC to evaluate long-term outcomes. In their long-term (16-year) CAPS study of 354 HRIs undergoing surveillance, Canto and colleagues[37] demonstrated that PDAC and/or high-grade dysplasia developed in 7% of the cohort (24 patients), with 71% of the PDACs detected at stages I and II. Outside of surveillance, patients with symptomatic PDAC have less than a 20% chance of having low-stage resectable disease.[1] The downstaging observed in the CAPS study was associated with better overall 3-year survival; 85% for the 10 PDACs detected in asymptomatic HRIs during surveillance versus 25% for the four symptomatic HRIs who developed PDAC after dropping out of surveillance ($P < 0.0001$).[37] Similarly, a prospective study following 178 *CKDN2A*/p16 Leiden mutation carriers in three expert European centers demonstrated that 75% of the PDACs detected during surveillance were resectable,[19] and a much higher proportion than the 15% reported for historical controls.[54] Furthermore, the 5-year survival rate was markedly higher (24%) than that previously described for individuals with symptomatic sporadic PDAC (4% to 7%) in the Dutch Cancer Registry.[55]

Early detection could be improved if it was possible to identify features on imaging or other characteristics to better tailor surveillance interval recommendations. Based on what has been estimated about the growth rate of pancreatic tumor masses[56] and the experience gained from surveillance of HRIs, most patients are recommended to undergo annual surveillance. Progression to PDAC occurs most often in those older than 60 years, those with numerous pancreatic cysts,[37] and in mutation carriers,[44] but these factors alone are not sufficiently discriminating of future PDAC risk to warrant changing surveillance intervals.

When worrisome features are detected on imaging, surveillance intervals should generally be adjusted.[36] The experience of surveillance of sporadic pancreatic cysts that led to the Sendai and Fukuoka International Consensus Guidelines for management of mucinous cysts are helpful: cyst size $\geq$ 3 cm, thickened/enhancing cyst walls, mural nodule in the cyst or main pancreatic duct (MPD), MPD dilation greater than 5 mm, abrupt change in MPD caliber, suspicious cytology for pancreatic malignancy, or rapid cyst growth rate greater than 2 mm in 6 months or greater than 4 mm in 1 year.[57] The ACG clinical guidelines acknowledge the difficulty in establishing clear-cut inclusion criteria for surgery and state that the decision should be individualized after multidisciplinary evaluation by experts of the field.[38] In fact, Dbouk and colleagues[58] assessed the diagnostic performance of the Fukuoka and CAPS guidelines for the management of pancreatic cysts in HRIs and showed that both would have failed to adequately recommend surgery for PDAC patients. They found that the Fukuoka criteria had a lower sensitivity (40%) for selection of HRIs for surgery compared with individuals with sporadic cysts, missing 60% of cysts with invasive carcinoma or IPMNs with high-grade dysplasia. The CAPS criteria also missed 40% of resected neoplastic IPMNs. Both consensus criteria might have recommended unnecessary surgery for 15% of HRIs.[58] One reason for the poor ability of imaging characteristics to predict the emergence of PDAC, especially in the familial/inherited risk setting, is the inability of current imaging tools to detect PanIN with high-grade dysplasia.

In the early years of pancreatic surveillance, patients were often sent for pancreatic resection for worrisome features, or other concerning abnormalities. For example, in their meta-analysis including 1,551 familial HRIs, Paiella and colleagues[59] reported a pooled proportion of overall surgery of 6% (95% CI 4.1–7.9, $P < 0.001$) and unnecessary surgery of 68.1% (95% CI 59.5–76.7, P < 0.001), with final pathology reports revealing diagnoses incompatible with screening goals in most cases. In addition, a review of such cases found that up to 15% of solid pancreatic lesions were benigns.[55] Nowadays, clinicians have learned to be more selective.

In summary, pancreatic surveillance of HRIs has been shown to detect PDAC with a high-resectability rate. Surgical resection in this setting is associated with acceptable morbidity, minimal mortality, and remarkable long-term survival.[60] There is some evidence that participation of HRIs in a screening program did not lead to an increase in cancer worry, as could have been previously presumed.[61] Instead, taking part in a surveillance plan procured a sense of control and even reduced anxiety in some patients.[62] The evaluation of long-term outcomes of HRIs should continue, but not without acknowledging that compliance to a surveillance program remains a territory that requires substantial exploration. Longitudinal studies should aim at identifying factors associated with poor surveillance compliance in HRIs.[63] In the United States, cost can be a barrier to being able to undertake annual EUS or MRI/MRCP surveillance, as insurance coverage for pancreatic surveillance is variable. Indeed, across the United States, among individuals diagnosed with PDAC (NCI SEER data-general population cases), having insurance is associated with a lower stage at diagnosis.[64]

THE POTENTIAL OF BIOMARKER TESTS TO IMPROVE PANCREAS SURVEILLANCE

Remarkable efforts have been made to identify HRIs who qualify for pancreas surveillance in the hope of optimizing early detection of pancreatic cancer in this unique population. Novel strategies are needed to better stratify PDAC risk in HRIs with the aim of increasing the number of eligible patients for pancreatic cancer surveillance.[65] Likewise, new tests are being evaluated to improve detection of high-grade precancerous lesions and early-stage invasive carcinomas not only in HRIs but also in the general population.

Improving the diagnostic accuracy of circulating tumor markers such as CA19-9 would be of great value. As a marker, CA19-9 is significantly influenced by common variants in the genes responsible for its synthesis (*FUT2* and *FUT3*). Abe and colleagues[66] found that classifying individuals into CA19-9 reference ranges based on these *FUT2/FUT3* variants significantly improved the accuracy of CA19-9 (and other tumor markers) for diagnosing pancreatic cancer. They showed that a tumor marker gene test combined with a CA19-9 test enhanced its diagnostic performance (particularly in patients with intact *FUT3*), with 66.4% sensitivity and 99.2% specificity for subjects with localized PDAC. To have the greatest impact, these tests need to detect stage I PDAC. A major challenge for the detection of stage I PDACs with a blood-based test is that smaller cancers generally shed fewer biomarkers into the bloodstream. Studying biomarkers from patients with stage I PDACs is similarly challenging because these cases are very rare,[66] and many newly diagnosed patients now receive neoadjuvant chemotherapy, obscuring assessment of their pathologic stage at presentation.[67]

Liquid biopsies have been used to evaluate circulating tumor DNA (ctDNA) as a noninvasive tool to detect early-stage pancreatic cancer. For pancreatic cancer detection, initial studies relied on mutated *KRAS* ctDNA. More recent studies have used pan-cancer ctDNA tests as part of multi-cancer detection approaches.[68] Further evidence is needed before considering its implementation in a clinical setting.

SUMMARY

Studies in recent years have provided a deeper understanding of the inherited predisposition to PDAC and its relationship to FPC. Experts have identified at present at least a dozen genes known to contribute to the development of PDAC in mutation carriers. Patients whose PDAC is localized to the pancreas have a better chance of survival than those with a more advanced form of the disease.[64,69] Individuals with familial and inherited risk of pancreatic cancer who undertake pancreas surveillance and are diagnosed with early-stage PDAC, especially stage I disease, have an excellent chance to achieve long-term survival.

CLINICS CARE POINTS

- Pancreatic ductal adenocarcinoma (PDAC) has an overall poor prognosis. Symptoms associated with PDAC commonly manifest late in the course of disease.

- Eligibility criteria for pancreas surveillance are based on age, germline mutation status, and family history. High-risk individuals (HRIs) with an estimated 5% or higher lifetime risk of developing PDAC are advised to undergo surveillance for PDAC.

- The accumulated evidence of pancreas surveillance studies demonstrates that pancreatic surveillance of HRIs can result in the diagnosis of early-stage PDAC, and this is associated with improved outcomes.

- Endoscopic ultrasound and/or magnetic resonance imaging/magnetic resonance cholangiopancreatography are considered the standard imaging modalities for screening to date. Computed tomography scan has been shown to be useful in characterizing concerning solid lesions found on surveillance but is not generally used as a first-line test.

- Blood-based biomarkers and circulating tumor DNA tests represent promising noninvasive tools to detect early-stage pancreatic cancer.

FUNDING

This work was supported by NIH grants U01210170, and R01CA176828). This work was also supported by a Stand Up To Cancer-Lustgarten Foundation Pancreatic Cancer Interception Translational Cancer Research Grant (Grant Number: SU2C-AACR-DT25-17). Stand Up To Cancer is a program of the Entertainment Industry Foundation. SU2C research grants are administered by the American Association for Cancer Research, the scientific partner of SU2C. MG is the Sol Goldman Professor of Pancreatic Cancer Research.

REFERENCES

1. Siegel RL, Miller KD, Fuchs HE, et al. Cancer statistics, 2022. CA Cancer J Clin 2022;72(1):7–33.
2. Rahib L, Wehner MR, Matrisian LM, et al. Estimated projection of US cancer incidence and death to 2040. JAMA Netw Open 2021;4(4):e214708.
3. Biller LH, Wolpin BM, Goggins M. Inherited pancreatic cancer syndromes and high-risk screening. Surg Oncol Clin N Am 2021;30(4):773–86.
4. Meza R, Jeon J, Moolgavkar SH, et al. Age-specific incidence of cancer: Phases, transitions, and biological implications. Proc Natl Acad Sci U S A 2008;105(42):16284–9.
5. Goggins M, Overbeek KA, Brand R, et al. Management of patients with increased risk for familial pancreatic cancer: updated recommendations from the International Cancer of the Pancreas Screening (CAPS) Consortium. Gut 2020; 69(1):7–17.

6. Klein AP, Brune KA, Petersen GM, et al. Prospective risk of pancreatic cancer in familial pancreatic cancer kindreds. Cancer Res 2004;64(7):2634–8.

7. Ngamruengphong S, Canto MI. Screening for pancreatic cancer. Surg Clin North Am 2016;96(6):1223–33.

8. Wood LD, Yurgelun MB, Goggins MG. Genetics of familial and sporadic pancreatic cancer. Gastroenterology 2019;156(7):2041–55.

9. Brune KA, Lau B, Palmisano E, et al. Importance of age of onset in pancreatic cancer kindreds. J Natl Cancer Inst 2010;102(2):119–26.

10. Rustgi SD, Hilfrank KJ, Kastrinos F. Familial predisposition and genetic risk factors associated with pancreatic cancer. Gastrointest Endosc Clin N Am 2022; 32(1):1–12.

11. Shindo K, Yu J, Suenaga M, et al. Deleterious germline mutations in patients with apparently sporadic pancreatic adenocarcinoma. J Clin Oncol 2017;35(30): 3382–90.

12. Yurgelun MB, Chittenden AB, Morales-Oyarvide V, et al. Germline cancer susceptibility gene variants, somatic second hits, and survival outcomes in patients with resected pancreatic cancer. Genet Med 2019;21(1):213–23.

13. Hu C, Hart SN, Polley EC, et al. Association between inherited germline mutations in cancer predisposition genes and risk of pancreatic cancer. JAMA 2018; 319(23):2401–9.

14. Daly MB, Pal T, Berry MP, et al. Genetic/familial high-risk assessment: breast, ovarian, and pancreatic, version 2.2021, nccn clinical practice guidelines in oncology. J Natl Compr Canc Netw 2021;19(1):77–102.

15. Tempero MA, Malafa MP, Al-Hawary M, et al. Pancreatic adenocarcinoma, version 2.2021, NCCN clinical practice guidelines in oncology. J Natl Compr Canc Netw 2021;19(4):439–57.

16. Stoffel EM, McKernin SE, Brand R, et al. Evaluating susceptibility to pancreatic cancer: ASCO provisional clinical opinion. J Clin Oncol 2019;37(2):153–64.

17. Li S, Silvestri V, Leslie G, et al. Cancer risks associated with BRCA1 and BRCA2 pathogenic variants. J Clin Oncol 2022;40(14):1529–41.

18. Hsu FC, Roberts NJ, Childs E, et al. Risk of pancreatic cancer among individuals with pathogenic variants in the ATM gene. JAMA Oncol 2021;7(11):1664–8.

19. Vasen H, Ibrahim I, Ponce CG, et al. Benefit of surveillance for pancreatic cancer in high-risk individuals: outcome of long-term prospective follow-up studies from three european expert centers. J Clin Oncol 2016;34(17):2010–9.

20. Vasen HF, Gruis NA, Frants RR, et al. Risk of developing pancreatic cancer in families with familial atypical multiple mole melanoma associated with a specific 19 deletion of p16 (p16-Leiden). Int J Cancer 2000;87(6):809–11.

21. Kastrinos F, Mukherjee B, Tayob N, et al. Risk of pancreatic cancer in families with Lynch syndrome. JAMA 2009;302(16):1790–5.

22. Yang X, Leslie G, Doroszuk A, et al. Cancer risks associated with germline PALB2 pathogenic variants: an international study of 524 families. J Clin Oncol 2020; 38(7):674–85.

23. Lowenfels AB, Maisonneuve P, DiMagno EP, et al. Hereditary pancreatitis and the risk of pancreatic cancer. International Hereditary Pancreatitis Study Group. J Natl Cancer Inst 1997;89(6):442–6.

24. Shelton CA, Umapathy C, Stello K, et al. Hereditary pancreatitis in the united states: survival and rates of pancreatic cancer. Am J Gastroenterol 2018; 113(9):1376.

25. Hearle N, Schumacher V, Menko FH, et al. Frequency and spectrum of cancers in the Peutz-Jeghers syndrome. Clin Cancer Res 2006;12(10):3209–15.

26. Giardiello FM, Brensinger JD, Tersmette AC, et al. Very high risk of cancer in familial Peutz-Jeghers syndrome. Gastroenterology 2000;119(6):1447–53.

27. Kawamoto M, Kohi S, Abe T, et al. Endoplasmic stress-inducing variants in CPB1 and CPA1 and risk of pancreatic cancer: A case-control study and meta-analysis. Int J Cancer 2022;150:1123–33. https://doi.org/10.1002/ijc.33883.

28. Neuhausen S, Gilewski T, Norton L, et al. Recurrent BRCA2 6174delT mutations in Ashkenazi Jewish women affected by breast cancer. Nat Genet 1996;13(1):126–8.

29. Tamura K, Yu J, Hata T, et al. Mutations in the pancreatic secretory enzymes CPA1 and CPB1 are associated with pancreatic cancer. Proc Natl Acad Sci U S A 2018;115(18):4767–72.

30. Jermusyk A, Zhong J, Connelly KE, et al. A 584 bp deletion in CTRB2 inhibits chymotrypsin B2 activity and secretion and confers risk of pancreatic cancer. Am J Hum Genet 2021;108(10):1852–65.

31. Lowenfels AB, Maisonneuve P, Whitcomb DC. Risk factors for cancer in hereditary pancreatitis. International Hereditary Pancreatitis Study Group. Med Clin North Am 2000;84(3):565–73.

32. Klein AP, Wolpin BM, Risch HA, et al. Genome-wide meta-analysis identifies five new susceptibility loci for pancreatic cancer. Nat Commun 2018;9(1):556.

33. Klein AP, Lindstrom S, Mendelsohn JB, et al. An absolute risk model to identify individuals at elevated risk for pancreatic cancer in the general population. PLoS One 2013;8(9):e72311.

34. Sharma S, Tapper WJ, Collins A, et al. Predicting pancreatic cancer in the UK Biobank cohort using polygenic risk scores and diabetes mellitus. Gastroenterology 2022;162(6):1665–74.e2. https://doi.org/10.1053/j.gastro.2022.01.016.

35. Canto MI, Harinck F, Hruban RH, et al. International Cancer of the Pancreas Screening (CAPS) Consortium summit on the management of patients with increased risk for familial pancreatic cancer. Gut 2013;62(3):339–47.

36. Aslanian HR, Lee JH, Canto MI. AGA clinical practice update on pancreas cancer screening in high-risk individuals: expert review. Gastroenterology 2020;159(1):358–62.

37. Canto MI, Almario JA, Schulick RD, et al. Risk of neoplastic progression in individuals at high risk for pancreatic cancer undergoing long-term surveillance. Gastroenterology 2018;155(3):740–51.e742.

38. Syngal S, Brand RE, Church JM, et al. ACG clinical guideline: genetic testing and management of hereditary gastrointestinal cancer syndromes. Am J Gastroenterol 2015;110(2):223–62 [quiz: 263].

39. Katona BW, Long JM, Ahmad NA, et al. EUS-based Pancreatic Cancer Surveillance in BRCA1/BRCA2/PALB2/ATM Carriers Without a Family History of Pancreatic Cancer. Cancer Prev Res (Phila) 2021;14(11):1033–40.

40. Kogekar N, Diaz KE, Weinberg AD, et al. Surveillance of high-risk individuals for pancreatic cancer with EUS and MRI: A meta-analysis. Pancreatology 2020;20(8):1739–46.

41. Corral JE, Mareth KF, Riegert-Johnson DL, et al. Diagnostic yield from screening asymptomatic individuals at high risk for pancreatic cancer: a meta-analysis of cohort studies. Clin Gastroenterol Hepatol 2019;17(1):41–53.

42. Overbeek KA, Levink IJM, Koopmann BDM, et al. Long-term yield of pancreatic cancer surveillance in high-risk individuals. Gut 2022;71:1152–60. https://doi.org/10.1136/gutjnl-2020-323611.

43. Jacobs EJ, Chanock SJ, Fuchs CS, et al. Family history of cancer and risk of pancreatic cancer: a pooled analysis from the Pancreatic Cancer Cohort Consortium (PanScan). Int J Cancer 2010;127(6):1421–8.

44. Abe T, Blackford AL, Tamura K, et al. Deleterious Germline Mutations Are a Risk Factor for Neoplastic Progression Among High-Risk Individuals Undergoing Pancreatic Surveillance. J Clin Oncol 2019;37(13):1070–80.

45. Harinck F, Konings IC, Kluijt I, et al. A multicentre comparative prospective blinded analysis of EUS and MRI for screening of pancreatic cancer in high-risk individuals. Gut 2016;65(9):1505–13.

46. Chu LC, Park S, Kawamoto S, et al. Current status of radiomics and deep learning in liver imaging. J Comput Assist Tomogr 2021;45(3):343–51.

47. Canto MI, Hruban RH, Fishman EK, et al. Frequent detection of pancreatic lesions in asymptomatic high-risk individuals. Gastroenterology 2012;142(4):796–804.

48. Brune K, Abe T, Canto M, et al. Multifocal neoplastic precursor lesions associated with lobular atrophy of the pancreas in patients having a strong family history of pancreatic cancer. Am J Surg Pathol 2006;30(9):1067–76.

49. Canto MI, Goggins M, Hruban RH, et al. Screening for early pancreatic neoplasia in high-risk individuals: a prospective controlled study. Clin Gastroenterol Hepatol 2006;4(6):766–81 [quiz: 665].

50. Shi C, Klein AP, Goggins M, et al. Increased prevalence of precursor lesions in familial pancreatic cancer patients. Clin Cancer Res 2009;15(24):7737–43.

51. Felsenstein M, Noe M, Masica DL, et al. IPMNs with co-occurring invasive cancers: neighbours but not always relatives. Gut 2018;67(9):1652–62.

52. Suenaga M, Yu J, Shindo K, et al. Pancreatic juice mutation concentrations can help predict the grade of dysplasia in patients undergoing pancreatic surveillance. Clin Cancer Res 2018;24(12):2963–74.

53. Hausner SH, Bold RJ, Cheuy LY, et al. Preclinical development and first-in-human imaging of the integrin $\alpha(v)\beta(6)$ with $[(18)F]\alpha(v)\beta(6)$-binding peptide in metastatic carcinoma. Clin Cancer Res 2019;25(4):1206–15.

54. Vasen HF, Wasser M, van Mil A, et al. Magnetic resonance imaging surveillance detects early-stage pancreatic cancer in carriers of a p16-leiden mutation. Gastroenterology 2011;140(3):850–6.

55. Integraal Kankercentrum Nederland: Dutch Cancer Registry. Available at: http://www.cijfersoverkanker.nl. Accessed February 1, 2022.

56. Yu J, Blackford A, Dal Molin M, et al. Time to progression of pancreatic ductal adenocarcinoma from low-to-high tumour stages. Gut 2015;64:1783–9.

57. Tanaka M, Fernández-Del Castillo C, Kamisawa T, et al. Revisions of international consensus Fukuoka guidelines for the management of IPMN of the pancreas. Pancreatology 2017;17(5):738–53.

58. Dbouk M, Brewer Gutierrez OI, Lennon AM, et al. Guidelines on management of pancreatic cysts detected in high-risk individuals: an evaluation of the 2017 Fukuoka guidelines and the 2020 International Cancer of the Pancreas Screening (CAPS) consortium statements. Pancreatology 2021;21(3):613–21.

59. Paiella S, Salvia R, De Pastena M, et al. Screening/surveillance programs for pancreatic cancer in familial high-risk individuals: A systematic review and proportion meta-analysis of screening results. Pancreatology 2018;18(4):420–8.

60. Canto MI, Kerdsirichairat T, Yeo CJ, et al. Surgical outcomes after pancreatic resection of screening-detected lesions in individuals at high risk for developing pancreatic cancer. J Gastrointest Surg 2020;24(5):1101–10.

61. Maheu C, Vodermaier A, Rothenmund H, et al. Pancreatic cancer risk counselling and screening: impact on perceived risk and psychological functioning. Fam Cancer 2010;9(4):617–24.

62. Konings IC, Sidharta GN, Harinck F, et al. Repeated participation in pancreatic cancer surveillance by high-risk individuals imposes low psychological burden. Psychooncology 2016;25(8):971–8.

63. Katona BW, Mahmud N, Dbouk M, et al. COVID-19 related pancreatic cancer surveillance disruptions amongst high-risk individuals. Pancreatology 2021;21(6): 1048–51.

64. Blackford AL, Canto MI, Klein AP, et al. Recent trends in the incidence and survival of stage 1A pancreatic cancer: a surveillance, epidemiology, and end results analysis. J Natl Cancer Inst 2020;112(11):1162–9.

65. Dudley B, Brand RE. Pancreatic cancer surveillance and novel strategies for screening. Gastrointest Endosc Clin N Am 2022;32(1):13–25.

66. Abe T, Koi C, Kohi S, et al. Gene variants that affect levels of circulating tumor markers increase identification of patients with pancreatic cancer. Clin Gastroenterol Hepatol 2020;18(5):1161–9.e1165.

67. Versteijne E, Dam Jlv, Suker M, et al. Neoadjuvant Chemoradiotherapy versus upfront surgery for resectable and borderline resectable pancreatic cancer: long-term results of the dutch randomized PREOPANC trial. Journal of Clinical Oncology 2022;40(11):1220–30.

68. Lennon AM, Buchanan AH, Kinde I, et al. Feasibility of blood testing combined with PET-CT to screen for cancer and guide intervention. Science 2020; 369(6499):eabb9601.

69. Gemenetzis G, Groot VP, Blair AB, et al. Survival in locally advanced pancreatic cancer after neoadjuvant therapy and surgical resection. Ann Surg 2019;270(2): 340–7.

Colorectal Cancer Screening in a Changing World

Robert S. Bresalier, MD

KEYWORDS

- Colorectal cancer screening • Guidelines • Underserved populations
- Early-onset colorectal cancer • Quality colonoscopy • Non-invasive screening tests
- Artificial intelligence

KEY POINTS

- Numerous professional societies have issued serial updates of CRC screening guidelines that have evolved to provide evidence-based recommendations, which include menus of options designed to maximize screening compliance.
- The incidence of CRC among adults younger than 50 years in the United States has nearly doubled since the early 1990s and continues to increase.
- Adherence to or uptake of CRC screening is especially poor among underserved populations, resulting in increased mortality.
- Quality metrics must be incorporated into CRC screening guidelines and practice.
- Overcoming multiple barriers to screening will require efficient use of multiple screening modalities, continued development of noninvasive screening tests, improved personal risk assessment to best risk-stratify patients, and development of organized screening programs to achieve target screening rates and reductions in CRC morbidity and mortality.

INTRODUCTION

Colorectal cancer (CRC) is the second leading cause of cancer death in industrialized nations, accounting for 10% of the total cancer burden with an individual lifetime risk of approximately 6% in western countries.[1–13] In 2022 it is estimated that 151,000 Americans will be diagnosed with CRC and 52,580 individuals will die of this disease.[1] Over 20 years of SEER data, US CRC incidence (all races, men, women) has decreased from 59.5 cases to 39.3 cases per 100,000 (35% reduction) with a corresponding mortality reduction over the same time period from 24 to 15.1 deaths per 100,000 (37% reduction).[2] However, although early detection by screening significantly reduces mortality and numerous screening options exist,[5–8]

Department of Gastroenterology, Hepatology and Nutrition, The University of Texas MD Anderson Cancer Center, 1515 Holcombe Boulevard Unit 1466, Houston, TX 77030, USA
E-mail address: rbresali@mdanderson.org

Gastroenterol Clin N Am 51 (2022) 577–591
https://doi.org/10.1016/j.gtc.2022.05.002
0889-8553/22/© 2022 Elsevier Inc. All rights reserved.

40% of guideline-eligible patients are not screened as recommended in the United States. Globally, 1.4 million new CRC cases and 700,000 related deaths occur yearly, and compliance with screening may even be lower. Guidelines for CRC screening from US and international professional societies most often provide menus of options based on strength of evidence,[5–8] but generally applied screening methods vary globally and even within the United States depending on access and resources. Consideration of screening options must take into account not only test performance but also issues of resources and individual versus population benefits (**Fig. 1**).

In the United States, colonoscopy is clearly the dominant method of CRC screening, but most of the developed countries recommend a 2-step approach (**Fig. 2**) and do not universally support first-step endoscopic screening. Universal implementation of colonoscopy for CRC screening for all persons ages 50 to 74 years would require a capacity to screen 250 million individuals over a 10-year period in North America and Europe, for example; this will increase substantially due to revisions in guidelines that recommend initiation of CRC screening at age 45 years.[6–8] Adherence to or uptake of CRC screening is especially poor among underserved populations, including those with low income and African American and Hispanic populations.[2,9–14] Novel strategies to improve screening uptake overall and efforts to deploy best practices to underserved populations is a high priority for health care and reducing CRC related morbidity and mortality. On the positive side, increased future adherence to screening guidelines in the United States may be driven by the profound changes in the organization of medical care including enhanced access via the Affordable Care Act, rigid guideline enforcement by payers with physician performance incentives and disincentives, and the rapid adaptation of electronic medical record systems enabling ease of referrals for screening, compliance reminders, and management tracking of compliance to care guidelines.

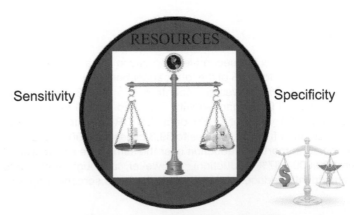

Fig. 1. The performance and success of a screening test in reducing colorectal cancer mortality does not simply depend on its test sensitivity and specificity at a single point in time, but programmatic benefit, including optimal use of available resources. (*Adapted from* Bresalier RS, Grady WM, Markowitz SD, et al. Biomarkers for early detection of colorectal cancer: The Early Detection Research Network, a framework for clinical translation. Cancer Epidemiol Biomarkers Prev 2020; 29:2431-2440; with permission.)

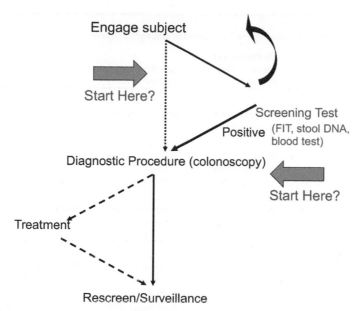

Fig. 2. Although in the United States colonoscopy represents a "first approach" to colorectal cancer screening, many countries that emphasize programmatic screening have taken a "2-step" approach where a less expensive, noninvasive test is first performed. If positive, this is then followed-up by colonoscopy.

The strength of evidence for individual CRC screening tests has been extensively reviewed in updated screening guideline recommendations.[5–8] Rather than duplicate this effort, this article discusses key issues that affect CRC screening in a changing world, including new test development.

SCREENING AND EARLY DETECTION: CURRENT GUIDELINES AND RECOMMENDED PRACTICE

Numerous professional societies have issued serial updates of CRC screening guidelines that have evolved to provide evidence-based recommendations, which include menus of options designed to maximize screening compliance.[5–8,15–17] Current guidelines for CRC screening and surveillance from major US societies are detailed in **Tables 1** and **2**, respectively. Although not all options have proved equivalence of efficacy and have different advantages and limitations, all societies conclude that there is a high certainty that screening for CRC in average-risk asymptomatic adults is of substantial net benefit. A broad set of screening choices for different levels of CRC risk is offered, thereby allowing greater flexibility in achieving screening goals.

The US Multi-Society Task Force on Colorectal Cancer (MSTF) representing the American College of Gastroenterology (ACG), the American Gastroenterological Association (AGA), and the American Society for Gastrointestinal Endoscopy (ASGE) in 2017 ranked CRC screening tests into 3 tiers based on performance features, cost, and practical considerations.[5] First-tier tests are colonoscopy every 10 years and annual fecal immunochemical tests (FIT), with colonoscopy offered first. Second-tier tests include computed tomography (CT) colonography every 5 years, FIT-fecal DNA every 3 years, and flexible sigmoidoscopy (FS) every 5 to 10 years. Capsule

Table 1
Guidelines for screening average-risk persons for colorectal cancer

Screening Tool	US Preventive Services Task Force[a]	American Cancer Society[b]	US Multi-Society Task Force[c]
Stool-Based Tests			
High-sensitivity FOBT (guaiac-based)	Recommended annually as an option	Recommended annually as an option	Not specifically recommended
Fecal immunochemical test (FIT)	Recommended annually as an option	Recommended annually as an option	Recommended annually as an option (tier 1 recommendation)
FIT-fecal DNA testing	Recommended every 3 y as an option	Recommended every 3 y as an option	Recommended every 3 y as a tier 2 option
Direct Visualization			
Colonoscopy	Recommended every 10 y as an option	Recommended every 10 y as an option	Recommended every 10 y as a tier 1 option
Flexible sigmoidoscopy	Recommended every 5 y or every 10 y plus FIT annually as an option	Recommended every 5 y as an option	Not recommended as an option
CT colonography	Recommended every 5 y as an option	Recommended every 5 y as an option	Recommended every 5 y as a tier 2 option
Colon capsule	Not recommended	Not recommended	Recommended every 5 y as a tier 3 option
Blood-based Tests			
Septin 9	Not recommended	Not recommended	Not recommended

Abbreviation: FOBT, fecal occult blood test.

[a] The US Preventive Services Task Force (USPSTF) recommends screening for adults aged 50 to 75 years (Grade A high certainty recommendation) and aged 45 to 49 years (Grade B moderate certainty recommendation). The decision to screening adults aged 76 to 85 years should be an individual one (selective screening), taking into account the patient's overall health and prior screening history. Adults in this age group who have never been screened for CRC are more likely to benefit. These guidelines discuss the strength of evidence for each modality and recommend individualized decision-making to the specific patient or situation. Cost is not considered by the USPSTF.

[b] The American Cancer Society recommends average-risk screening beginning at age 45 years as a qualified recommendation. Screening adults aged 76 to 85 years should be individualized based on patient preferences, life expectancy, health status, and prior screening history. Discussion is presented regarding the 2018 MISCAN modeling analysis with comparison of potential life years gained (LYG) for each screening scenario. Data from CA Cancer J Clin. 2018; 68:250-281.

[c] The US Multi-Society Task Force (MSTF) on Colorectal Cancer representing the American College of Gastroenterology (ACG), the American Gastroenterological Association (AGA), and the American Society for Gastrointestinal Endoscopy (ASGE) recommends average-risk screening beginning at age 45 years. Discontinuation should be considered when individuals up to date with screening and who have prior negative screening reach age 75 years or have less than 10 years life expectancy. For individuals ages 76 to 85 years the decision to start or continue screening should be individualized based on prior screening history, life expectancy, CRC risk, and personal preference. Screening is not recommended after age 85 years. The MSTF ranks screening tests by

recommended tiers. In a separate document the ACG discussed one-step screening (colonoscopy) versus a 2-step approach and examined the quality of evidence for each test. The recommendation to begin average-risk screening at age 50 years was considered a strong recommendation based on moderate-quality evidence, whereas the recommendation to begin screening at age 45 years was considered to be a conditional recommendation based on very low-quality evidence.

Data from Refs.[5–7]

colonoscopy every 5 years is a third-tier test. It is suggested that the Septin9 blood test not be used for screening. Tools for enhancing colonoscopy quality are stressed. These guidelines were updated in 2022, with a consensus statement focusing on when to start and when to stop CRC screening.[6] The MSTF now recommends that average-risk screening begin at age 45 years. In a separate document the ACG discussed 1-step screening (colonoscopy) versus a 2-step approach and examined the quality of evidence for each test. The recommendation to begin average-risk screening at age 50 years was considered a strong recommendation based on moderate-quality evidence, whereas the recommendation to begin screening at age 45 years was considered to be a conditional recommendation based on very low-quality evidence.[17]

The American Cancer Society (ACS) updated its guidelines in 2018 and recommended that average-risk individuals undergo regular screening beginning at age 45 years with either a high-sensitivity stool-based test (FIT or high-sensitivity guaiac-based fecal occult blood test annually, multitarget stool DNA test every 3 years) or a structural examination (colonoscopy every 10 years, CT colonography every 5 years, FS every 5 years).[8] All positive results on noncolonoscopy screening tests should be followed by timely colonoscopy.

The US Preventive Services Taskforce (USPSTF) commissioned a systematic review to evaluate the benefits and harms of CRC screening. In an updated recommendation statement in 2021, the USPSTF concluded with "high certainty" that CRC screening in average-risk asymptomatic adults aged 50 to 75 years has "substantial" net benefit and concluded with "moderate certainty" that screening in adults aged 45 to 49 years has "moderate net benefit." The USPSTF indicated that multiple strategies are available to choose from with different levels of evidence to support their effectiveness, as well as unique advantages and limitations. Eight screening strategies were recommended with details of evidence of efficacy and discussion of considerations including stool-based tests and direct visualization tests. Stool-based tests include high-sensitivity guaiac-based fecal occult blood testing, FIT, and a multitarget stool DNA test, which includes an FIT component. Direct visualization tests include colonoscopy, CT colonography, flexible sigmoidoscopy, and flexible sigmoidoscopy with FIT. Numerous international CRC screening programs have been initiated, as evidence grows for an impact of CRC screening on mortality.[18]

CHANGING DEMOGRAPHICS, UNDERSERVED POPULATIONS, AND THE IMPACT ON COLORECTAL CANCER SCREENING
Early Onset Colorectal Cancer

Although the incidence of CRC continues to decline in older populations, the incidence among adults younger than 50 years in the United States has nearly doubled since the early 1990s and continues to increase. Similar increases in incidence of early onset CRC (EoCRC) have been observed in Europe, Canada, Australia, as well as in some countries in Asia. Time trends demonstrate that incidence of young-onset CRC has continued to increase across successive birth cohorts[2,13] of individuals born after 1960, suggesting that exposures accumulated over the life course may increase the

Table 2
Guidelines for surveillance after high-quality colonoscopy

Risk Category	Time or Age to Begin Surveillance	Recommended Test	Comment
Persons with Adenomas at Colonoscopy			
Persons with 1 or 2 tubular adenomas <10 mm	7–10 y after initial polypectomy	Colonoscopy	Precise timing is based on clinical factors and on patient and physician preferences
Persons with 3–4 tubular adenomas < 10 mm	3–5 y after initial polypectomy	Colonoscopy	—
Persons with 5–10 adenomas or 1 adenoma ≥10 mm or any adenoma with villous features or high-grade dysplasia	3 y after initial polypectomy	Colonoscopy	If the follow-up examination is normal or shows 1 or 2 small tubular adenomas, subsequent examination at 5 y
Persons with >10 adenomas on a single examination	1 y after initial polypectomy	Colonoscopy	Consider familial syndrome
Persons with serrated polyps at colonoscopy			
Persons with sessile adenomas or sessile serrated polyps ≥20 mm that are removed piecemeal	6 mo after initial colonoscopy	Colonoscopy	Surveillance individualized based on clinical judgment
Persons with 1–2 sessile serrated polyps/lesions < 10 mm without dysplasia	5–10 y after initial polypectomy	Colonoscopy	—
Persons with 3–4 sessile serrated polyps/lesions < 10 mm without dysplasia	3–5 y after initial polypectomy	Colonoscopy	—
Persons with 5–10 sessile serrated polyps/lesions, sessile serrated polyps ≥10 mm or with dysplasia or traditional serrated adenoma	3 y after initial polypectomy	Colonoscopy	—
Hyperplastic polyp ≥ 10 mm	3–5 y after initial polypectomy	Colonoscopy	—
Persons with CRC			

Persons undergoing curative resection for CRC	Colonoscopy	Preoperatively or 3–6 mo after surgery in the case of obstructive CRC, then 1 y after surgery (or 1 y after the clearing perioperative colonoscopy)	Persons with CRC should undergo high-quality perioperative clearing of the colon. For nonobstructing tumors, examination can be done preoperatively; for obstructing cancer, CTC can be used to detect proximal neoplasms If the examination at 1 y is normal, perform the next examination at 3 y (ie, 4 y after surgery or perioperative colonoscopy). If that examination is normal, then perform the next examination at 5 y (ie, 9 y after surgery or perioperative colonoscopy), and then at 5-y intervals. Periodic examination of the rectum with FS or EUS (3- to 6-mo intervals for the first 2–3 y) may be considered after resection of rectal cancer in those at high risk for recurrence (in addition to colonoscopy surveillance for metachronous neoplasia)
—		—	
Persons with a Family History of CRC			
CRC or an advanced adenoma in 2 first-degree relatives diagnosed at any age OR colorectal cancer or an advanced adenoma in a single first-degree relative <60 y	Colonoscopy	Age 40 y, or 10 y before the youngest case in the immediate family	For those in whom no significant neoplasia appears by age 60 years, consider offering an expanded interval between colonoscopies

(continued on next page)

Table 2
(continued)

Risk Category	Time or Age to Begin Surveillance	Recommended Test	Comment
CRC or an advanced adenoma in a single first-degree relative ≥ age 60 y	Age 40 y	Screening options at intervals recommended for average-risk persons	Screening should begin at an earlier age, but patients may be screened with any recommended form of testing
Persons at High Risk			
Lynch syndrome	Age 20–25 y or 2–5 y before the youngest case in the immediate family, whichever comes first	Colonoscopy every 1–2 y	For MSH6 mutation carriers, consider a later age of onset for colonoscopy
Family colon cancer syndrome X	Age 10 y before the age of diagnosis of the youngest affected relative	Colonoscopy every 5 y	—
BMMRD syndrome	Age 6 y	Colonoscopy annually	—
IBD (UC and Crohn colitis)	8 y after the onset of pancolitis	Colonoscopy (chromoendoscopy) with targeted biopsies every 1–3 y	Surveillance interval depends on clinical history and colonoscopy findings

Patients with cumulative greater than 20 hyperplastic polyps of any size throughout the colon with at least 5 proximal to the rectum, as well as those with 5 serrated polyps proximal to the rectum greater than 5 mm, with at least two ≥10 mmm meet criteria for serrated polyposis syndrome and may require specialized management.

Abbreviations: BMMRD, biallelic mismatch deficiency syndrome; CTC, CT colonography; FS, flexible sigmoidoscopy; IBD, inflammatory bowel disease; UC, ulcerative colitis.

Data from Rex DK, Boland CR, Dominitz JA et al. Colorectal cancer screening: recommendations for physicians and patients from the U.S. Multi-Society Taskforce on Colorectal Cancer. Gastroenterology 2017;153:307-323; Gupta S, Lieberman DA, Anderson JC et al, Guidelines for colonoscopy surveillance after screening and polypectomy: Recommendations for follow-up after colonoscopy and polypectomy: A consensus update by the US Multi-Society Taskforce on Colorectal Cancer. Gastroenterology 2020; 158:1131-1153; Kahi CJ, Boland CR, Dominitz JA et al. Colonoscopy surveillance after colorectal cancer. Gastroenterology 2016; 150:758-768.

risk of CRC. Many have suggested that changes in diet, alterations in gut microbiota, and increases in obesity may contribute to colorectal carcinogenesis.[19,20] Interestingly, the increase in incidence rates of EoCRC has been driven primarily by increases in rectal (vs colon) cancer. Racial disparities, described in detail later, also exist in EoCRC, with blacks experiencing higher incidence of CRC and worse CRC survival when compared with non-Hispanic whites.[21,22]

Studies have demonstrated that 16% to 20% of individuals diagnosed with EoCRC carry pathogenic germline variants in genes associated with cancer susceptibility.[23] Lynch syndrome and familial adenomatous polyposis are implicated in 3% and 1% of unselected CRC diagnoses overall, with pathogenic germline variants in other cancer susceptibility genes found in an additional 5% to 6%. Importantly, a significant proportion of patients with CRC who carry pathogenic germline variants associated with cancer susceptibility do not meet clinical diagnostic criteria for the corresponding genetic diagnosis, which presents challenges to identifying individuals at increased risk for early onset colorectal neoplasia.

The approach to CRC screening in asymptomatic individuals ideally takes into account risk stratification and the likelihood of developing the disease. Compared with individuals with no family history of CRC, the relative risk of developing CRC when at least one first-degree relative has CRC is 2.24. Among individuals with more than 1 first-degree relative with CRC diagnosed younger than 50 years, the relative risk of CRC is 3.55. Current CRC risk assessment algorithms consider patient's age, family history, and personal history of CRC. However, more than two-thirds of individuals diagnosed with EoCRC report no family history of CRC in first-degree relatives. As noted earlier, the USPSTF, the ACS, and the MSTF have all made qualified recommendations to expansion of CRC screening to individuals aged 45 to 49 years. EoCRCs, however, are also diagnosed in those older than 45 years (especially rectal cancers), and a high index of suspicion is warranted in individuals presenting with a family history of CRC and/or suggestive histories.

Underserved Populations

Adherence to or uptake of CRC screening is especially poor among underserved populations, including those with low income and African American and Hispanic populations.[9–12] CRC incidence and mortality rates are also higher in non-Hispanic blacks compared with non-Hispanic whites, whereas insurance coverage is disproportionately lower. This problem will continue to grow with shifting demographics in the United States. Texas, for example, is a high population state with substantial racial and ethnic diversity. It is home to the second largest population of African Americans in the United States and is projected to be a Hispanic-majority state by 2022. Over the last 4 decades CRC incidence rates for all ages have dropped 33.9% in US whites but only 6.6% in African Americans. Novel strategies to improve screening uptake and deploy best practices to underserved populations is a high priority for health care in the nation. Black Americans have the highest incidence of CRC (45.7 per 100,000), followed by Native Americans (43.3), Whites (38.6), Hispanics (34.1), and Asians (30.0). Racial/ethnic variation in deaths due to CRC show similar patterns.[13] Compared with whites, incidence rates are 24% higher in African American men and 19% higher in African American women.[24] Stage-adjusted CRC mortality is also disproportionately higher in African Americans, with rates being 47% higher in African American men and 34% higher in African American women compared with whites.[25] The reasons for these differences are not entirely clear but disparities in care, such as lower rates of screening, diagnostic follow-up, and treatment are postulated. One study estimates that 19% of the racial disparity in CRC mortality rates can be attributed to lower screening rates and 36% to lower stage-specific survival among African Americans.[26] Access barriers to screening disproportionality affect racial/ethnic, low socioeconomic status, recent immigrants, and uninsured/Medicaid populations, whom all have lower colonoscopy rates compared with white, high socioeconomic status, and private/Medicare groups.[13] Screening rates are lowest among individuals with low education attainment, lack of health insurance, poor access to care, low socioeconomic status, and from racial/ethnicity minority backgrounds. Safety-net populations, similar to those served in community health centers (CHCs), have among the lowest rates of CRC screening.[27] Although results from modeling studies such as CIS-NET do not specifically support different screening strategies by race,[28,29] the MSTF beginning in 2017 recommended initiation of screening in Black adults at age 45 years while starting screening at age 50 years for other races. Current guidelines from the MSTF, USPSTF, and ACS recommend starting screening for everyone at age 45 years, removing this differentiation. Access to colonoscopy is a major barrier to CRC screening, particularly in community settings, including federally qualified health centers and community health centers.[30,31] In CHCs, similar to other settings where screening colonoscopy may not be feasible or easily accessible, stool-based screening (ie, FIT and s-DNA-FIT) has emerged as a common, noninvasive screening strategy.[32–35]

Quality Metrics

As the number of colonoscopies (and endoscopists) have increased, quality-assurance measures have been adopted and are included in the most recent CRC screening guidelines.[5] Quality metrics and standardization included in the Affordable Care Act mandate that the Center for Medicare and Medicaid Services change reimbursement to a value-based system. Adenoma detection rate (ADR) is defined by the percentage of screening colonoscopies of average-risk patients with at least one adenoma and is the most commonly used quality measure in practice. Benchmarks for adequate ADRs set in 2015 by the ASGE suggested ADR requirements of at least 20% for women and 30% for men ($\geq$30% overall),[36] but progressive technical and quality improvements in colonoscopy suggest that a higher bar be set with updated benchmarks. The ADR is considered by the ASGE/ACG Task Force on Quality in Endoscopy and the MSTF to be the best neoplasia-related indicator of quality performance for screening colonoscopy. The ADR has been demonstrated to be an independent predictor of the risk of interval CRC after screening colonoscopy, and increased ADR is associated with reduced risk of CRC-related mortality.[37] The recent qualified recommendations from the USPSTF, ACS, and MSTF to initiate average-risk CRC screening at age 45 years may require age-adjusted ADRs.[38] Increasing knowledge regarding sessile serrated lesions or sessile serrated polyps has led to the suggestion of inclusion of a separate criteria for recognition of these lesions, but this has not yet been universally adopted. A measure of adenomas per colonoscopy (APC) has also been suggested,[39] as it measures the quality of colonoscopy over a complete examination. Performance indicators of other CRC screening modalities such as FIT in organized screening programs have also been suggested.[40] Endoscopist characteristics (volume, polypectomy and completion rate, specialization, and setting) derived from administrative data are correlated with the development of postcolonoscopy CRC and have potential use as quality indicators. Other quality measures include quality of bowel preparation and completeness of polyp resection. The MSTF recommended in 2014 that at least 85% of outpatient colonoscopies should have adequate bowel preparation, but increasing standardization and quantitative clinical grading scales such as the Boston Bowel Preparation Scale may lead to improvements in practice.

The incomplete resection rate in the Complete Adenoma Resection study was 10.1% overall and varied broadly among endoscopists.[41] A physician performance measurement set for endoscopy and surveillance has been proposed in a joint document by the ASGE, the AGA, the Physician Consortium for Performance Improvement, and the National Committee for Quality Assurance. Quality measures also have been stressed by European quality control programs.

New Screening Tests and Technology

One-third of guideline eligible individuals in the United States do not access CRC screening as recommended. In addition, the paradigm for CRC screening worldwide outside the United States is often a 2-step process whereby an initial positive screening test then triggers colonoscopy as a diagnostic test (see **Fig. 2**). Although this is especially important in resource-limited countries, it is also the model in many countries with organized CRC screening programs such as the United Kingdom, Canada, Australia, Denmark, the Netherlands, and many other countries in Europe and Asia. As a result, development of, and clinical interest in noninvasive screening tests for CRC using "biomarkers" has been high, including various forms of stool- and blood-based tests.[42] Patient-friendly approaches that improve patient uptake are needed to achieve the CRC screening goal of high compliance but must also demonstrate high performance characteristics (sensitivity and specificity) for detection of early stage cancer and high-risk precursor lesions and must have broad acceptability to the general population, health care providers, regulatory agencies, and third-party payers. Consistent with this goal, adoption of cost-effective noninvasive methodologies designed to improve overall acceptance of the screening process are highly desirable.

Stool-based tests such as fecal immunochemical tests and the multitarget FIT-DNA test (commercially Cologuard, Exact Sciences, Madison, WI) are relatively sensitive and specific for the detection of CRC (up to 90%) but less so for advanced adenomas (28% for FIT and 40% for FIT-DNA in one pivotal trial).[43,44] Successful use of these tests highly depends on compliance. FIT is the most commonly used noninvasive stool test world-wide and is often the first step in 2-step population-based screening; this is to some extent due to its relatively low cost per test. Threshold for test positivity and test performance over multiple rounds of screening is important in evaluating overall performance in these population-based screening programs.[45] FIT is currently recommended as a first-tier test by the MSTF and is the comparator for many studies aimed at validating other noninvasive markers. Single-application FIT tests have moderate-to-high sensitivity for detecting CRC, depending on the threshold for positivity used, but sensitivity for advanced adenomas is low.

A molecular approach to CRC screening is attractive because it targets biological changes that are fundamental to the neoplastic process. The feasibility of detecting altered DNA in stool has been demonstrated using a multitarget assay panel of molecular markers. The multitargeted stool FIT-DNA test (Cologuard, Exact Sciences) is approved by Food and Drug Administration (FDA) and Centers for Medicare and Medicaid Services (CMS) as a CRC screening test and is included as part of USMSTF guidelines (every 3 years; tier 2 recommendation). The false-positive rate for CRC approaches 14%, however, and a second-generation test is currently under evaluation.

Serum or plasma markers have been considered an important "next step" for the successful implementation of population-based screening for colorectal neoplasia,[42] but blood-based markers have, to date, proved inadequate for this purpose. Although any screening test must demonstrate high positive and negative predictive values in clinically relevant settings, blood-based markers are attractive in several ways.

Specimens are easy to sample and control for reproducibility, can be combined to enhance performance, and should lead to high-compliance, cost-effective tests. Blood-based biomarkers also have good potential for use in low-compliance or underserved populations and in some cases may lead to easily administered point-of-care tests. Blood tests are also noninvasive compared with colonoscopy and are likely to prove more socially acceptable compared with stool-based tests. An integrated signal in blood should make it possible to detect both proximal (right-sided) and distal lesions. Noninvasive tests have proved useful in individuals refusing other forms of screening and may be valuable as reflex tests following inadequate colonoscopy. Although existence of an acceptable blood-based biomarker would of course not result in 100% compliance by screen-eligible individuals, the target of unscreened individuals is substantial.

A large number of blood-based markers have been proposed for early detection of colorectal neoplasia, but few have been evaluated in adequately powered prospective screening trials. An assay for methylated Septin 9 (Epi proColon, Epigenomics AG, Berlin, Germany) is commercially available and FDA approved for individuals refusing other screening tests but is not guideline recommended, nor reimbursed by the CMS due to limited performance in detecting early stage lesions. Several promising blood-based marker assays are on the horizon, either as CRC limited tests or as multicancer detection tests. Many are based on measurement of aberrantly methylated circulating DNA, and the term "liquid biopsy" is often used to describe the use of circulating cell-free DNA to detect neoplasia. "Multi-omics" tests that include panels of both circulating DNA and protein markers are also being evaluated. CMS has recently introduced metrics for coverage of blood-based biomarker tests for average-risk individuals, which include FDA marker authorization, proven test performance of sensitivity for detecting CRC equal to 74% and specificity greater than 90%, and inclusion as a recommended routine CRC screening test in at least one professional society guideline or consensus statement or recommendation by the USPSTF.[46]

Deep learning systems with real-time computer-aided polyp detection have been recently introduced as a means of increasing adenoma detection rates. Incorporation of artificial intelligence during colonoscopy as an aid for detection of neoplastic lesions resulted in increases in ADR and APC in recent studies,[47] especially in the hands of less experienced examiners.[48] Such systems are now commercially available, but at the moment do not differentiate polyp histology.

Knowledge Gaps and a Roadmap for Future Colorectal Cancer Screening

An expert consensus conference held by the AGA recently suggested that a once-size-fits-all approach to CRC screening was unlikely to result in increased screening uptake or desired outcomes and that overcoming the multiple barriers to screening will require efficient use of multiple screening modalities, continued development of noninvasive screening tests, and improved personal risk assessment to best risk-stratify patients. Furthermore, organized screening programs will ultimately be needed to achieve target screening rates and reductions in CRC morbidity and mortality.[49]

Knowledge gaps will ultimately need to be provided by research aimed at understanding what affects uptake and adherence to individual screening tests, improved risk-stratification, performance of screening tests not simply at one point in time but in programmatic screening, factors that affect incidence and mortality in underserved populations, and screening approaches to young-onset CRC. Acceptable approaches that allow new screening tests to proceed from discovery to clinical practice at an accelerated pace will need to be determined, including whether it is necessary to directly compare the effectiveness of new tests in head-to-head randomized trials.

CLINICS CARE POINTS

- Colorectal cancer screening reduces cancer-related mortality.
- Quality metrics are key to improving outcomes of colorectal cancer screening and reducing the occurrence of interval cancers.
- Uptake and adherence to colorectal cancer screening guidelines are key to reducing colorectal cancer mortality, especially in underserved populations.

FUNDING

The work was supported in part by grants from the National Cancer Institute (U01CA086400) and the National Institutes of Health (NIH P30DK056338, the Texas Medical Center Digestive Disease Center).

DISCLOSURE

The author has nothing to disclose.

REFERENCES

1. Siegel RL, Miller KD, Fuchs HE, et al. Cancer Statistics, 2022. CA Cancer J Clin 2022;72:7–33.
2. Siegel R, Fedewa SA, Anderson WF, et al. Colorectal cancer incidence patterns in the United States, 1974-2013. J Natl Cancer Instit 2017;109:1–6.
3. Cronin KA, Lake AJ, Scott S, et al. Annual report to the nation on the status of cancer, Part I: National statistics. Cancer 2018;124:785–800.
4. Arahgi M, Soerjomataram I, Jenkine M, et al. Global trends in colorectal cancer mortality: projections to the year 2035. J Cancer 2019;144:2992–3000.
5. Rex DK, Boland CR, Dominitz JA, et al. Colorectal cancer screening: recommendations for physicians and patients from the U.S. Multi-society task force on colorectal cancer. Gastroenterology 2017;53:307–23.
6. Patel SG, May FP, Anderson JC, et al. Update on age to start and stop colorectal cancer screening: recommendations from the US Multi-Society Task Force on Colorectal Cancer. Gastroenterology 2022;162:285–9.
7. US Preventive Services Task Force. Screening for colorectal cancer. US Preventive Services Task Force recommendations statement. JAMA 2022;325:1965–77.
8. Wolf A, Fontham ETH, Church TR, et al. Colorectal cancer screening for average-risk adults: 2018 guideline update from the American Cancer Society. CA Cancer J Clin 2018;68:250–81.
9. Araghi M, Fidler MM, Arnold M, et al. The future burden of colorectal cancer among US blacks and whites. J Natl Cancer Instit 2018;110:791–3.
10. Carethers JM. Screening for colorectal cancer in African Americans: Determinants and rationale for an earlier age to commence screening. Dig Dis Sci 2015;60:711–21.
11. Sineshaw HM, Ng K, Flanders WD, et al. Factors that contribute to differences in survival of black vs white patients with colorectal cancer. Gastroenterology 2018; 154:906–15.
12. Fedewa SA, Flanders WD, Ward KC, et al. Racial and ethnic disparities in interval colorectal cancer incidence. A population-based cohort study. Ann Intern Med 2017;166:857–66.

13. Murphy CC, Singal AG, Baron JA, et al. Decrease in incidence of young-onset colorectal cancer before recent increase. Gastroenterology 2018;155:1716–9.
14. Miller KD, Ortiz AP, Pinheiro PS, et al. Cancer statistics for US Hispanic/Latino population, 2021. CA Cancer J Clin 2021;71:466–87.
15. Senore C, Basu P, Anttila A, et al. Performance of coloretcal cancer screening in the European Union member stes:dta from the second European screning report. Gut 2019;68:1232–44.
16. Sung JJ, Ng SC, Chan FKL, et al. An ipdated Asia Pacific Consensus Tecommendations on colorectal cancer screening. Gut 2015;64:121–32.
17. Shaukat A, Kahi C, Burke C, et al. ACG Clinical Guidelines: Colorectal Cancer Screening 2021. Am J Gastroenterol 2021;116:458–79.
18. Rabeneck L, Chiu H-M, Senore C. International perspective on the burden of colorectal cancer and public health effects. Gastroenterology 2020;158:447–52.
19. Song M, Chan AT. Environmental Factors, Gut Microbiota, and Colorectal Cancer Prevention. Clin Gastroenterol Hepatol 2019;275–89.
20. Song M, Chan AT. Diet, Gut Microbiota, and Colorectal Cancer Prevention: A Review of Potential Mechanisms and Promising Targets for Future Research. Curr Colorectal Cancer Rep 2017;13:429–39.
21. Murphy CC, Wallace K, Sandler RS, et al. Racial Disparities in Incidence of Young-Onset Colorectal Cancer and Patient Survival. Gastroenterology 2018;155(6):1716–9.
22. Murphy CC, Sanoff HK, Stitzenberg KB, et al. Patterns of Sociodemographic and Clinicopathologic Characteristics of Stages II and III Colorectal Cancer Patients by Age: Examining Potential Mechanisms of Young-Onset Disease. J Cancer Epidemiol 2017;2017:4024580.
23. Stoffel E, Koeppe E, Everett J, et al. Germline genetic features of younf individuals with colorectal cancer. Gastroenterology 2018;154:897–905.
24. American Cancer Society. Cancer Facts and Figures for African Americans 2019–2021, vol. 2019. Atlanta (GA): American Cancer Society; 2019. Available at: https://www.cancer.org/content/dam/cancer-org/research/cancer-facts-and-statistics/cancer-facts-and-figures-for-african-americans/cancer-facts-and-figures-for-african-americans-2019-2021.pdf.
25. Centers for Disease Control and Prevention (CDC). Vital signs: Colorectal cancer screening, incidence, and mortality—United States, 2002–2010. MMWR Morb Mortal Wkly Rep 2011;60:884–9.
26. Lansdorp-Vogelaar I, Kuntz KM, Knudsen AB, et al. Contribution of screening and survival differences to racial disparities in colorectal cancer rates. Cancer Epidemiol Biomarkers Prev 2012;21:728–36.
27. Gupta S, Tong L, Allison JE, et al. Screening for colorectal cancer in a safety-net health care system: access to care is critical and has implications for screening policy. Cancer Epidemiol Biomarkers Prev 2009;18:2373–9.
28. Knudsen AB, Rutter CM, Peterse EFP, et al. A decision analysis for the US Preventive Services Taskforce. Agency foe Healthcare Research and Quality; 2021. AHRQ publication 20-05271-EF-2.
29. Knudesen AB, Rutter CM, Peterse EFP, et al. Colorectal cancer screening:a collaborative modeling study for the US preventive Services Taskforce. JAMA 2021;325(19):1998–2011.
30. Inadomi JM, Vijan S, Janz NK, et al. Adherence to colorectal cancer screening: a randomized clinical trial of competing strategies. Arch Intern Med 2012;172(7):575–82.

31. Montminy EM, Karlitz JJ, Landreneau SW. Progress of colorectal cancer screening in United States: Past achievements and future challenges. Prev Med 2019;120:78–84.
32. Lee JK, Liles EG, Bent S, et al. Accuracy of fecal immunochemical tests for colorectal cancer: systematic review and meta-analysis. Ann Intern Med 2014;160:171.
33. Zorzi M, Fedeli U, Schievano E, et al. Impact on colorectal cancer mortality of screening programmes based on the faecal immunochemical test. Gut 2015; 64:784–90.
34. Chiu HM, Chen SL, Yen AM, et al. Effectiveness of fecal immunochemical testing in reducing colorectal cancer mortality from the One Million Taiwanese Screening Program. Cancer 2015;121(18):3221–9.
35. Chiang TH, Chuang SL, Chen SL, et al. Difference in performance of fecal immunochemical tests with the same hemoglobin cutoff concentration in a nationwide colorectal cancer screening program. Gastroenterology 2014;147:1317–26.
36. Rex DK, Scheonfeld PS, Cohen J, et al. Quality indicators for colonoscopy. Gastrointest Endosc 2015;81:31–53.
37. Kaminski MF, Wieszczy P, Rupinki P, et al. Increased adenoma detection associates with reduced risk of colorectal cancer death. Gastroenterology 2017;153:98–105.
38. Crockett SD, Lauderbaum U. Potential effects of lowering colorectal cancer screening age to 45 years on colonoscopy demand, case mix, and adenoma detection rate. Gastroenterology 2022;162:984–6.
39. Kaminski MF, Robertson DJ, Senore C, et al. Optimizing the quality of colorectal screening world-wide. Gastroenterology 2020;158:404–17.
40. Ding H, Lin J, Xu Z, et al. A global evaluation of the performance indicators of colorectal cancer screening with fecal immunochemical tets and colonoscopy: A systematic review and meta-analysis. Cancers 2022;14:1073.
41. Pohl H, Srivastava A, Nenson SP, et al. Incomplete polyp resection during colonoscopy—Results of the Complete Adenoma Resection (CARE) study. Gastroenterology 2013;144:74–80.
42. Bresalier RS, Grady WM, Markowitz SD, et al. Biomarkers for early detection of colorectal cancer: The Early Detection Research Network, a framework for clinical translation. Cancer Epidemiol Biomarkers Prev 2020;29:2431–40.
43. Imperiale TF, Gruber RN, Stump TE, et al. Performance characteristics of fecal immunochemical tests for colorectal cancer and advanced adenomatous polyps. A systematic review and meta-analysis. Ann Intern Med 2019;170:319–29.
44. Impariale TF, Ransohoff DF, Itzkowitz SH, et al. Multitarget stool DNA testing for colorctal-cancer screening. N Engl J Med 2014;370:1287–97.
45. Kooyker AI, Toes-Zoutendijk E, Opstal-van Winden AWJ, et al. The second round of the Dutch colorectal cancer screening program: Impact of an increased fecal immunochemical test cut-off on yield of screening. Int J Cancer 2020;147:1098–106.
46. Centers for Medicare and Medicaid Services. Screening for Colorectal Cancer - Blood-Based Biomarker Tests. CAG-00454N. 2021. Available at: www.CMS.gov.
47. Repici A, Spadaccini M, Antonelli G, et al. Artificial intelligence and colonoscopy experience:lesons from tworandomised trials. Gut 2022;71:757–65.
48. Cesare Hassan M, Spadaccini M, Iannone A, et al. Performance of artificial intelligence in colonoscopy for adenoma and polyp detection: a systematic review and meta-analysis. Gastrointest Endosc 2021;93:77–85.
49. Melson JE, Imperiale TF, Itzkowitz SH, et al. AGA white paper: Roadmap for the future of colorectal cancer screening in the United States. Clin Gastroenterol Hepatol 2020;18:2667–78.

Approach to Familial Predisposition to Colorectal Cancer

Veroushka Ballester, MD, MSc[a,b], Marcia Cruz-Correa, MD, PhD[a,b],*

KEYWORDS

- Colorectal cancer • Familial colorectal cancer
- Hereditary colorectal cancer syndromes • Polyposis syndromes
- Nonpolyposis syndromes • Lynch syndrome • Familial adenomatous polyposis

KEY POINTS

- Approximately 20% to 30% of patients with colorectal cancer have a potentially definable inherited cause.
- Our understanding of familial predisposition to colorectal cancer and colorectal cancer syndromes has significantly increased due to advances in next-generation sequencing technologies.
- A personalized approach to colorectal cancer prevention requires appropriate assessment of familial and genetic risk of colorectal cancer development.

INTRODUCTION

Approximately 20% to 30% of patients with colorectal cancer (CRC) have a potentially definable inherited cause. Most families with a history of CRC and/or adenomas do not carry genetic variants associated with cancer syndromes; this is called common familial CRC. Individuals with a family history of CRC are at increased risk for developing CRC; the magnitude of risk depends on the number of relatives with CRC, whether the relatives are first-degree relatives (FDR) versus second-degree relatives, and the age at which their relatives were diagnosed with CRC. Studies have reported an estimated 2-fold increase in risk of CRC in individuals with 1 or more FDR with CRC compared with individuals without a family history.[1–5] Furthermore, the age of CRC diagnosis in a relative affects the risk of CRC. A systematic review found that in

[a] University of Puerto Rico Comprehensive Cancer Center, PMB 711 89 De Diego, De Diego Avenue 105, Rio Piedras, PR 00927-6346, USA; [b] Department of Medicine, Biochemistry and Surgery, University of Puerto Rico Medical Sciences Campus, PO BOX 365067, San Juan, PR 00936, USA
* Corresponding author. University of Puerto Rico Comprehensive Cancer Center, PMB 711 89 De Diego, De Diego Avenue 105, Rio Piedras, PR 00927-6346.
E-mail address: marcia.cruz1@upr.edu

Gastroenterol Clin N Am 51 (2022) 593–607
https://doi.org/10.1016/j.gtc.2022.06.001
0889-8553/22/© 2022 Elsevier Inc. All rights reserved.

persons with an FDR who were diagnosed with CRC at an age of 50 years or younger, the relative risk of CRC was 3.55 (95% confidence interval [CI], 1.84–6.83) compared with 2.18 (95% CI, 1.56–3.04) for individuals with an FDR who were diagnosed with CRC at an age older than 50 years.[1]

Approximately 3% to 5% of CRCs are associated with hereditary cancer syndromes. Our understanding of familial predisposition to CRC and inherited CRC syndromes has significantly improved due to advances in next-generation sequencing technology, which has led to more effective identification of individuals with germline pathogenic variants and tailored management for the proband and at-risk family members to effectively decrease CRC incidence and mortality. Hereditary CRC syndromes are a group of conditions that are associated with an increased lifetime risk of colorectal adenocarcinoma and extraintestinal malignancies. There are several hereditary CRC syndromes, assigned to categories of polyposis or nonpolyposis syndromes. Criteria to be considered in differentiating the various hereditary cancer syndromes include polyp distribution throughout the gastrointestinal (GI) tract, polyp number, the presence of extraintestinal manifestations or malignancy, and family history. Identification of relevant causative genes has improved our understanding of specific hereditary cancer syndromes including phenotypic characteristics and associated cancer risks.

Nonpolyposis Colorectal Cancer Syndromes

Lynch syndrome

Lynch syndrome is the most common CRC syndrome, accounting for approximately 3% of all newly diagnosed CRC cases.[6,7] In addition, it accounts for nearly 10% of CRC diagnosed at the age of 50 years. Lynch syndrome is an autosomal dominant disorder caused by germline pathogenic variants in the mismatch repair (MMR) genes *MLH1, MSH2, MSH6*, or *PMS2*, as well as the *EPCAM* gene, in which deletions in *EPCAM* cause epigenetic silencing of *MSH2*. Although CRC is the most common cancer, Lynch syndrome is also associated with a predisposition for developing extracolonic cancers, including cancers of the endometrium, ovaries, stomach, small intestine, hepatobiliary system, pancreas, and brain, as well as transitional cell carcinoma of the ureters and renal pelvis.[8] Specific MMR gene alterations are associated with different phenotypes and cancer risks. The risk of CRC associated with pathogenic variants in *MLH1* and *MSH2* ranges from 58% to 82%, with mean age of diagnosis ranging from 44 to 61 years.[9–14] A weaker phenotype is associated with pathogenic variants in the more prevalent genes, *MSH6* and *PMS2*, with CRC risks of 10% to 22% with mean age of 55 to 66 years.[9,10,12,14–17] Pathogenic variants in *MSH6* and *PMS2* might be more commonly detected in individuals with CRC (regardless of age at diagnosis, family history, or results of tumor testing), than *MLH1* and *MSH2* variants, which are more commonly identified in individuals at high risk for CRC. In an international population–based study of 5744 CRC cases, the pathogenic variant in *MLH1* was estimated to occur in 1 in every 1946 persons with CRC, pathogenic variants in *PMS2* were estimated to be 1 in 714, and 1 in 758 for those with pathogenic variants in *MSH6*.[18]

Diagnosis

The genetics of both the tumor and the germline have an important role in the diagnosis of Lynch syndrome. Approximately 90% of colorectal and extraintestinal tumors from patients with Lynch syndrome exhibit microsatellite instability (MSI). In addition, most of the Lynch syndrome tumors exhibit a unique histopathology characterized by the absence of expression of one of the MMR proteins on immunohistochemistry

(IHC)[19–23]; therefore, tumor testing is a key component in the diagnosis of Lynch syndrome, in addition to family history. Universal tumor testing of all individuals with newly diagnosed CRCs at the the age of 70 years or younger for MMR deficiency is a recommended strategy to screen for Lynch syndrome, in order to identify those individuals who will need germline genetic testing. If there is no tissue available for MSI or IHC testing, it is reasonable to begin with germline genetic testing in a patient with cancer.

Several computer-based clinical prediction models based on personal and family history have been developed as alternative modalities to provide systematic genetic risk assessment for Lynch syndrome. These risk models include the prediction of MMR gene mutations (PREMM),[24–26] MMRPredict,[27] and MMRpro.[28] The PREMM model has been most extensively validated and has been updated to include all 5 genes associated with Lynch syndrome (PREMM5 model).[25]

Screening and management

Intensive cancer screening and surveillance strategies, including frequent colonoscopy and risk-reducing surgeries for the prevention of endometrial and ovarian cancer, are mainstays in the clinical management of individuals with Lynch syndrome. Surveillance of other organs, such as small intestine, pancreatic and biliary systems, or brain, is not supported by evidence although recommendations by expert consensus panels may vary.

The Colorectal Adenoma/Carcinoma Prevention Programme (CAPP2) was a double-blind, placebo-controlled, randomized trial to determine the role of aspirin in preventing CRC in patients with Lynch syndrome.[29] Results from this study supported the use of aspirin for prevention of CRC in Lynch syndrome without significant differences in adverse events between the aspirin and placebo groups. However, experts believe the evidence is not sufficiently robust to recommend its standard use.[14]

Results from a recent study support the concept of frameshift peptide neoantigen vaccination as a promising strategy for the immunoprevention of intestinal mismatch repair deficiency (MMRD) tumors, particularly for individuals with Lynch syndrome.[30] These results were limited to a mouse model, and clinical effectiveness needs to be demonstrated in clinical trials.

Lynch-like syndrome

Lynch-like syndrome (LLS) relates to MMR-deficient CRC cases that are not caused by germline MMR mutations (or *MLH1* hypermethylation). LLS is observed in 2.5% to 4% of individuals with CRC.[31,32] The incidence of CRC in patients with LLS is increased (standard incidence ratio, 2.12; 95% CI, 1.16–3.56) compared with patients with colorectal tumors that have not lost MMR proteins (0.48; 95% CI, 0.27–0.79).[31] These individuals have a lower incidence of cancer in their families than patients with Lynch syndrome and have low rates of synchronous and metachronous CRC. The implications of this recently identified colorectal tumor phenotype on screening and surveillance recommendations are unclear. Recommendations for CRC screening are based on family history of CRC.[33]

Familial colorectal cancer type X

Familial CRC type X refers to individuals suspected of having Lynch syndrome based on family history of CRC (Amsterdam criteria: 3 relatives in 2 generations) and young-onset CRC diagnosed before the age of 50 years but do not carry pathogenic MMR gene variants and whose colorectal tumors are MMR proficient.[34] The risk of CRC in patients with familial CRC syndrome X is estimated to be twice that of the general population (standard incidence ratio, 2.3, 95% CI, 1.7–3.0) and modest compared with Lynch syndrome with defects in MMR (standard incidence ratio, 6.1, 95% CI, 5.7–7.2).

CRC surveillance recommendations are similar to those with family history of CRC with colonoscopy every 5 years.

Polymerase proofreading–associated polyposis

Polymerase proofreading–associated polyposis (PPAP) is an autosomal dominant disorder associated with pathogenic variants in the DNA polymerase epsilon, catalytic subunit gene (POLE) and DNA polymerase delta 1, catalytic subunit gene (POLD1) that cause an oligo-polyposis phenotype, in which polyps are often fewer than those in patients with familial adenomatous polyposis (FAP).[35] PPAP is rare, only 0.12% to 0.25% of patients suspected of having FAP or familial CRC are found to have PPAP. Although the precise risk and mean age of CRC development are still not clear, a study found patients with mutations in POLE to have a 28% risk and patients with POLD1 mutations to have an 82% to 90% risk of CRC by age 70 years. The spectrum of cancer increases with age and includes, but is not limited to, endometrial, ovarian, small bowel, and central nervous system.[36–38]

The AXIN2 gene regulates degradation of beta-catenin in the Wnt pathway. Pathogenic variants in AXIN2 have been associated with autosomal-dominant colorectal adenomatous polyposis. The phenotype seems similar to attenuated FAP. Tooth agenesis is related to pathogenic variants in this gene and possibly breast and liver cancer.

Polyposis Syndromes

Familial adenomatous polyposis

FAP is one of the most clearly defined polyposis syndromes and is estimated to occur in one of 10,000 births. FAP is caused by pathogenic variants in the APC gene, on chromosome 5q21, with nearly complete penetrance.[39] Up to 25% to 30% of new FAP cases are de novo, without any known clinical or genetic evidence of FAP in the family.[40] Individuals with classic FAP develop hundreds to thousands of colonic adenomatous polyps at young ages, usually in the mid- to late teens and early 20s.[41] CRC risk approaches 100% by age 50 years without intervention, which involves prophylactic colectomy in young adulthood or when polyp burden becomes too high to be managed endoscopically. Without treatment, 7% of patients with FAP have CRC by age 21 years, 50% by age 39 years, and 90% by age 50 years.

The FAP mutation spectrum has been studied in a limited number of Hispanic countries. Most mutations identified in Hispanic patients from both Latin America, Portugal, and Spain have been in exon 15 of the APC gene.[42] This exon comprises more than 75% of the coding sequence and is the most commonly mutated region of the APC gene.[43]

Clinical manifestations

In addition to a high risk of colon adenomas in patients with FAP, various extracolonic manifestations have also been described, including upper GI tract adenomas and adenocarcinomas. Fundic gland polyps occur in 50% or more of persons with FAP but gastric cancer is uncommon, occurring in about 1% of patients. Duodenal adenomas are found in up to 90% of patients with FAP, and cancer risk increases with age, reaching 10%. In addition, there is a 0.5% to 2.0% risk of cancers of the thyroid, pancreas, brain, and liver in the first decade of life. Benign growths are also a common feature of FAP; there is a 20% to 30% incidence of osteoma and epidermoid cysts and a smaller incidence of pilomatricomas, supernumerary teeth, and odontomas. Congenital hypertrophy of the retinal pigment epithelium is common and relates to the location of mutation in the APC gene. Desmoid tumors occur in 20% to 30% of patients with FAP and although benign, are associated with significant morbidity and mortality.

A low-penetrance *APC* variant, I1307K is found in approximately 7% of Ashkenazi Jews and is associated with a 2-fold increase in CRC risk without colonic polyposis.[44–46] There is little difference in the clinical presentation of individuals with sporadic CRC and those with the *APC* I1307K variant. It is not clear whether risk of CRC is further affected by family history of CRC in individuals with this mutation. Based on available data, it is unclear whether the I1307K carrier state should guide decisions regarding age to initiate screening or the frequency of screening.

Management

Management of FAP involves intensive endoscopic surveillance and appropriately timed colectomy. Patients with attenuated FAP (AFAP) can delay initiation of endoscopy for several years, with intensive surveillance intervals based on polyp burden.

Currently, there are no Food and Drug Administration–approved drugs for chemoprevention in FAP. Celecoxib, a specific cyclooxygenase 2 (COX-2) inhibitor, and sulindac, a nonspecific COX-2 inhibitor, have been associated with a decrease in polyp size and number in patients with FAP, suggesting a potential role as chemopreventive agents.[47,48] However, some issues regarding the use of COX-2 inhibitors for the treatment of colonic and duodenal polyps in patients with FAP include partial elimination of polyps, complications from COX-2 inhibitors including cardiac-related events, and loss of effect after the medication is discontinued.[49] A study that evaluated the efficacy of the combination of nonprescription supplements curcumin and quercetin to regress adenomas in patients with FAP found that the combination seems to reduce the number and size of ileal and rectal adenomas without appreciable toxicity. Randomized controlled trials are needed to validate these findings.[50] Additional chemoprevention strategies are currently under study.[51]

Attenuated familial adenomatous polyposis

AFAP is a less severe form of FAP associated with particular *APC* pathogenic variants, including pathogenic variants at the 5' end of the *APC* gene and exon 4 in which patients can present with 2 to more than 500 adenomas, pathogenic variants at the 3' region in which patients have less than 50 adenomas, and exon 9–associated phenotypes in which patients may have 1 to 150 adenomas without upper GI manifestations.[52,53] Patients with AFAP have fewer colonic adenomas than those with classic FAP and are predominantly located in the proximal colon. The emergence of adenomas is believed to occur to patients in their mid- to late 20s.[54] The average age at diagnosis is greater than in classic FAP, at age 56 years.[52,55,56] Patients with attenuated FAP may present with extracolonic manifestations including gastric and duodenal adenomas; however, these occur less often than in patients with classic FAP. AFAP may be challenging to diagnose without genetic testing. *APC* testing is pivotal in the evaluation of these patients, as the differential diagnosis is broad and includes *MUTYH,* Lynch syndrome, biallelic mismatch repair deficiency, and polymerase proofreading–associated polyposis (*POLD1* and *POLE*).

Autosomal Recessive Polyposis Syndromes

MUTYH-associated polyposis

MUTYH-associated polyposis (MAP) is an autosomal recessive attenuated polyposis syndrome caused by biallelic germline variants in *MUTYH,* a gene involved in DNA oxidative damage repair. The phenotype of MAP is similar to that of AFAP. Individuals with MAP can develop duodenal adenomas and cancer, as well as sebaceous gland carcinomas and benign extraintestinal findings similar to patients with FAP. Biallelic *MUTYH* pathogenic variants are found in 7% (95% CI, 6%–8%) of patients with 20 to 99 adenomas and 7% (95% CI, 6%–8%) of patients with 100 to 999 adenomas.[57]

Although the predominant polyp type is adenoma, serrated adenomas and hyperplastic polyps may also be seen in patients with MAP. Full gene sequencing of *MUTYH* is recommended in individuals with polyposis without a pathogenic variant in the *APC* gene. Specific mutations in the *MUTYH* gene that give rise to polyposis vary among individuals from different countries. In Caucasians of northern European descent, 2 variants, Y179C and G396D, account for 70% of biallelic pathogenic variants in patients with MAP.[58] CRC associated with MAP is predominantly right sided, may present with synchronous lesions at presentation, and have a better prognosis compared with sporadic CRC.[59] Recommendations for colonic surveillance range between yearly to every 3 years beginning at age 18 to 30 years.[60,61] If polyp burden cannot be managed endoscopically or if there is evidence of advanced histology, total colectomy with ileorectal anastomosis or subtotal colectomy should be considered depending on polyp burden.

Monoallelic pathogenic variants in *MUTYH* are detected in up to 2% of the general population. Monoallelic *MUTYH* pathogenic variants do not have much effect on CRC risk (odds ratio 1.15;95% CI, 0.98–1.36) in the absence of family history of CRC.[62] The risk of CRC in monoallelic *MUTYH* carriers with a family history of CRC is approximately 2-fold compared with the general population.[17] Similar to individuals with family history of an FDR with CRC diagnosed before the age of 50 years, MUTYH heterozygotes with an FDR with CRC warrant more intensive surveillance compared with the general population.[17,63]

Constitutional mismatch repair deficiency syndrome

Constitutional mismatch repair deficiency syndrome (CMMRDS) is a rare autosomal recessive polyposis syndrome caused by homozygous pathogenic variants in MMR genes associated with Lynch syndrome.[64] PMS2 gene is markedly overrepresented in cases of CMMRD. This syndrome is characterized by early childhood onset of malignancies (hematologic, brain, small bowel, colorectal, ureter, bone/soft tissues) and features of neurofibromatosis *NF1,* most notably café-au-lait macules.[65] GI manifestations include colonic polyposis, predominantly adenomas, and CRC, which typically presents before the age of 20 years.[64] The likelihood of CMMRD involving homozygous MMR gene pathogenic variants is higher among consanguineous unions. No consensus has been reached regarding surveillance guidelines for CMMRDS. Annual colonoscopy, esophagogastroduodenoscopy (EGD), and capsule endoscopy starting in the first decade of life is recommended by the International Biallelic MMR Deficiency (BMMRD) Consortium and the European Consortium for the Care of CMMRD.[66,67]

NTHL1

The *NTHL1* gene is associated with an autosomal recessive adenomatous polyposis phenotype with an increased risk of CRC. Carriers of biallelic germline *NTHL1* pathogenic variants have extracolonic malignancies, including breast and endometrial cancer.[68] Currently, there is no known risk of cancer for individuals with a single monoallelic germline pathogenic variant in *NTHL1*. Cumulative cancer risk is uncertain, and there is minimal data on optimal surveillance approach.

Other Polyposis Syndromes

Hereditary mixed polyposis syndrome

Hereditary mixed polyposis syndrome (HMPS) is a rare syndrome caused by pathogenic variants in the *GREM1* gene, a bone morphogenetic protein antagonist. This syndrome has been associated with *GREM1* pathogenic variants among Ashkenazi Jews. The phenotype of HMPS is characterized by oligopolyposis, which includes a variety of histology including adenomas, serrated adenomas, atypical juvenile polyps, and hyperplastic polyps. It is also characterized by early onset CRC. There is high degree of variability in polyp number, histology, and age of onset. Extracolonic malignancies have been described in a small number of carriers.

Serrated polyposis syndrome

Serrated polyposis syndrome (SPS), previously referred to as hyperplastic polyposis syndrome, is characterized by a predisposition to sessile serrated polyps. SPS is diagnosed based on clinical criteria, as the genetic cause remains elusive. Rarely, families with SPS can be identified to harbor a germline pathogenic variant in the *RNF43* gene.[69,70] The World Health Organization diagnostic criteria for SPS include any one of the following[1]: at least 5 serrated polyps proximal to the sigmoid colon with 2 or more of them larger than 10 mm in diameter[2]; any number of serrated polyps proximal to the sigmoid colon in an individual who has an FDR with SPS; or[3] more than 20 serrated polyps of any size distributed throughout the colon. Approximately half of the SPS cases have a positive family history of CRC.[71] The prevalence of CRC in patients who meet criteria for SPS is 50% or more.[71] Very limited data exist as to whether extracolonic polyps or cancers are associated with SPS. Management includes colonoscopy with polypectomy. Removal of all polyps is preferred but not always feasible. Colonoscopy should be repeated every 1 to 3 years, depending on the number, size, and histology of polyps. Subtotal colectomy with ileorectal anastomosis should be considered if polyposis cannot be controlled endoscopically or if there is evidence of histologically advanced polyps or colon cancer. Data do not support extracolonic cancer screening at this time. The National Comprehensive Cancer Network recommends that FDR should have colonoscopy at the earliest of the following[1]: age 40 years[2]; same age as the youngest SPS diagnosis in the family[3]; 10 years before CRC in the family in a patient with SPS.[60] Further work is ongoing to better define the cancer risks in probands and their relatives so that more accurate risk stratification and screening recommendations can be made.

Hamartomatous Polyposis Syndromes

Peutz-Jeghers syndrome

Peutz-Jeghers syndrome (PJS) is an autosomal dominantly inherited syndrome caused by pathogenic variants in the *STK11/LKB1* gene. Patient's with this syndrome develop histologically distinctive hamartomatous polyps of the GI tract and characteristic melanocytic macules on the lips, perioral region, and buccal region.[72,73] A high risk for GI and non-GI cancers is integral to this condition, including malignancies in the colon, stomach, pancreas, breast, and ovary. More than half of PJS cases have colon polyps, and the risk for CRC is 39% at a mean age of 46 years.[40] The cumulative risks for breast cancer is estimated to be 32% to 54% and 21% for ovarian cancer.[74] For pancreatic cancer, the risk has been estimated to be more than 100-fold higher than for the general population.[74]

Diagnosis

Diagnosis is made based on evaluating for the presence of any one of the following: (1) 2 or more histologically confirmed PJS polyps; (2) any number of PJS polyps detected in 1 individual who has a family history of PJS in close relatives; (3) characteristic mucocutaneous pigmentation in an individual who has a family history of PJS in close relatives; (4) any number of PJS polyps in an individual who also has characteristic mucocutaneous pigmentation.[75] In addition to these criteria, genetic testing is a standard part of clinical practice. Surveillance guidelines for PJS are empiric and based on the risk for GI complications and cancer. A consortium review group has recommended EGD and colonoscopy starting at age 8 years.[76]

Management

Treatment involves endoscopic removal of polyps. Colectomy is sometimes necessary if colonic polyp burden cannot be controlled endoscopically or if histology shows neoplastic changes. Intussusception is the primary complication of small bowel polyps, starting at a young age, and continuing throughout life. Surveillance and treatment of the small bowel are based on prevention of this complication. Surveillance for other extraintestinal cancers including breast, pancreas, and ovarian is recommended.

Juvenile polyposis syndrome

Juvenile polyposis syndrome (JPS) is a rare autosomal dominantly inherited condition characterized by hamartomatous polyposis throughout the GI tract, predominantly in the colon with childhood to early adult onset. JPS is caused by germline pathogenic variants in the *SMAD4* gene (also called the *MADH4/DPC4*), in approximately 15% to 60% of cases,[77] and pathogenic variants in the gene encoding bone morphogenic protein receptor 1A, *BMPR1A* in approximately 25% to 40% of cases.[78,79] A clinical diagnosis of JPS is done when individuals fulfill one or more of the following criteria[1]: more than 5 juvenile polyps in the colon or rectum[2]; juvenile polyps in other parts of the GI tract[3]; any number of juvenile polyps in a person with a known family history of juvenile polyps.[80] Colon polyps begin to develop in the first decade of life and if left untreated, CRC incidence approaches 68%, with a mean age of occurrence of 34 years. Colorectal screening consists of colonoscopy starting at age 12 years and is repeated every 1 to 3 years depending on polyp burden.[77] Similarly, upper GI endoscopy should be done every 1 to 3 years beginning at age 12 years or earlier if symptoms present. The small bowel should be examined if duodenal polyposis is present.

Phosphatase and Tensin homology hamartoma tumor syndrome

PTEN hamartoma tumor syndrome includes several autosomal dominant disorders that arise from mutations of the Phosphatase and Tensin homology (*PTEN*) gene. The clinical phenotypes overlap considerably, and the conditions seem to be a spectrum of a single disease. The disorders include Cowden syndrome, Bannayan-Riley-Ruvalcaba syndrome (BRRS), and adult-onset dysplastic gangliocytoma of the cerebellum (Lhermitte–Duclos disease). Approximately 85% of patients diagnosed with Cowden syndrome and approximately 60% of patients with BRRS have a pathogenic variant in the *PTEN* gene.[81] Primary features include multiple hamartomas of the skin, mucous membranes, GI tract, and other organs, as well as an increased risk of cancers of several sites, including CRC risk, which is modestly increased. Polyps of multiple histologic types, including ganglioneuromas, occur throughout the GI tract. Screening and surveillance recommendations are based on expert opinion.

Identifying High-Risk Individuals: Who Is a Candidate for Genetic Evaluation and Testing?

Referral for genetic evaluation for hereditary CRC syndromes is largely underused. Many questions remain regarding the integration of a multigene panel into a screening strategy and eligibility criteria to direct testing with multigene panels. Genetic evaluation is an integral part of the risk assessment process, and referral to genetic specialists is recommended for high-risk individuals. Genetic specialists help to identify the appropriate genetic testing options and educate patients on cancer risks attributed to inherited susceptibility. They also provide tailored screening (**Table 1**) and surveillance recommendations for the proband and at-risk family members based on the interpretation of genetic test results.

Table 1
Recommendations for colorectal cancer screening for individuals with hereditary cancer syndromes

Condition	Gene	Age to Initiate Screening	Screening Interval	Comments
Lynch syndrome	MMR genes: MLH1, MSH2, MSH6, PMS2	20–25 y	1–2 y	—
FAP	APC	10–15 y	1 y	—
AFAP	APC	25–30 y	1–3 y based on polyp burden	—
MAP	Biallelic variants in MUTYH	25–30 y	1–3 y based on polyp burden	—
	Monoallelic variants in MUTYH	40 y	5 y	Based on presence of CRC in family
Juvenile polyposis syndrome	SMAD4 and BMPR1A	15 y	1–3 based on polyp burden	—
PJS	STK11/LKB1	15 y	2–3 y based on polyp burden	—
PTEN hamartomatous tumors or Cowden disease	PTEN	35 y	3–5 y based on polyp burden	—
Polymerase proofreading–associated polyposis	POLE, POLD1	25–30 y	2–3 y; 1–2 y if polyps	—
	AXIN2, GREM1, and biallelic variants in NTHL1	25–30 y	2–3 y; 1–2 y if polyps	—
Familial colorectal cancer type X	Unknown	5–10 y before earliest CRC diagnosis in family	5 y	Defined as 3 relatives with CRC, in 2 generations, 1 diagnosis before age 50 y, with negative results from germline testing for Lynch syndrome; consider germline testing, such as multi-gene panel testing
Family history CRC (≥1 FDR)	None	40 y	5 y	Consider referral for genetic evaluation; evaluate if PREMM5 of 2.5% or more

Data from Refs.[45,60,85]

Box 1
How to identify individuals with a high-risk personal and/or family history of cancer

- Colon cancer diagnosed < 50 years of age
- Multiple colonic malignancies present either synchronous or metachronous
- Multiple primary cancers diagnosed, either colonic or extracolonic
- Over a lifetime, ≥10 adenomas present or ≥2 histologically characteristic hamartomatous polyps
- Colon cancer in more than one generation of the individual's family
- Clustering of extracolonic cancers in family members

To decrease morbidity and mortality, institutions are adopting universal Lynch syndrome colorectal tumor testing, which has been endorsed by the National Comprehensive Cancer Network. This strategy has been shown to maximize sensitivity for identifying individuals with Lynch syndrome compared with selection based on clinical criteria.[10] In addition, to try to systemize the evaluation of inherited CRC, risk assessment tools have been developed, including the PREMM5 model to help identify which individuals would benefit from germline testing for Lynch syndrome.[82] These strategies can be implemented in clinical practice to help recognize individuals at increased risk based on phenotype and family history who will benefit from referral for genetic evaluation and genetic testing.

Genetic evaluation of individuals with high colorectal polyp burden is often triggered by the number of cumulative polyps (≥10 cumulative adenomas), the presence of multiple hamartomatous polyps, extracolonic cancers, and other manifestations of polyposis syndromes. Identification of these patients is important because they may require personalized interventions including frequent surveillance colonoscopies, EGDs, and risk-reducing surgery such as prophylactic colectomy or colectomy for polyp burden that cannot be managed endoscopically.

Taking a detailed history is pivotal in identifying patients with high-risk personal and family history of cancer (**Box 1**).[83,84] Assessing risk of CRC requires evaluation of cancer history in multiple generations and extends beyond CRC. Clinicians should obtain a detailed history of CRC and extracolonic cancers (including, but not limited to uterine, ovarian, gastric, and pancreatic cancers), age at diagnosis of any affected family member, and personal and family history of colon polyps (in particular the number of polyps they have had throughout their lifetime), to be able to differentiate polyposis syndromes from nonpolyposis syndromes.

SUMMARY

To optimize our ability to identify individuals with pathogenic genetic variants before CRC develops requires effective implementation of strategies for genetic risk assessment and testing, followed by tailored screening and surveillance recommendations. The introduction into clinical practice of next-generation sequencing technology has changed the traditional paradigm to hereditary cancer risk assessment, which was based on phenotype-driven genetic testing. We have now transitioned to multigene panel testing, which has the advantage of detecting germline mutations that would not have been discovered based on phenotype and clinical guidelines. This change in approach has led to more effective management of patients with potentially high-risk CRC and a decrease in CRC incidence and mortality.

CLINICS CARE POINTS

- Taking a detailed history, including history of CRC and extracolonic cancers, age at diagnosis of any affected family member, and personal and family history of colon polyps is pivotal in identifying patients with high-risk personal and family history of cancer.

- Universal tumor screening is recommended to identify high-risk individuals by testing all CRC tumors for molecular features suggestive of Lynch Syndrome.

DISCLOSURE

Dr V. Ballester has nothing to disclose. Dr M. Cruz-Correa—pharmaceutical industry research support: Merck, Bristol, SeaGen, QED, Abbvie, Janssen, Regeneron, MIR-ATI, Gilead, and Pfizer. Chief Medical Officer and stock ownership, Pan American Center for Oncology Trials. Governing board memberships (voluntary): American Association for Cancer Research, Precision Oncology Alliance, American Association for Cancer Institutes, and Foundation for Clinical Oncology.

REFERENCES

1. Butterworth AS, Higgins JP, Pharoah P. Relative and absolute risk of colorectal cancer for individuals with a family history: a meta-analysis. Eur J Cancer 2006;42(2):216–27.
2. Johns LE, Houlston RS. A systematic review and meta-analysis of familial colorectal cancer risk. Am J Gastroenterol 2001;96(10):2992–3003.
3. Johnson CM, Wei C, Ensor JE, et al. Meta-analyses of colorectal cancer risk factors. Cancer Causes Control 2013;24(6):1207–22.
4. Lowery JT, Ahnen DJ, Schroy PC 3rd, et al. Understanding the contribution of family history to colorectal cancer risk and its clinical implications: A state-of-the-science review. Cancer 2016;122(17):2633–45.
5. Baglietto L, Jenkins MA, Severi G, et al. Measures of familial aggregation depend on definition of family history: meta-analysis for colorectal cancer. J Clin Epidemiol 2006;59(2):114–24.
6. Hampel H, Frankel W, Panescu J, et al. Screening for Lynch syndrome (hereditary nonpolyposis colorectal cancer) among endometrial cancer patients. Cancer Res 2006;66(15):7810–7.
7. Pinol V, Castells A, Andreu M, et al. Accuracy of revised Bethesda guidelines, microsatellite instability, and immunohistochemistry for the identification of patients with hereditary nonpolyposis colorectal cancer. JAMA 2005;293(16):1986–94.
8. Umar A, Boland CR, Terdiman JP, et al. Revised Bethesda Guidelines for hereditary nonpolyposis colorectal cancer (Lynch syndrome) and microsatellite instability. J Natl Cancer Inst 2004;96(4):261–8.
9. Bonadona V, Bonaiti B, Olschwang S, et al. Cancer risks associated with germline mutations in MLH1, MSH2, and MSH6 genes in Lynch syndrome. JAMA 2011; 305(22):2304–10.
10. Giardiello FM, Allen JI, Axilbund JE, et al. Guidelines on genetic evaluation and management of Lynch syndrome: a consensus statement by the US Multisociety Task Force on colorectal cancer. Am J Gastroenterol 2014;109(8): 1159–79.
11. Hendriks YM, Wagner A, Morreau H, et al. Cancer risk in hereditary nonpolyposis colorectal cancer due to MSH6 mutations: impact on counseling and surveillance. Gastroenterology 2004;127(1):17–25.

12. Moller P, Seppala T, Bernstein I, et al. Cancer incidence and survival in Lynch syndrome patients receiving colonoscopic and gynaecological surveillance: first report from the prospective Lynch syndrome database. Gut 2017;66(3):464–72.

13. Stoffel E, Mukherjee B, Raymond VM, et al. Calculation of risk of colorectal and endometrial cancer among patients with Lynch syndrome. Gastroenterology 2009;137(5):1621–7.

14. Syngal S, Brand RE, Church JM, et al. ACG clinical guideline: Genetic testing and management of hereditary gastrointestinal cancer syndromes. Am J Gastroenterol 2015;110(2):223–62, quiz 63.

15. Baglietto L, Lindor NM, Dowty JG, et al. Risks of Lynch syndrome cancers for MSH6 mutation carriers. J Natl Cancer Inst 2010;102(3):193–201.

16. Senter L, Clendenning M, Sotamaa K, et al. The clinical phenotype of Lynch syndrome due to germ-line PMS2 mutations. Gastroenterology 2008;135(2):419–28.

17. Win AK, Dowty JG, Cleary SP, et al. Risk of colorectal cancer for carriers of mutations in MUTYH, with and without a family history of cancer. Gastroenterology 2014;146(5):1208–11.e1-5.

18. Win AK, Jenkins MA, Dowty JG, et al. Prevalence and Penetrance of Major Genes and Polygenes for Colorectal Cancer. Cancer Epidemiol Biomarkers Prev 2017; 26(3):404–12.

19. Vilar E, Gruber SB. Microsatellite instability in colorectal cancer-the stable evidence. Nat Rev Clin Oncol 2010;7(3):153–62.

20. Boland CR, Thibodeau SN, Hamilton SR, et al. A National Cancer Institute Workshop on Microsatellite Instability for cancer detection and familial predisposition: development of international criteria for the determination of microsatellite instability in colorectal cancer. Cancer Res 1998;58(22):5248–57.

21. Grady WM, Carethers JM. Genomic and epigenetic instability in colorectal cancer pathogenesis. Gastroenterology 2008;135(4):1079–99.

22. Lindor NM, Burgart LJ, Leontovich O, et al. Immunohistochemistry versus microsatellite instability testing in phenotyping colorectal tumors. J Clin Oncol 2002; 20(4):1043–8.

23. Boland CR, Goel A. Microsatellite instability in colorectal cancer. Gastroenterology 2010;138(6):2073–87, e3.

24. Kastrinos F, Steyerberg EW, Mercado R, et al. The PREMM(1,2,6) model predicts risk of MLH1, MSH2, and MSH6 germline mutations based on cancer history. Gastroenterology 2011;140(1):73–81.

25. Kastrinos F, Uno H, Ukaegbu C, et al. Development and Validation of the PREMM5 Model for Comprehensive Risk Assessment of Lynch Syndrome. J Clin Oncol 2017;35(19):2165–72.

26. Balmana J, Stockwell DH, Steyerberg EW, et al. Prediction of MLH1 and MSH2 mutations in Lynch syndrome. JAMA 2006;296(12):1469–78.

27. Barnetson RA, Tenesa A, Farrington SM, et al. Identification and survival of carriers of mutations in DNA mismatch-repair genes in colon cancer. N Engl J Med 2006;354(26):2751–63.

28. Chen S, Wang W, Lee S, et al. Prediction of germline mutations and cancer risk in the Lynch syndrome. JAMA 2006;296(12):1479–87.

29. Burn J, Gerdes AM, Macrae F, et al. Long-term effect of aspirin on cancer risk in carriers of hereditary colorectal cancer: an analysis from the CAPP2 randomised controlled trial. Lancet 2011;378(9809):2081–7.

30. Gebert J, Gelincik O, Oezcan-Wahlbrink M, et al. Recurrent Frameshift Neoantigen Vaccine Elicits Protective Immunity With Reduced Tumor Burden and

Improved Overall Survival in a Lynch Syndrome Mouse Model. Gastroenterology 2021;161(4):1288–302, e13.

31. Rodriguez-Soler M, Perez-Carbonell L, Guarinos C, et al. Risk of cancer in cases of suspected lynch syndrome without germline mutation. Gastroenterology 2013; 144(5):926–932 e1, quiz e13-14.

32. Boland CR. The mystery of mismatch repair deficiency: lynch or lynch-like? Gastroenterology 2013;144(5):868–70.

33. Pearlman R, Haraldsdottir S, de la Chapelle A, et al. Clinical characteristics of patients with colorectal cancer with double somatic mismatch repair mutations compared with Lynch syndrome. J Med Genet 2019;56(7):462–70.

34. Lindor NM, Rabe K, Petersen GM, et al. Lower cancer incidence in Amsterdam-I criteria families without mismatch repair deficiency: familial colorectal cancer type X. JAMA 2005;293(16):1979–85.

35. Palles C, Cazier JB, Howarth KM, et al. Germline mutations affecting the proof-reading domains of POLE and POLD1 predispose to colorectal adenomas and carcinomas. Nat Genet 2013;45(2):136–44.

36. Bellido F, Pineda M, Aiza G, et al. POLE and POLD1 mutations in 529 kindred with familial colorectal cancer and/or polyposis: review of reported cases and recommendations for genetic testing and surveillance. Genet Med 2016;18(4):325–32.

37. Church DN, Briggs SE, Palles C, et al. DNA polymerase epsilon and delta exonuclease domain mutations in endometrial cancer. Hum Mol Genet 2013;22(14): 2820–8.

38. Rohlin A, Zagoras T, Nilsson S, et al. A mutation in POLE predisposing to a multi-tumour phenotype. Int J Oncol 2014;45(1):77–81.

39. Burt R, Neklason DW. Genetic testing for inherited colon cancer. Gastroenterology 2005;128(6):1696–716.

40. Jasperson KW, Tuohy TM, Neklason DW, et al. Hereditary and familial colon cancer. Gastroenterology 2010;138(6):2044–58.

41. Galiatsatos P, Foulkes WD. Familial adenomatous polyposis. Am J Gastroenterol 2006;101(2):385–98.

42. Cruz-Correa M, Perez-Mayoral J, Dutil J, et al. Hereditary cancer syndromes in Latino populations: genetic characterization and surveillance guidelines. Hered Cancer Clin Pract 2017;15:3.

43. Daly MB, Pilarski R, Axilbund JE, et al. Genetic/familial high-risk assessment: breast and ovarian, version 1.2014. J Natl Compr Canc Netw 2014;12(9): 1326–38.

44. Ma X, Zhang B, Zheng W. Genetic variants associated with colorectal cancer risk: comprehensive research synopsis, meta-analysis, and epidemiological evidence. Gut 2014;63(2):326–36.

45. Katona BW, Yurgelun MB, Garber JE, et al. A counseling framework for moderate-penetrance colorectal cancer susceptibility genes. Genet Med 2018;20(11): 1324–7.

46. Boursi B, Sella T, Liberman E, et al. The APC p.I1307K polymorphism is a significant risk factor for CRC in average risk Ashkenazi Jews. Eur J Cancer 2013; 49(17):3680–5.

47. Steinbach G, Lynch PM, Phillips RK, et al. The effect of celecoxib, a cyclooxygenase-2 inhibitor, in familial adenomatous polyposis. N Engl J Med 2000;342(26):1946–52.

48. Giardiello FM, Yang VW, Hylind LM, et al. Primary chemoprevention of familial adenomatous polyposis with sulindac. N Engl J Med 2002;346(14):1054–9.

49. Phillips RK, Wallace MH, Lynch PM, et al. A randomised, double blind, placebo controlled study of celecoxib, a selective cyclooxygenase 2 inhibitor, on duodenal polyposis in familial adenomatous polyposis. Gut 2002;50(6):857–60.

50. Cruz-Correa M, Hylind LM, Marrero JH, et al. Efficacy and Safety of Curcumin in Treatment of Intestinal Adenomas in Patients With Familial Adenomatous Polyposis. Gastroenterology 2018;155(3):668–73.

51. Samadder NJ, Kuwada SK, Boucher KM, et al. Association of Sulindac and Erlotinib vs Placebo With Colorectal Neoplasia in Familial Adenomatous Polyposis: Secondary Analysis of a Randomized Clinical Trial. JAMA Oncol 2018;4(5):671–7.

52. Spirio L, Olschwang S, Groden J, et al. Alleles of the APC gene: an attenuated form of familial polyposis. Cell 1993;75(5):951–7.

53. Soravia C, Berk T, Madlensky L, et al. Genotype-phenotype correlations in attenuated adenomatous polyposis coli. Am J Hum Genet 1998;62(6):1290–301.

54. Burt RW. Gastric fundic gland polyps. Gastroenterology 2003;125(5):1462–9.

55. Brensinger JD, Laken SJ, Luce MC, et al. Variable phenotype of familial adenomatous polyposis in pedigrees with 3' mutation in the APC gene. Gut 1998; 43(4):548–52.

56. Giardiello FM, Brensinger JD, Luce MC, et al. Phenotypic expression of disease in families that have mutations in the 5' region of the adenomatous polyposis coli gene. Ann Intern Med 1997;126(7):514–9.

57. Grover S, Kastrinos F, Steyerberg EW, et al. Prevalence and phenotypes of APC and MUTYH mutations in patients with multiple colorectal adenomas. JAMA 2012; 308(5):485–92.

58. Nielsen M, Joerink-van de Beld MC, Jones N, et al. Analysis of MUTYH genotypes and colorectal phenotypes in patients With MUTYH-associated polyposis. Gastroenterology 2009;136(2):471–6.

59. Nielsen M, Morreau H, Vasen HF, et al. MUTYH-associated polyposis (MAP). Crit Rev Oncol Hematol 2011;79(1):1–16.

60. Network NCC. National comprehensive cancer Network: NCCN clinical practice guidelines in Oncology: genetic/familial high-risk assessment: colorectal. Plymouth Meeting, PA: National Comprehensive Cancer Network; 2019. Available at: https://www.nccn.org/professionals/physician_gls/default.aspx#genetics_colon.

61. Nieuwenhuis MH, Vogt S, Jones N, et al. Evidence for accelerated colorectal adenoma–carcinoma progression in MUTYH-associated polyposis? Gut 2012;61(5): 734–8.

62. Morak M, Laner A, Bacher U, et al. MUTYH-associated polyposis - variability of the clinical phenotype in patients with biallelic and monoallelic MUTYH mutations and report on novel mutations. Clin Genet 2010;78(4):353–63.

63. Jones N, Vogt S, Nielsen M, et al. Increased colorectal cancer incidence in obligate carriers of heterozygous mutations in MUTYH. Gastroenterology 2009; 137(2):489–94.e1, quiz 725-726.

64. Herkert JC, Niessen RC, Olderode-Berends MJ, et al. Paediatric intestinal cancer and polyposis due to bi-allelic PMS2 mutations: case series, review and follow-up guidelines. Eur J Cancer 2011;47(7):965–82.

65. Wimmer K, Etzler J. Constitutional mismatch repair-deficiency syndrome: have we so far seen only the tip of an iceberg? Hum Genet 2008;124(2):105–22.

66. Durno CA, Aronson M, Tabori U, et al. Oncologic surveillance for subjects with biallelic mismatch repair gene mutations: 10 year follow-up of a kindred. Pediatr Blood Cancer 2012;59(4):652–6.

67. Weston BR, Helper DJ, Rex DK. Positive predictive value of endoscopic features deemed typical of gastric fundic gland polyps. J Clin Gastroenterol 2003;36(5): 399–402.
68. Weren RD, Ligtenberg MJ, Kets CM, et al. A germline homozygous mutation in the base-excision repair gene NTHL1 causes adenomatous polyposis and colorectal cancer. Nat Genet 2015;47(6):668–71.
69. Quintana I, Mejias-Luque R, Terradas M, et al. Evidence suggests that germline RNF43 mutations are a rare cause of serrated polyposis. Gut 2018;67(12): 2230–2.
70. Taupin D, Lam W, Rangiah D, et al. A deleterious RNF43 germline mutation in a severely affected serrated polyposis kindred. Hum Genome Var 2015;2:15013.
71. Chow E, Lipton L, Lynch E, et al. Hyperplastic polyposis syndrome: phenotypic presentations and the role of MBD4 and MYH. Gastroenterology 2006; 131(1):30–9.
72. Jeghers H, Mc KV, Katz KH. Generalized intestinal polyposis and melanin spots of the oral mucosa, lips and digits; a syndrome of diagnostic significance. N Engl J Med 1949;241(26):1031–6.
73. Spigelman AD, Williams CB, Talbot IC, et al. Upper gastrointestinal cancer in patients with familial adenomatous polyposis. Lancet 1989;2(8666):783–5.
74. Giardiello FM, Brensinger JD, Tersmette AC, et al. Very high risk of cancer in familial Peutz-Jeghers syndrome. Gastroenterology 2000;119(6):1447–53.
75. Latchford A, Cohen S, Auth M, et al. Management of Peutz-Jeghers Syndrome in Children and Adolescents: a position paper from the ESPGHAN polyposis working group. J Pediatr Gastroenterol Nutr 2019;68(3):442–52.
76. Beggs AD, Latchford AR, Vasen HF, et al. Peutz-Jeghers syndrome: a systematic review and recommendations for management. Gut 2010;59(7):975–86.
77. Latchford AR, Neale K, Phillips RK, et al. Juvenile polyposis syndrome: a study of genotype, phenotype, and long-term outcome. Dis Colon Rectum 2012;55(10): 1038–43.
78. Howe JR, Bair JL, Sayed MG, et al. Germline mutations of the gene encoding bone morphogenetic protein receptor 1A in juvenile polyposis. Nat Genet 2001; 28(2):184–7.
79. Zhou XP, Woodford-Richens K, Lehtonen R, et al. Germline mutations in BMPR1A/ ALK3 cause a subset of cases of juvenile polyposis syndrome and of Cowden and Bannayan-Riley-Ruvalcaba syndromes. Am J Hum Genet 2001;69(4): 704–11.
80. Jass JR, Williams CB, Bussey HJ, et al. Juvenile polyposis–a precancerous condition. Histopathology 1988;13(6):619–30.
81. Zhou XP, Waite KA, Pilarski R, et al. Germline PTEN promoter mutations and deletions in Cowden/Bannayan-Riley-Ruvalcaba syndrome result in aberrant PTEN protein and dysregulation of the phosphoinositol-3-kinase/Akt pathway. Am J Hum Genet 2003;73(2):404–11.
82. Idos G, Gupta S. When Should patients undergo genetic testing for hereditary colon cancer syndromes? Clin Gastroenterol Hepatol 2018;16(2):181–3.
83. Kaz AM, Brentnall TA. Genetic testing for colon cancer. Nat Clin Pract Gastroenterol Hepatol 2006;3(12):670–9.
84. Ballester V, Cruz-Correa M. How and when to consider genetic testing for colon cancer? Gastroenterology 2018;155(4):955–9.
85. Valle L, Vilar E, Tavtigian SV, et al. Genetic predisposition to colorectal cancer: syndromes, genes, classification of genetic variants and implications for precision medicine. J Pathol 2019;247(5):574–88.

A Gastroenterologist's Approach to the Diagnosis and Management of Gastrointestinal Stromal Tumors

Raquel E. Davila, MD

KEYWORDS

- Gastrointestinal stromal tumors • GIST • GI stromal tumors • Subepithelial lesions
- Endoscopic ultrasound • Endoscopic ultrasound fine-needle aspiration
- Endoscopic ultrasound fine-needle biopsy • Endoscopic biopsy

KEY POINTS

- Gastrointestinal stromal tumors (GISTs) are mesenchymal tumors of the gastrointestinal (GI) tract, omentum, mesentery, and peritoneum.
- The majority of GISTs harbor gain-of-function mutations of the c-KIT proto-oncogene which encodes a tyrosine kinase receptor that regulates cell growth.
- Mutations of c-KIT lead to constitutive activation of the tyrosine kinase receptor, which in turn leads to oncogenic cell transformation.
- Tumor location, size, and mitotic index are factors used to predict the risk of malignant behavior.
- Endoscopy and endoscopic ultrasound play a critical role in the evaluation and diagnosis of GISTs, and can significantly impact the management of these tumors.

DEFINITION, PROPOSED PATHOGENESIS, AND IMMUNOHISTOCHEMISTRY OF GASTROINTESTINAL STROMAL TUMORS

Gastrointestinal stromal tumors (GISTs) are the most common mesenchymal tumors of the gastrointestinal (GI) tract. These tumors were previously misclassified as smooth muscle tumors of the GI tract, including leiomyomas and leiomyosarcomas, but are now defined as soft tissue sarcomas of the digestive system.[1] Although GISTs are typically found within the bowel wall, some tumors can also arise in the omentum, mesentery or peritoneum, and are described as extragastrointestinal stromal tumors.[2]

GISTs are characterized by almost universal expression of the c-KIT proto-oncogene protein.[3,4] The c-KIT proto-oncogene is located in the long arm of chromosome 4, and it encodes a 145 kD transmembrane receptor that has internal tyrosine

University of Texas at Dallas, 4500 S. Lancaster Road, Dallas, TX 75216-7167, USA
E-mail address: rdavila.1996@gmail.com

Gastroenterol Clin N Am 51 (2022) 609–624
https://doi.org/10.1016/j.gtc.2022.06.009
0889-8553/22/© 2022 Elsevier Inc. All rights reserved.

kinase activity known as c-kit (receptor) or CD117. The binding of ligand known as stem cell factor, causes dimerization and activation of the c-kit receptor. Once the receptor is activated, a series of intracellular signals are turned on resulting in cell growth. In a landmark study published in Science in 1998, Hirota and colleagues reported the finding of gain-of-function mutations in the c-KIT proto-oncogene in the large majority of GISTs.[5] These mutations result in the constitutive activation of the c-kit receptor without ligand binding, leading to uncontrolled cell proliferation, inhibition of normal apoptotic cell death, and oncogenic cell transformation.[5–7] Subsequently, the development of gain-of-function mutations of the c-KIT proto-oncogene has been proposed as a key step in the pathogenesis of GISTs. A small minority of GISTs harbor mutations of the platelet-derived growth factor receptor alpha (PDGFRA), which result in ligand-independent activation of the receptor and similar intracellular signal transduction.

Immunohistochemical analysis of tissue specimens can help differentiate GISTs from other mesenchymal tumors of the GI tract. CD117 is an antigen on the extracellular portion of the c-kit tyrosine kinase receptor and has become a term interchangeable with the c-kit receptor. More than 95% of GISTs stain positive for CD117 on immunohistochemical analysis.[8,9] (**Fig. 1**) Leiomyomas, leiomyosarcomas, and other mesenchymal tumors of the GI tract do not express the c-kit protein and are CD117 negative. DOG1 (Discovered On Gastrointestinal Stromal Tumors 1) is another marker expressed in GISTs and can be found in greater than 95% of cases.[10] (**Fig. 1**) Positive staining for DOG1 is most helpful in identifying GIST cases where the tumor stains negative for CD117.[11] Approximately 60% to 70% of GISTs are positive for CD34, a

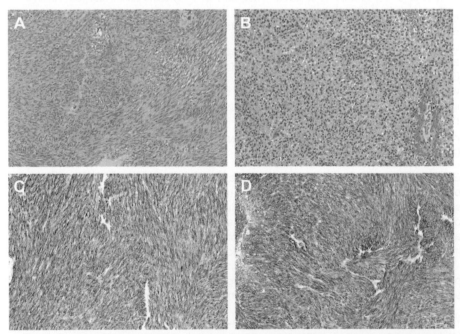

Fig. 1. (*A*) H & E stain of a GIST specimen showing spindle cell type histology with eosinophilic cytoplasm and ovoid, elongated nuclei. (*B*) H & E stain of a GIST specimen showing epithelioid type histology with round, irregular cells, and uniform, round nuclei. (*C*) Immunohistochemical staining for CD117 demonstrating diffuse uptake. (*D*) Immunohistochemical staining for DOG1 demonstrating diffuse uptake.

sialylated transmembrane glycoprotein and hematopoietic progenitor cell antigen found in mesenchymal cells. In a study of 300 GIST cases, 90% of gastric, esophageal, and rectal GISTs were found to stain positive for CD34, whereas only 50% of small intestinal GISTs were CD34 positive.[9] Although a small subset of small intestinal GISTs can stain positive for smooth muscle actin (SMA), the majority of GISTs are negative for SMA. GISTs are also typically negative for desmin and S100. Leiomyomas usually stain positive for SMA and desmin, and are negative for CD117 and CD34. Similarly, schwannomas, another class of benign mesenchymal tumors of the GI tract, stain negative for CD117 and CD34, and are positive for S100 protein.

It has been proposed that GISTs arise from the interstitial cells of Cajal (ICCs) which are a complex network of cells found within the muscle layers of the gastrointestinal wall. The ICCs serve as a pacemaker system within the GI tract wall that regulates gut motility.[12] The development of ICCs appears to be dependent on normal c-kit activity, with animal studies showing the inhibition of the normal development of ICCs and disruption of gut motility in the setting of genetic mutations of c-KIT.[12] Immunohistochemical studies of ICCs have shown identical patterns of staining to a range of antigens compared with GISTs, including strong CD117 staining.[13,14] Subsequently, it is thought that GISTs may originate from the ICCs or may evolve from a precursor pluripotential stem cell that differentiates toward a pacemaker cell phenotype.[13,15] Since the ICCs are normally found within the GI tract wall, it has been suggested that rare ICCs may migrate to other sites during embryologic development and can lead to extragastrointestinal stromal tumors.

EPIDEMIOLOGY

In a systematic review of 29 studies of more than 13,550 patients with GIST from 19 countries, the incidence of GISTs was estimated to be 10 to 15 cases per million population year.[16] In the same study, the median age at presentation was in the mid 60's and there was no gender difference. In an analysis of GIST cases from the United States Cancer Statistics database from 2001 to 2015, the overall incidence of GISTs was 0.70 per 100,000 people per year.[17] Furthermore, the incidence in blacks increased with an annual percent change of 6.27 from 2001 to 2015.[17] In a study of the Surveillance, Epidemiology, and End Results (SEER) database for GISTs from 2002 to 2015, the incidence rate of GIST was 0.75 per 100,000 and was found to be twice as high in African Americans compared to white patients.[18] Overall, patients with GIST tend to be older, and typically present in their 6th decade. In general, GISTs are rarely seen in patients younger than 40, and are very rare in children. Hereditary forms of GIST due to genetic alterations and germline mutations can occur in up to 5% of patients including primary familial GIST syndrome; neurofibromatosis type 1; Carney–Stratakis syndrome; and Carney triad.

CLINICAL PRESENTATION

Up to 30% of GIST may be asymptomatic and can be identified incidentally at the time of endoscopy, imaging, or surgery for other indications.[3,19] The clinical presentation of patients with symptomatic GIST depends on tumor location. Approximately 60% to 70% of GISTs occur in the stomach, 20% to 30% in the small intestine, 5% in the colon and rectum, and less than 5% can be found in the esophagus and other sites (appendix, gallbladder, mesentery, omentum, retroperitoneum).[4,20] In the stomach, tumors are more commonly found in the cardia and fundus rather than in the body and antrum. Small intestinal tumors tend to occur in the jejunum more than in the ileum and are relatively rare in the duodenum. Rectal tumors are typically more common than colonic GISTs. The majority of the gastric, small intestinal, and colonic GISTs present with gastrointestinal bleeding (occult or overt), anemia, abdominal pain, or a palpable mass on physical examination. Larger tumors can present with acute gastrointestinal bleeding, tumor rupture with ascites, small bowel obstruction, and perforation. Other presentations of gastrointestinal and extragastrointestinal tumors have been described elsewhere.[21]

TUMOR HISTOPATHOLOGY

There are three main types of GISTs on histopathology including spindle cell type (70%–80% of tumors), epithelioid type (20%–30%), and mixed type (<10%) (**Fig. 1**). The spindle cell type consists of uniform eosinophilic cells arranged in short fascicles or whorls, with pale eosinophilic cytoplasm, and uniform nuclei in an ovoid shape. The epithelioid type has round or irregular cells with variable eosinophilic to clear cytoplasm. These cells have uniform nuclei which can be round or ovoid. The epithelioid type can sometimes have a carcinoid-like appearance. The mixed type can have histologic features of both the spindle cell and epithelioid types. The addition of immunohistochemical staining of tissue specimens with antibodies against CD117, CD34, and other markers can confirm the diagnosis of GIST and can differentiate GISTs from other mesenchymal tumors.

TUMOR BEHAVIOR AND PREDICTORS OF MALIGNANCY

Malignancy or malignant behavior is defined by: direct invasion to adjacent organs; metastasis to extra-intestinal organs or the abdominal wall; omental, mesenteric, or peritoneal seeding; and tumor recurrence after surgical resection.[3,19] The majority of metastases occur in the liver (50%), followed by the peritoneum, mesentery, and omentum (<25%), lung (<10%), and bone (<10%). Lymph node metastases are extremely rare, but have been reported in wild-type GISTs (<10% of all tumors) which have no detectable c-KIT or PDGFRA mutations. Up to 30% of GISTs are considered to be clinically malignant,[3] although all GISTs have the potential to behave in a malignant fashion. When tumors are intact without evidence of malignancy, the clinical challenge becomes accurately predicting which tumors are at risk of postoperative recurrence or metastasis, so that surgical planning can be performed and selected tumors can be targeted with medical therapy using tyrosine kinase inhibitors (see Management section).

Tumor size and mitotic index, or the number of mitoses seen per 50 high power field (HPF), are the most widely used pathologic features for the risk stratification of GISTs.[22] In 2001, the NIH GIST Workshop developed a guideline for predicting malignant behavior based on tumor size and mitotic index.[23] In general, tumors that are small (<5 cm) and have a low mitotic index (≤5 per 50 HPF) have a low risk for malignancy, whereas large tumors (>5 cm) or tumors with high mitotic index (>5 per 50 HPF) are associated with a high risk. However, the Workshop recommended considering decreasing the size threshold for small intestinal tumors by 1 cm to 2 cm in each category, as these tumors can exhibit more aggressive behavior compared with gastric tumors. In 2006, a new risk stratification scheme was developed based on the Armed Forces Institute of Pathology data on more than 1600 intestinal GISTs.[24] (**Table 1**) This scheme takes into account tumor size, mitotic index, and tumor location. Based on this scheme, small GISTs that are ≤2 cm in size and have a low mitotic index (≤5 per 50 HPF) have no risk of malignant behavior, irrespective of tumor location. However, intestinal and rectal tumors >2 cm in size with a mitotic index of ≤5 per 50 HPF have a significantly higher risk of malignancy compared to gastric tumors with the

Table 1
Risk stratification of GIST by mitotic index, tumor size, and tumor location based on data from the Armed Forces Institute of Pathology

Tumor Parameters			Risk of Progressive Disease[a] (%)			
Mitotic Index	Size	Stomach	Duodenum	Jejunum/ Ileum	Rectum
≤5 per 50 hpf	≤ 2 cm	None (0%)	None (0%)	None (0%)	None (0%)
≤5 per 50 hpf	>2 ≤ 5 cm	Very low (1.9%)	Low (4.3%)	Low (8.3%)	Low (8.5%)
≤5 per 50 hpf	>5 ≤ 10 cm	Low (3.6%)	Moderate (24%)	(Insuff. data)	(Insuff. data)
≤5 per 50 hpf	>10 cm	Moderate (10%)	High (52%)	High (34%)	High (57%)
>5 per 50 hpf	≤ 2 cm	None[b]	High[b]	(Insuff. data)	High (54%)
>5 per 50 hpf	>2 ≤ 5 cm	Moderate (16%)	High (73%)	High (50%)	High (52%)
>5 per 50 hpf	>5 ≤ 10 cm	High (55%)	High (85%)	(Insuff. data)	(Insuff. data)
>5 per 50 hpf	>10 cm	High (86%)	High (90%)	High (86%)	High (71%)

Abbreviations: GIST, gastrointestinal stromal tumor; hpf, high power field; Insuff, Insufficient.
[a] Defined as metastases or tumor-related death.
[b] Denotes small number of cases.
Adapted from Miettinen M, Lasota J. Gastrointestinal stromal tumors: pathology and prognosis at different sites. Semin Diagn Pathol. 2006;23(2):70-83; with permission.

same features. A modified scheme taking into account tumor size, mitotic index, tumor location, and tumor rupture has also been proposed for the risk stratification of patients with GIST.[25]

GENETIC MUTATIONS

More than 80% of GISTs harbor mutations of the c-KIT proto-oncogene which result in constitutive activation of the c-kit tyrosine kinase without the binding of ligand.[4,7,26,27] Mutations involving exon 11 of c-KIT are the most common, and occur in up to 70% to 85% of GISTs in a variety of locations throughout the GI tract.[28–30] These mutations affect the intracellular portion of the tyrosine kinase receptor in the juxtamembrane domain. In a study of 124 patients with GIST, patients with exon 11 mutations had a worse prognosis compared to mutation-negative cases, with a statistically significant increase in tumor recurrence and decreased 5-year survival.[31] Mutations of exon 9 are found in 5% to 13% of GISTs and affect the extracellular dimerization domain of the tyrosine kinase, which lead to the dimerization and activation of the receptor independent of ligand.[30] Exon 9 mutations are predominantly found in small intestinal tumors and are associated with a more aggressive clinical behavior.[32,33] Mutations affecting exons 13, 14, 17, and 18 have also been described and are rare, occurring in less than 2% of cases. These mutations are seen more often as secondary mutations that develop after treatment with tyrosine kinase inhibitors. Interestingly, c-KIT mutations (predominantly exon 11 mutations) have been found in small incidental GISTs measuring ≤1 cm.[34] This supports the view that c-KIT mutations may be acquired early in the development of GISTs.

PDGFRA mutations occur in 5% to 10% of GISTS and result in ligand-independent activation of a tyrosine kinase receptor resulting in an intracellular signal transduction pathway similar to what is seen with the c-kit receptor.[35] c-KIT and PDGFRA mutations are mutually exclusive in GISTs. Exon 18 mutations account for more than 80% of PDGFRA mutations and have 2 forms: D842V and non-D842V. The D842V exon 18 mutation is more common (>60% of PDGFRA mutations), and has important implications for tumor response to tyrosine kinase inhibitors (see Management section).[36] Exon 12 mutations comprise approximately 9% of PDGFRA mutations, whereas exon 10 and 14 mutations are very rare.

There is a small subset of GISTs (5%) that do not harbor c-KIT or PDGFRA mutations and are referred to as "wild-type." These tumors may express mutations in the genes encoding for subunits of the enzymes in the succinate dehydrogenase (SDH) enzyme family.[37] Mutations result in functional loss or deficiency of one of several enzymes in the SDH enzyme family. These mutations have been associated with Carney–Stratakis syndrome (GIST and paragangliomas) and Carney triad (GIST, pulmonary chondromas, and paragangliomas) in pediatric patients. Other genetic mutations found in wild-type GIST may affect BRAF, NF-1 (neurofibromatosis type 1), and NTRK (neurotrophic tyrosine kinase receptor).

IMAGING IN THE INITIAL EVALUATION OF GISTs

Radiologic imaging of GISTs can be used to characterize primary tumors, determine location and size, rule out extension to other organs or adjacent structures, and rule out metastatic disease. Computer tomography (CT) is the preferred modality for suspected GISTs; however, magnetic resonance imaging (MRI) may be a reasonable alternative.[38–40] (**Fig. 2**) MRI may be considered in cases of rectal tumors.[41] Positron emission tomography (PET) is typically not used during the initial evaluation of patients presenting with GIST; however, it may be used to establish a baseline prior to treatment with tyrosine kinase inhibitors.

ENDOSCOPY AND ENDOSCOPIC ULTRASOUND

On endoscopic evaluation, GISTs usually appear as a subepithelial lesion (also known as "submucosal" lesion) or a smooth bulge in the lumen of the GI tract. Lesions usually have normal overlying mucosa, although there can be central ulceration or umbilication (**Fig. 3**). The differential diagnosis of a suspected GIST or subepithelial lesion on endoscopy includes leiomyoma, lipoma, duplication cyst, granular cell tumor, pancreatic rest, neuroendocrine tumor, glomus tumor, schwannoma, inflammatory fibroid polyp, varices, endometriosis, metastatic cancer, lymphoma, or extrinsic compression from an adjacent extramural structure.[42,43] Probing of a suspected

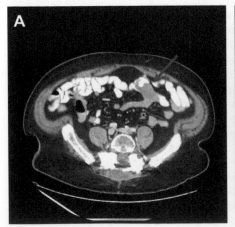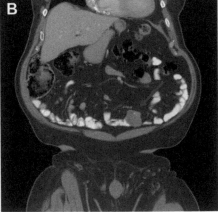

Fig. 2. (*A*) Axial CT image of an ileal GIST. (*B*) Coronal CT image of the same ileal tumor.

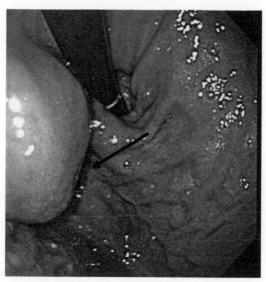

Fig. 3. Endoscopic image of a gastric GIST appearing as a subepithelial lesion with central ulceration.

GIST lesion with closed biopsy forceps can be done and may demonstrate a firm consistency.[42] Forceps biopsies are usually nondiagnostic as they typically cannot reach deeper to the mucosa. Use of large capacity jumbo biopsy forceps with a bite-on-bite or tunnel technique has been shown to have a low diagnostic yield.[44,45] When ulceration is present, forceps biopsies of the ulcerated area should be considered as it may be diagnostic, although this may not be recommended in the setting of GI bleeding.[46]

Video capsule endoscopy (VCE) and deep enteroscopy (DE) can be used to evaluate small-bowel tumors including GISTs (**Fig. 4**). In a large European multicenter study including 5,129 patients undergoing VCE, 124 (2.4%) had small-bowel tumors, including 112 primary tumors and 12 metastatic tumors.[47] Nearly a third of the primary small-bowel tumors (32%) were found to be GIST. In general, the diagnostic yield of double-balloon enteroscopy (DBE) for small-bowel tumors is 9% to 14%.[48] In a retrospective Japanese multicenter study of DBE in 1,035 consecutive cases, 144 small-bowel tumors were identified, including 27 (18.8%) GISTs.[49] In a meta-analysis comparing VCE to DBE in patients with suspected small-bowel disorders, there was no difference in the overall diagnostic yield or detection of small-bowel tumors.[50] The advantage of deep enteroscopy is that it allows for biopsies of tumors, tattoo placement for subsequent localization during surgery, and therapeutic interventions. VCE can miss up to 18.9% of small-bowel tumors,[51] and in this setting, DE can successfully detect tumors missed by VCE.[52,53] However, GIST may be subtle, especially if exophytic, and can be missed on VCE followed by DE.[54]

Endoscopic ultrasound (EUS) is critical in the evaluation, characterization, and diagnosis of GISTs. Typically on EUS, GISTs appear as a hypoechoic mass lesion arising from the fourth hypoechoic layer or muscularis propria.[55–58] A subset of GIST can arise within the muscularis mucosa and can be seen within the second wall layer. Some GISTs can be found in the submucosa (third wall layer), and in these cases, it has been suggested that these tumors originated from the muscularis propria or muscularis mucosa and grew into the submucosa.[59] GISTs are typically ovoid or elliptical in shape, although they can be pedunculated or multilobular. In a study of CD117

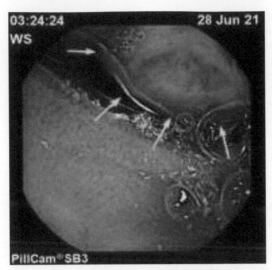

Fig. 4. Video capsule endoscopy image of an ulcerated GIST in the ileum.

positive versus CD117 negative mesenchymal tumors of the upper GI tract, large size greater than 4 cm, ulceration, cystic spaces, and nonesophageal location were EUS features associated with a diagnosis of GIST.[44] Overall, EUS has a sensitivity of 64.7% to 95% and specificity of 72% to 91.7%.[60]

EUS features may be helpful in identifying malignant tumors. In a study of 35 GISTs, tumor size greater than 4 cm, irregular border, echogenic foci, and cystic spaces were independent risk factors associated with malignancy.[61] In cases where 2 out of 3 features (irregular borders, echogenic foci, and cystic spaces) were present, the sensitivity of EUS for detecting malignant GISTs was 80% to 100%. In a retrospective study of 56 GISTs, the presence of cystic spaces and irregular margins were independent predictors of malignancy.[62] The combined presence of 2 out of 3 EUS features (cystic spaces, irregular borders, and lymph nodes) had a positive predictive value of 100% for malignant or borderline stromal cell tumors. Furthermore, size ≤ 3 cm, homogeneous echo pattern, and regular margins were EUS features associated with benign GISTs. The presence of all 3 features combined had a specificity of 100% for benign tumors. Additional retrospective studies have suggested that large tumor size (>3 cm), ulceration, irregular tumor margins, and cystic spaces are associated with malignant behavior.[63–65] However, conflicting results have been reported, with some studies showing no correlation between EUS features and risk of malignancy.[66,67] Further prospective studies are needed to determine the value of EUS features in predicting malignancy.

More recently, enhanced EUS imaging with contrast-enhanced EUS (CE-EUS) or elastography, and artificial intelligence (AI)-based applications have been used to improve the accuracy of EUS in the diagnosis of GIST, and increase the predictive value of EUS in determining malignancy. In a study of 157 patients with submucosal lesions of the upper GI tract evaluated with CE-EUS, 84.5% of GISTs had hyperenhancement compared to 26.7% of non-GISTs.[68] Furthermore, 36.2% of GISTs showed inhomogeneous contrast enhancement compared to 13.3% of non-GISTs. If hyperenhancement was considered to indicate GISTs, the sensitivity, specificity, and accuracy were 84.5%, 73.3%, and 82.2%, respectively. In a study of 29 resected GISTs, CE-EUS identified irregular vessels and thereby, predicted malignant GIST with a sensitivity, specificity, and accuracy of 100%, 63%, and 83%, respectively.[69] Tsuji and colleagues studied the diagnostic utility of EUS elastography in 25 gastric submucosal tumors.[70] Higher Giovannini elasticity scores (4–5) correlated with a diagnosis of GIST, whereas lower scores (2–3) correlated with a diagnosis of leiomyoma. In a study of 631 subepithelial lesions (SELs) and 16,110 images, an AI-based diagnostic system had an accuracy of 86.1% for differentiating SELs (GIST, leiomyoma, schwannoma, neuroendocrine tumor, and ectopic pancreas).[71] The sensitivity, specificity, and accuracy of the AI system for differentiating GISTs from non-GISTs were 98.8%, 67.6%, and 89.3%, respectively.

In general, EUS-guided fine-needle aspiration (EUS-FNA) is the preferred method of diagnosis of GISTs. In a systematic review of 46 studies of EUS including 4,534 cases of GISTs, the diagnostic yield of EUS-FNA was 84% (73.8%–100%) compared to 68.7% (40%–100%) for EUS alone. Some studies have suggested that certain factors may influence the diagnostic yield of EUS-FNA including lesion location (gastric location being more favorable); tumor size (>2 cm more favorable); tumor shape (oval or round more favorable than irregular); wall layer of origin (3rd or 4th layers more favorable); and the presence of on-site cytopathologist.[72,73] Factors such as needle size and number of needle passes do not appear to influence diagnostic yield.

In addition to cytologic analysis, FNA specimens are normally evaluated with immunohistochemical staining for CD117 and other markers to make the diagnosis of GIST.[74] In general, EUS-FNA alone is not helpful for predicting tumor behavior, as the mitotic index is inconsistently present on FNA specimens.[75] The addition of immunohistochemical staining for Ki-67 (a labeling index that denotes mitotic activity and cell proliferation) to FNA specimens may be helpful for predicting tumor risk of malignancy. In a study of 23 GISTs, the use of Ki-67 combined with EUS-FNA cytology had a sensitivity and specificity of 100% for malignant GIST.[76]

The addition of EUS-guided core biopsy to EUS-FNA is performed to increase the diagnostic yield, and provide mitotic index, which can be used to risk-stratify GISTs and potentially guide patient management. Initial studies on the use of EUS-guided (Trucut core) biopsy, known as EUS-TCB, were performed using a 19 gauge Tru-cut needle which is no longer available on the market. Although initial studies showed an increase in diagnostic yield with EUS-TCB, other studies showed that EUS-TCB had either no improvement or only modest improvement in diagnostic yield compared with EUS-FNA, mainly due to the high rate of failure of EUS-TCB.[77–79] In the past decade, a variety of needles have been introduced to the market which have been effectively used for EUS fine-needle biopsy (EUS-FNB) of subepithelial lesions and suspected GISTs. In a study of 229 patients with subepithelial lesions, the sensitivity and accuracy of EUS-FNB were superior to EUS-FNA (79.4% vs 51.9%, and 88% vs 77.2%, respectively).[80] In a multicenter study of 147 suspected GISTs, the diagnostic yield of EUS-FNB was 89% compared to 37% seen with EUS-FNA.[81]

Several studies have now demonstrated the utility of EUS-FNB for mutational analysis to detect c-KIT and PDGFRA mutations prior to neoadjuvant treatment with tyrosine kinase inhibitors. DNA sequencing of FNB specimens is successful in 95% to 98% of cases.[82–84] The detection of c-KIT and PDGFRA mutations allows for individualized, targeted therapy with tyrosine kinase inhibitors. (See Management section).

MANAGEMENT

A detailed review of the surgical and medical management of GISTs is beyond the scope of this article and is outlined elsewhere.[1]

Surgical resection is the primary treatment for patients with localized tumors ≥2 cm or potentially resectable lesions without evidence of metastasis.[1] The goal is to achieve complete resection. Segmental or wedge resection is recommended, and wide margins of resection do not appear to be necessary. Lymphadenectomy does not need to be performed as lymph node metastases are rare. Resection of pathologically enlarged nodes should be considered in cases of SDH-deficient tumors. Laparoscopic approach is preferred in select cases (tumors in the stomach anterior wall, jejunum, and ileum), and may be associated with low recurrence, short hospital duration, and low morbidity.[1,85]

Imatinib is a selective inhibitor of several tyrosine kinases including c-KIT and PDGFRA. The FDA approved imatinib in 2002 for the treatment of unresectable and metastatic GIST. The optimal dose is 400 mg daily. Currently, imatinib is indicated in the treatment of advanced diseases including tumors that are metastatic, and locally invasive tumors. Imatinib is also indicated as adjuvant therapy for resected tumors with high-risk features. Neoadjuvant therapy with imatinib is indicated in patients with potentially resectable tumors with significant perioperative morbidity, locally advanced unresectable tumors, borderline resectable tumors, and rectal tumors.

The presence and type of c-KIT or PDGFRA mutation have been identified as predictors of response to imatinib.[1,86] Subsequently, genetic analysis for mutations or genotyping, should be considered in patients undergoing neoadjuvant or adjuvant therapy. In a study by Blanke and colleagues, response to imatinib was found to be dependent on c-KIT mutation.[87] Exon 11 mutations were associated with better survival.[87] Furthermore, exon 9 mutations were associated with lower survival, and increasing the dose of imatinib to 800 mg a day resulted in a benefit in progression-free survival.[87] Several randomized trials have shown that the presence of c-KIT exon 11 mutation is associated with better response rates, progression-free survival, and overall survival compared to exon 9 mutations or wild-type tumors.[1] GISTs with D842V exon 18 PDGFRA mutation are resistant to imatinib and should be treated with alternative tyrosine kinase inhibitors. SDH deficient GISTs are poorly responsive to imatinib and have higher probability of responding to sunitinib, another tyrosine kinase inhibitor. Sunitinib is indicated in patients who are intolerant to imatinib, or who are shown to have disease progression on imatinib. Other tyrosine kinase inhibitors can be used in the setting of advanced GISTs with resistance to imatinib and sunitinib, including regorafenib, sorafenib, nilotinib, dasatinib, and pazopanib.[1]

The management of small <2 cm, incidentally found, asymptomatic GISTs is controversial. Surveillance with EUS can be considered in stomach GISTs less than 2 cm with no high-risk EUS features (irregular border, heterogeneous echo pattern, presence of cystic spaces, and echogenic foci).[1,88] The frequency of EUS surveillance is not known, but every 12 months may be considered.[88]

Endoscopic resection of GISTs using a variety of endoscopic techniques has been described.[60] It can be performed in small (<2 cm) lesions of the stomach located within the muscularis mucosa or submucosa. Resection of tumors in the muscularis propria and tumors >2 cm in size has been reported with variable follow-up and is associated with expected risk of perforation and bleeding. If performed, this should be done in expert, high-volume centers. Additional studies are needed to determine the role of endoscopic resection in the management of GIST.

SUMMARY

GISTs are mesenchymal tumors of the gastrointestinal tract that harbor oncogenic mutations of c-KIT and PDGFRA. All GISTs have the potential to behave in a malignant fashion. Several models have been proposed to risk stratify tumors based on location, size, and mitotic index. EUS-FNA is the most reliable method of obtaining tissue diagnosis. EUS-guided fine-needle biopsy can be used to obtain core tissue specimens which can then be analyzed for genetic mutations of c-KIT and PDGFRA. This information can help determine neoadjuvant therapy in select patients. Current management of patients includes surgical resection and tyrosine kinase inhibitors. Gastroenterologists currently play a critical role in the care of these patients.

CLINICS CARE POINTS

- All GISTs have the potential to behave in a malignant fashion.
- EUS with FNA and FNB are essential in the diagnosis and risk-stratification of GISTs.
- Surgical resection is the mainstay of treatment.
- Tyrosine kinase inhibitors can be used as neoadjuvant therapy in potentially resectable and locally advanced unresectable GISTs. They are also indicated in the treatment of recurrent or metastatic disease.

DISCLOSURE

The authors have nothing to disclose.

REFERENCES

1. National Comprehensive Cancer Network Guidelines Version 1.2022 Gastrointestinal Stromal Tumors (GISTs). Available at: http://www.nccn.org/professionals/physician_gls/pdf/sarcoma.pdf. Accessed May 31, 2022.
2. Reith JD, Goldblum JR, Lyles RH, et al. Extragastrointestinal (soft tissue) stromal tumors: an analysis of 48 cases with emphasis on histologic predictors of outcome. Mod Pathol 2000;13:577–85.
3. Miettinen M, Sarlomo-Rikala M, Lasota J. Gastrointestinal stromal tumors: Recent advances in understanding of their biology. Hum Pathol 1999;30:1213–20.
4. Miettinen M, Lasota J. Gastrointestinal stromal tumors – Definition, clinical, histological, immunohistochemical, and molecular genetic features and differential diagnosis. Virchows Arch 2001;438:1–12.
5. Hirota S, Isozaki K, Moriyama Y, et al. Gain-of-function mutations of c-kit in human gastrointestinal stromal tumors. Science 1998;279:577–80.
6. Nakahara M, Isozaki K, Hirota S, et al. A novel gain-of-function mutation of c-kit gene in gastrointestinal stromal tumors. Gastroenterology 1998;115:1090–5.
7. Hirota S, Nishida T, Isozaki K, et al. Gain-of-function mutation at the extracellular domain of KIT in gastrointestinal stromal tumours. J Pathol 2001;193:505–10.
8. Sarlomo-Rikala M, Kovatich AJ, Barusevicius A, et al. CD117: A sensitive marker for gastrointestinal stromal tumors that is more specific than CD34. Mod Pathol 1998;11:728–34.
9. Miettinen M, Sobin LH, Sarlomo-Rikala M. Immunohistochemical spectrum of GISTs at different sites and their differential diagnosis with a reference to CD117 (KIT). Mod Pathol 2000;13:1134–42.
10. Miettinen M, Wang ZF, Lasota J. DOG1 antibody in the differential diagnosis of gastrointestinal stromal tumors: a study of 1840 cases. Am J Surg Pathol 2009;33:1401–8.

11. Liegl B, Hornick JL, Corless CL, et al. Monoclonal antibody DOG1.1 shows higher sensitivity than KIT in the diagnosis of gastrointestinal stromal tumors, including unusual subtypes. Am J Surg Pathol 2009;33:437–46.

12. Sanders KM. A case for interstitial cells of Cajal as pacemakers and mediators of neurotransmission in the gastrointestinal tract. Gastroenterology 1996;111: 492–515.

13. Kindblom LG, Remotti HE, Aldenborg F, et al. Gastrointestinal pacemaker cell tumor (GIPACT): gastrointestinal stromal tumors show phenotypic characteristics of the interstitial cells of Cajal. Am J Pathol 1998;152:1259–69.

14. Sakurai S, Fukasawa T, Chong JM, et al. Embryonic form of smooth muscle myosin heavy chain (SMemb/MHC-B) in gastrointestinal stromal tumor and interstitial cells of Cajal. Am J Pathol 1999;154:23–8.

15. Wang L, Vargas H, French SW. Cellular origin of gastrointestinal stromal tumors: a study of 27 cases. Arch Pathol Lab Med 2000;124:1471–5.

16. Søreide K, Sandvik OM, Søreide JA, et al. Global epidemiology of gastrointestinal stromal tumours (GIST): A systematic review of population-based cohort studies. Cancer Epidemiol 2016;40:39–46.

17. Patel N, Benipal B. Incidence of gastrointestinal stromal tumors in the United States from 2001-2015: A United States Cancer Statistics analysis of 50 states. Cureus 2019;11:e4120.

18. Ulanja MB, Rishi M, Beutler BD, et al. Racial disparity in incidence and survival for gastrointestinal stromal tumors (GISTs): an analysis of SEER database. J Racial Ethn Health Disparities 2019;6:1035–43.

19. Miettinen M, Sarlomo-Rikala M, Lasota J. Gastrointestinal stromal tumours. Ann Chir Gynaecol 1998;87:278–81.

20. Tran T, Davila JA, El-Serag HB. The epidemiology of malignant gastrointestinal stromal tumors: an analysis of 1,458 cases from 1992-2000. Am J Gastroenterol 2005;100:162–8.

21. Davila RE, Faigel DO. GI stromal tumors. Gastrointest Endosc 2003;58:80–8.

22. Miettinen M, El-Rifai W, Sobin LH, et al. Evaluation of malignancy and prognosis of gastrointestinal stromal tumors: A review. Hum Pathol 2002;33:478–83.

23. Fletcher CD, Berman JJ, Corless C, et al. Diagnosis of gastrointestinal stromal tumors: A consensus approach. Hum Pathol 2002;33:459–65.

24. Miettinen M, Lasota J. Gastrointestinal stromal tumors: pathology and prognosis at different sites. Semin Diagn Pathol 2006;23:70–83.

25. Joensuu H. Risk stratification of patients diagnosed with gastrointestinal stromal tumor. Hum Pathol 2008;39:1411–9.

26. Lux ML, Rubin BP, Biase TL, et al. KIT extracellular and kinase domain mutations in gastrointestinal stromal tumors. Am J Pathol 2000;156:791–5.

27. Rubin BP, Singer S, Tsao C, et al. KIT activation is a ubiquitous feature of gastrointestinal stromal tumors. Cancer Res 2001;61:8118–21.

28. Moskaluk CA, Tian Q, Marshall CR, et al. Mutations of c-kit JM domain are found in a minority of human gastrointestinal stromal tumors. Oncogene 1999;18: 1897–902.

29. Ernst SI, Hubbs AE, Przygodzki RM, et al. KIT mutation portends poor prognosis in gastrointestinal stromal/smooth muscle tumors. Lab Invest 1998;78:1633–6.

30. Hirota S, Isozaki K. Pathology of gastrointestinal stromal tumors. Pathol Int 2006; 56:1–9.

31. Taniguchi M, Nishida T, Hirota S, et al. Effect of c-kit mutation on prognosis of gastrointestinal stromal tumors. Cancer Res 1999;59:4297–300.

32. Lasota J, Wozniak A, Sarlomo-Rikala M, et al. Mutations in exons 9 and 13 of KIT gene are rare events in gastrointestinal stromal tumors. A study of 200 cases. Am J Pathol 2000;157:1091–5.
33. Sakurai S, Oguni S, Hironaka M, et al. Mutations in c-kit gene exons 9 and 13 in gastrointestinal stromal tumors among Japanese. Jpn J Cancer Res 2001;92: 494–8.
34. Corless CL, McGreevey L, Haley A, et al. KIT mutations are common in incidental gastrointestinal stromal tumors one centimeter or less in size. Am J Pathol 2002; 160:1567–72.
35. Heinrich MC, Corless CL, Duensing A, et al. PDGFRA activating mutations in gastrointestinal stromal tumors. Science 2003;299:708–10.
36. Corless CL, Schroeder A, Griffith D, et al. PDGFRA mutations in gastrointestinal stromal tumors: frequency, spectrum and in vitro sensitivity to imatinib. J Clin Oncol 2005;23:5357–64.
37. Janeway KA, Kim SY, Lodish M, et al. Defects in succinate dehydrogenase in gastrointestinal stromal tumors lacking KIT and PDGFRA mutations. Proc Natl Acad Sci U S A 2011;108:314–8.
38. Tateishi U, Hasegawa T, Satake M, et al. Gastrointestinal stromal tumor. Correlation of computer tomography findings with tumor grade and mortality. J Comput Assist Tomogr 2003;27:792–8.
39. Levy AD, Remotti HE, Thompson WM, et al. Gastrointestinal stromal tumors: radiologic features with pathologic correlation. Radiographics 2003;23:283–304.
40. Xu J, Zhou J, Wang X, et al. A multi-class scoring system based on CT features for preoperative prediction in gastric gastrointestinal stromal tumors. Am J Cancer Res 2020;10:3867–81.
41. Levy AD, Remotti HE, Thompson WM, et al. Anorectal gastrointestinal stromal tumors: CT and MR imaging features with clinical and pathologic correlation. AJR Am J Roentgenol 2003;180:1607–12.
42. Hwang JH, Rulyak SD, Kimmey MB. American Gastroenterological Association Institute technical review on the management of gastric subepithelial masses. Gastroenterology 2006;130:2217–28.
43. Standards of Practice Committee, Faulx AL, Kothari S, et al. The role of endoscopy in subepithelial lesions of the GI tract. Gastrointest Endosc 2017;85: 1117–32.
44. Hunt GC, Smith PP, Faigel DO. Yield of tissue sampling for submucosal lesions evaluated by EUS. Gastrointest Endosc 2003;57:68–72.
45. Cantor MJ, Davila RE, Faigel DO. Yield of tissue sampling for subepithelial lesions evaluated by EUS: a comparison between forceps biopsies and endoscopic submucosal resection. Gastrointest Endosc 2003;64:29–34.
46. Hoda KM, Rodriguez SA, Faigel DO. EUS-guided sampling of suspected GI stromal tumors. Gastrointest Endosc 2009;69:1218–23.
47. Rondonotti E, Pennazio M, Toth E, et al. Small-bowel neoplasms in patients undergoing video capsule endoscopy: a multicenter European study. Endoscopy 2008; 40:488–95.
48. ASGE Standards of Practice Committee, Khashab MA, Pasha SF, Muthusamy VR, et al. The role of deep enteroscopy in the management of small-bowel disorders. Gastrointest Endosc 2015;82:600–7.
49. Mitsui K, Tanaka S, Yamamoto H, et al. Role of double-balloon endoscopy in the diagnosis of small-bowel tumors: the first Japanese multicenter study. Gastrointest Endosc 2009;70:498–504.

50. Pasha SF, Leighton JA, Das A, et al. Double-balloon enteroscopy and capsule endoscopy have comparable diagnostic yield in small-bowel disease: a meta-analysis. Clin Gastroenterol Hepatol 2008;6:671–6.
51. Lewis BS, Eisen GM, Friedman S. A pooled analysis to evaluate results of capsule endoscopy trials. Endoscopy 2005;37:960–5.
52. Ross A, Mehdizadeh S, Tokar J, et al. Double balloon enteroscopy detects small bowel mass lesions missed by capsule endoscopy. Dig Dis Sci 2008;53:2140–3.
53. Chong AKH, Chin BWK, Meredith CG. Clinically significant small-bowel pathology identified by double-balloon enteroscopy but missed by capsule endoscopy. Gastrointest Endosc 2006;64:445–9.
54. Jonanovic I, Krivokapic Z, Nenkovic N, et al. Ineffectiveness of capsule endoscopy and total double-balloon enteroscopy to elicit the cause of obscure overt gastrointestinal bleeding: think GIST! Endoscopy 2011;43(Suppl 2 UCTN):E91–2.
55. Caletti G, Zani L, Bolondi L, et al. Endoscopic ultrasonography in the diagnosis of gastric submucosal tumor. Gastrointest Endosc 1989;35:413–8.
56. Tio TL, Tytgat GN, den Hartog Jager FC. Endoscopic ultrasonography for the evaluation of smooth muscle tumors in the upper gastrointestinal tract: An experience with 42 cases. Gastrointest Endosc 1990;36:342–50.
57. Boyce GA, Sivak MV, Rösch T, et al. Evaluation of submucosal upper gastrointestinal tract lesions by endoscopic ultrasound. Gastrointest Endosc 1991;37: 449–54.
58. Kameyama H, Niwa Y, Arisawa T, et al. Endoscopic ultrasonography in the diagnosis of submucosal lesions of the large intestine. Gastrointest Endosc 1997;46: 406–11.
59. Savides TJ. Gastrointestinal submucosal masses. In: Gress FG, Battacharya I, editors. Endoscopic Ultrasonography. Malden: Blackwell Science; 2001. p. 92–102.
60. Faigel DO, Abulhawa S. Gastrointestinal stromal tumors: the role of the gastroenterologist in diagnosis and risk stratification. J Clin Gastroenterol 2012;46:629–36.
61. Chak A, Canto MI, Rösch T, et al. Endosonographic differentiation of benign and malignant stromal cell tumors. Gastrointest Endosc 1997;45:468–73.
62. Palazzo L, Landi B, Cellier C, et al. Endosonographic features predictive of benign and malignant gastrointestinal stromal cell tumours. Gut 2000;46:88–92.
63. Shah P, Gao F, Edmundowicz SA, et al. Predicting malignant potential of gastrointestinal stromal tumors using endoscopic ultrasound. Dig Dis Sci 2009;54: 1265–9.
64. Jeon SW, Park YD, Chung YJ, et al. Gastrointestinal stromal tumors of the stomach: endosonographic differentiation in relation to histological risk. J Gastroenterol Hepatol 2007;22:2069–75.
65. Chen TH, Hsu CM, Chu YY, et al. Association of endoscopic ultrasonographic parameters and gastrointestinal stromal tumors (GISTs): can endoscopic ultrasonography be used to screen gastric GISTs for potential malignancy? Scand J Gastroenterol 2016;51:374–7.
66. Kim MN, Kang SJ, Kim SG, et al. Prediction of risk of malignancy of gastrointestinal stromal tumors by endoscopic ultrasonography. Gut and Liver 2013;7:642–7.
67. Seven G, Arici DS, Senturk H. Correlation of endoscopic ultrasonography features with the mitotic index in 2- to 5-cm gastric gastrointestinal stromal tumors. Dig Dis 2022;40:14–22.
68. Kamata K, Takenaka M, Kitano M, et al. Contrast-enhanced harmonic endoscopic ultrasonography for differential diagnosis of submucosal tumors of the upper gastrointestinal tract. J Gastroenterol Hepatol 2017;32:1686–92.

69. Sakamoto H, Kitano M, Matsui S, et al. Estimation of malignant potential of GI stromal tumors by contrast-enhanced harmonic EUS (with videos). Gastrointest Endosc 2011;73:227–37.

70. Tsuji Y, Kusano C, Gotoda T, et al. Diagnostic potential of endoscopic ultrasonography-elastography of gastric submucosal tumors: A pilot study. Dig Endosc 2016;28:173–8.

71. Hirai K, Kuwahara T, Furukawa K, et al. Artificial intelligence-based diagnosis of upper gastrointestinal subepithelial lesions on endoscopic ultrasonography images. Gastric Cancer 2022;25:382–91.

72. Sepe P, Moparty B, Pitman MB, et al. EUS-guided FNA for the diagnosis of GI stromal cell tumors: sensitivity and cytology yield. Gastrointest Endosc 2009; 70:254–61.

73. Watson RR, Binmoeller KF, Hamerski CM, et al. Yield and performance characteristics of endoscopic ultrasound-guided fine needle aspiration for diagnosing upper GI tract stromal tumors. Dig Dis Sci 2011;56:1757–62.

74. Gu M, Ghafari S, Nguyen PT, et al. Cytologic diagnosis of gastrointestinal stromal tumors of the stomach by endoscopic ultrasound-guided fine-needle aspiration biopsy. Cytomorphologic and immunohistochemical study of 12 cases. Diagn Cytopathol 2001;25:343–50.

75. Rader AE, Avery A, Wait CL, et al. Fine-needle aspiration biopsy diagnosis of gastrointestinal stromal tumors using morphology, immunocytochemistry, and mutational analysis of c-kit. Cancer Cytopathol 2001;93:269–75.

76. Ando N, Goto H, Niwa Y, et al. The diagnosis of GI stromal tumors with EUS-guided fine needle aspiration with immunohistochemical analysis. Gastrointest Endosc 2002;55:37–43.

77. Dewitt J, Emerson RE, Sherman S, et al. Endoscopic ultrasound-guided Trucut biopsy of gastrointestinal mesenchymal tumor. Surg Endosc 2011;25:2192–202.

78. Fernández-Esparrach G, Sendino O, Solé O, et al. Endoscopic ultrasound-guided fine-needle aspiration and trucut biopsy in the diagnosis of gastric stromal tumors, a randomized crossover study. Endoscopy 2010;42:292–9.

79. Polkowski M, Gerke W, Jarosz D, et al. Diagnostic yield and safety of endoscopic ultrasound-guided trucut [corrected] biopsy in patients with gastric submucosal tumors: a prospective study. Endoscopy 2009;41:329–34.

80. De Moura DTH, McCarty TR, Jirapinyo P, et al. EUS-guided fine-needle biopsy sampling versus FNA in the diagnosis of subepithelial lesions: a large multicenter study. Gastrointest Endosc 2020;92:108–19.

81. Trindade AJ, Benias PC, Alshelleh M, et al. Fine-needle biopsy is superior to fine-needle aspiration of suspected gastrointestinal stromal tumors: a large multicenter study. Endosc Int Open 2019;7:E931–6.

82. Hedenström P, Nilsson B, Demir A, et al. Characterizing gastrointestinal stromal tumors and evaluating neoadjuvant imatinib by sequencing of endoscopic ultrasound-biopsies. World J Gastroenterol 2017;23:5925–35.

83. Funasaka K, Miyahara R, Furukawa K, et al. Mutation analysis of gastrointestinal stromal tumors using RNA obtained via endoscopic ultrasound-guided fine-needle aspiration. Transl Oncol 2020;13:1–7.

84. Hedenström P, Andersson C, Slovall H, et al. Pretreatment tumor DNA sequencing of KIT and PDGFRA in endosonography-guided biopsies optimizes the preoperative management of gastrointestinal stromal tumors. Mol Diagn Ther 2020;24:201–14.

85. Demetri GD, von Mehren M, Antonescu CR, et al. NCCN Task Force report; update on the management of patients with gastrointestinal stromal tumors. J Natl Compr Canc Netw 2010;8(Suppl 2):S1–41.
86. Lasota J, Miettinen M. Clinical significance of oncogenic *KIT* and *PDGFRA* mutations in gastrointestinal stromal tumours. Histopathology 2008;53:245–66.
87. Blanke CD, Demetri GD, von Mehren M, et al. Long-term results from a randomized phase II trial of standard- versus higher-dose imatinib mesylate for patients with unresectable or metastatic gastrointestinal stromal tumors expressing KIT. J Clin Oncol 2008;26:620–5.
88. ASGE Standards of Practice Committee, Evans JA, Chandrasekhara V, Chathadi KV, et al. The role of endoscopy in the management of premalignant and malignant conditions of the stomach. Gastrointest Endosc 2015;82:1–8.

Gastroenteropancreatic Neuroendocrine Tumors

Conrad J. Fernandes, MD[a], Galen Leung, MD[b], Jennifer R. Eads, MD[c], Bryson W. Katona, MD, PhD[b],*

KEYWORDS

- Gastroenteropancreatic neuroendocrine tumor • Endoscopy
- Functional neuroendocrine tumor • Carcinoid syndrome

KEY POINTS

- The incidence of neuroendocrine tumors of the gastrointestinal tract and the pancreas (GEP-NETs) is increasing.
- GEP-NETs are oftentimes discovered incidentally on imaging or during endoscopic evaluation for other indications.
- Upon diagnosis, it is critical to classify GEP-NETs based on their location, grade, stage, and functionality, because these factors are important for prognosis and management.
- Management of GEP-NETs depends on multiple tumor-specific factors and can involve surveillance alone, endoscopic therapy, surgery, somatostatin analogues, peptide receptor radionuclide therapy (PRRT), liver-directed therapies, and systemic therapy with targeted agents or chemotherapy.
- Gastroenterologists play a major role in the diagnosis, treatment, and surveillance of GEP-NETs and should therefore be an integral part of all comprehensive GEP-NET management teams.

INTRODUCTION

Neuroendocrine tumors (NETs) are an uncommon, heterogeneous group of tumors arising from cells of neuroendocrine origin, which can be found at multiple sites throughout the body. Although NETs have classically been considered more indolent

[a] Department of Medicine, Hospital of the University of Pennsylvania, 3400 Civic Center Boulevard, 751 South Pavilion, Philadelphia, PA 19104, USA; [b] Division of Gastroenterology and Hepatology, Department of Medicine, Perelman School of Medicine at the University of Pennsylvania, 3400 Civic Center Boulevard, 751 South Pavilion, Philadelphia, PA 19104, USA; [c] Division of Hematology/Oncology, Department of Medicine, Perelman School of Medicine at the University of Pennsylvania, 3400 Civic Center Boulevard, 751 South Pavilion, Philadelphia, PA 19104, USA
* Corresponding author. Perelman Center for Advanced Medicine, University of Pennsylvania Perelman School of Medicine, 3400 Civic Center Boulevard 751 South Pavilion, Philadelphia, PA 19104.
E-mail address: bryson.katona@pennmedicine.upenn.edu

Gastroenterol Clin N Am 51 (2022) 625–647
https://doi.org/10.1016/j.gtc.2022.06.002
0889-8553/22/© 2022 Elsevier Inc. All rights reserved.

than many other tumor types, there is now growing recognition that some NETs can be aggressive, leading to substantial morbidity and mortality.[1]

EPIDEMIOLOGY

The incidence of NETs has increased in the last few decades, with the Surveillance, Epidemiology, and End Results (SEER) database showing a 6.4-fold increase in the age-adjusted incidence rate of NETs in the United States from 1973 to 2012, now totaling 6.98 per 100,000.[2] Similar trends are noted in other countries and across different primary NET sites.[3–7] Although some of this increased incidence may be due to improved detection of earlier-stage asymptomatic lesions and an aging population, there are likely other unknown factors contributing as well.[2,5,8] The overall survival of patients with NETs has also improved over the last few decades.[2] Although increased detection of asymptomatic and indolent NETs likely plays a role in this trend, the observed improved overall survival in metastatic NETs also results from improvements in NET treatment modalities.[2]

NETs originate from multiple primary sites as illustrated in **Fig. 1**. Most NETs are found in the luminal gastrointestinal (GI) tract or pancreas (55%–70%), collectively known as gastroenteropancreatic NETs (GEP-NETs).[9,10] The remainder of this review focuses primarily on the diagnosis and management of GEP-NETs.

CLASSIFICATION
Location

GEP-NETs themselves are heterogeneous and can be located throughout the GI tract. These tumors can be subgrouped based on location and classified as gastric, small bowel (including duodenal/ampullary and jejunal/ileal), pancreatic, and colonic (including colonic, rectal, and appendiceal) NETs. The relative proportions of these subgroups are shown in **Fig. 1**. GEP-NET location is important in diagnosis and management and may help define prognosis because overall survival varies by location, with pancreatic NETs having the worst median overall survival and rectal NETs having the best.[1,7] GEP-NET location is also particularly important for management because pancreatic NETs (pNETs) have some unique treatment options that are not used for luminal NETs.[11]

Grading

GEP-NET grade is assigned as G1, G2, or G3 as outlined by the most recent World Health Organization definitions from 2019.[12] Grade is based on histologic characteristics of the tumor including differentiation, mitotic rate, and Ki-67 indices as outlined in **Table 1**. Tumor grading should be performed on all newly diagnosed GEP-NETs, because NET grade is important for management and prognosis.[13] While NETs are by definition well-differentiated tumors, neuroendocrine carcinomas (NECs) are poorly differentiated tumors with distinct molecular differences from NETs.[14] Collectively, NETs and NECs fall under the umbrella term of neuroendocrine neoplasms (NENs). GEP-NECs are divided into large-cell type and small-cell type based on histology, with approximately 60% of GEP-NECs being large-cell type.[15] Overall survival of GEP-NECs is poor, with a median survival ranging from 5 months in metastatic disease to 38 months in localized disease.[16] Given the scope of this article, the remainder of this review focuses only on GEP-NETs.

Functional Versus Nonfunctional

NETs can also be classified as functional or nonfunctional based on their ability to secrete hormones. Most GEP-NETs are nonfunctional (approximately 60%), although

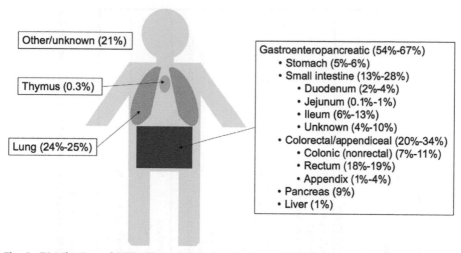

Fig. 1. Distribution of NETs. The relative distribution of NETs based on data from the SEER database. (*Data from* Modlin IM, Lye KD, Kidd M. A 5-decade analysis of 13,715 carcinoid tumors. *Cancer.* 2003;97(4):934-959 and Sackstein PE, O'Neil DS, Neugut AI, Chabot J, Fojo T. Epidemiologic trends in neuroendocrine tumors: an examination of incidence rates and survival of specific patient subgroups over the past 20 years. Semin Oncol. 2018;45(4):249-258)

the incidence of functional GEP-NETs may be increasing.[17] Functional GEP-NETs can present with a wide variety of clinical syndromes that depend on the site of origin of the tumor. Functional pNETs include insulinomas, gastrinomas, VIPomas, glucagonomas, and somatostatinomas, which are found mainly in the pancreas, and also sometimes in the duodenum (**Table 2**). NETs arising in the intestinal tract, especially those of small bowel origin, are known to cause carcinoid syndrome. Carcinoid syndrome is associated with secretory diarrhea (58%–100%), skin flushing (45%–96%), wheezing (3%–18%), pellagra-like skin lesions (1%), and right-sided heart disease (11%–70%),

Table 1
Classification and grading criteria of neuroendocrine neoplasms of the gastrointestinal tract and pancreas

Classification	Differentiation	Grade	Mitotic Rate (Mitoses/ 2 mm² or Mitoses/ 10HPFs)	Ki-67 Index
Grade 1 NET (G1)	Well differentiated	Low	<2	<3%
Grade 2 NET (G2)	Well differentiated	Intermediate	2–20	3%–20%
Grade 3 NET (G3)	Well differentiated	High	>20	>20%
NEC	Poorly differentiated	High	>20	>20%

Characteristics used to classify NENs, including NETs and NECs.
Abbreviations: HPFs, high-power fields; NEC, neuroendocrine carcinoma; NEN, neuroendocrine neoplasm.
Adapted from Nagtegaal ID, Odze RD, Klimstra D, et al. The 2019 WHO classification of tumors of the digestive system. Histopathology. 2020;76(2):182–188; with permission.

Table 2
Most common functional pancreatic neuroendocrine tumors

Tumor Type	Incidence per 100,000/year	Primary Tumor Location	Malignant	Secreted Hormone	Important Clinical Associations	Clinical Syndrome
Insulinoma	1–3	Pancreas	5%–15%	Insulin	Hypoglycemia, neuroglycopenic symptoms (visual changes, confusion, seizures), autonomic symptoms (diaphoresis palpitations)	N/A
Gastrinoma	0.5–1.5	Duodenum (70%), pancreas (25%), gastrinoma triangle	60%–90%	Gastrin	Peptic ulcer disease, esophagitis, diarrhea, abdominal pain	Zollinger-Ellison syndrome
VIPoma	0.05–2	Pancreas	70%–90%	VIP	Diarrhea, achlorhydria/hypochlorhydria, hypokalemia, dehyration	Verner-Morrison syndrome, WDHA syndrome, pancreatic cholera syndrome
Glucagonoma	0.01–0.1	Pancreas	60%–75%	Glucagon	Diabetes mellitus, necrolytic migratory erythema (rash), weight loss	N/A
Somatostatinoma	<0.1%	Pancreas	40%–60%	Somatostatin	Diabetes mellitus, cholelithiasis, diarrhea (steatorrhea)	N/A

Incidence and clinical characteristics of the more common functional pNETs.

Abbreviations: N/A, not applicable; VIP, vasoactive intestinal peptide; WDHA, watery diarrhea-hypokalemia-achlorhydria.

Adapted from Ito T, Igarashi H, Jensen RT. Pancreatic neuroendocrine tumors: clinical features, diagnosis and medical treatment: advances. Best Pract Res Clin Gastroenterol. 2012;26(6):737–753; with permission.

also known as cardiac carcinoid. Carcinoid syndrome can be present in up to 20% of patients with a small bowel NET.[18–20] Symptoms of carcinoid syndrome result from NET secretion of multiple vasoactive products, including serotonin and serotonin metabolites.[18] Oftentimes carcinoid syndrome only arises from NETs with substantial liver metastases, because hepatic metabolism normally neutralizes vasoactive substances secreted by NETs into the portal circulation before they reach the systemic circulation. However, carcinoid syndrome can arise in the absence of extensive hepatic disease, particularly in patients with a large tumor burden.[18,21–24]

PRESENTATION AND DIAGNOSIS OF GASTROENTEROPANCREATIC NEUROENDOCRINE TUMORS

There are differences in the presentation and diagnosis of GEP-NETs based on primary tumor site; therefore, each primary tumor site is reviewed separately. Diagnosis of GEP-NETs often relies on multiple different modalities, including endoscopy, surgery, laboratory tests, and imaging. The widespread use of endoscopy has led to an increase in the diagnosis of early-stage GEP-NETs.[25] In addition, although traditional cross-sectional imaging modalities such as computed tomography (CT) and MRI are frequently used in NET diagnosis, there have also been great improvements in functional somatostatin-receptor-based imaging using ^{68}Ga-DOTATATE, ^{68}Ga-DOTATOC, and ^{64}Cu-DOTATATE that have substantially improved the ability to image GEP-NETs.[26,27]

Gastric

Presentation
Gastric NETs (gNETs) can present with nonspecific symptoms such as abdominal pain, anemia, or GI bleeding but can also be identified incidentally on endoscopy. gNETs are divided into 3 subtypes with different characteristics, mechanisms of tumorigenesis, and metastatic potential as outlined in **Table 3**.[28,29] Type 1 gNETs typically arise in the setting of chronic atrophic gastritis, resulting from either autoimmune gastritis or *Helicobacter pylori*-associated atrophic gastritis, which leads to loss of parietal cells, an increase in gastrin levels, and resulting hypertrophy of enterochromaffin-like cells. There is emerging evidence that long-term treatment with proton pump inhibitors (PPIs) can also lead to elevated gastrin levels, which can be associated with the development of type 1 gNETs.[30,31] Type 2 gNETs are typically associated with Zollinger-Ellison syndrome, a rare syndrome in which a gastrinoma leads to elevated gastrin levels, and which can be associated with multiple endocrine neoplasia type 1 (MEN1) syndrome.[32] Although localized gNETs are most frequently asymptomatic, individuals with Zollinger-Ellison syndrome-associated type 2 gNETs may have substantial upper GI symptoms resulting from reflux esophagitis and peptic ulcer disease due to acid hypersecretion.[28] Type 3 gNETs develop independently of hypergastrinemia and occur sporadically, yet these gNETs are the most aggressive and are associated with the worst prognosis.

Diagnosis
gNETs are most frequently identified incidentally on esophagogastroduodenoscopy (EGD) being performed for other indications, and will most often present as polypoid lesions predominantly found in the fundus or body of the stomach.[28] Type 1 gNETs will typically be associated with flattened gastric folds and atrophic-appearing gastric mucosa, often coupled with an elevated gastric pH (while off acid suppression therapy).[28,33] In contrast, type 2 gNETs are found along with hypertrophied gastric folds, and can be associated with a low gastric pH (while off acid suppression

Table 3
Comparison of gastric neuroendocrine tumor subtypes

	Type 1	Type 2	Type 3
Proportion of all gastric NETs	70%–80%	5%–10%	15%–20%
Location	Body and fundus	Body and fundus	Body and fundus
Size	Small (<2 cm)	Small (<2 cm)	Large (>2 cm)
Number of tumors	Frequently multiple	Frequently multiple	Single lesion
Associated conditions	Chronic atrophic gastritis, possibly chronic PPI use	Gastrinoma (Zollinger-Ellison syndrome), MEN1 syndrome	None
Fasting serum gastrin level	↑	↑	Normal
Gastric pH	↑	↓	Normal
Gastric mucosa appearance	Atrophic	Hypertrophic	Normal
Invasion	Rare	Intermediate	Common
Lymph node metastases	5%–10%	10%–20%	50%–100%
Prognosis	Excellent	Very good	Similar to gastric adenocarcinoma

Characteristics, distinguishing features, and prognostic features of the subtypes of gastric NETs.
Abbreviations: ↑, Increase; ↓, decrease; MEN1, multiple endocrine neoplasia type 1; PPI, proton pump inhibitor.
Adapted from Grozinsky-Glasberg S, Alexandraki KI, Angelousi A, Chatzellis E, Sougioultzis S, Kaltsas G. Gastric carcinoids. Endocrinol Metab Clin North Am. 2018;47(3):645-660; with permission.

therapy), especially in the setting of Zollinger-Ellison syndrome.[33] Endoscopically, type 1 and 2 gNETs, which arise from the mucosa or muscularis mucosa and may invade into the submucosa, generally appear as multiple smooth round subepithelial or polypoid lesions.[34] There may also be a red or yellow mucosal hue with central depression.[34] Type 3 gNETs usually appear as a single lesion with signs of ulceration, indicating deeper invasion.[35] Type 1 and 2 gNETs are also usually smaller in size (<1–2 cm) compared with type 3 gNETs, which can often be greater than 2 cm.[28] Diagnosis of a gNET is typically made endoscopically via forceps biopsy or after gastric polypectomy. If suspicion for a gNET is high on the index EGD, biopsies should be obtained from the antrum and body to assess for underlying atrophic gastritis, intestinal metaplasia, and *H pylori*. In addition, a gastric pH and fasting serum gastrin level should be obtained.[28] Gastric pH and fasting gastrin levels can both be altered by chronic PPI use, therefore, ideally a PPI should be stopped for 1 to 2 weeks before testing if clinically safe to do so.[36]

Once a histologic diagnosis of a gNET is made, other ancillary data are critical to determine the type of gNET. Elevated serum gastrin levels can help differentiate between type 1/2 (elevated gastrin) and type 3 (normal gastrin). Gastric biopsies showing atrophic gastritis, an elevated gastric pH (off acid suppression therapy), and positive anti-parietal cell and anti-intrinsic factor antibodies would be consistent with a type 1 gNET in the setting of chronic autoimmune atrophic gastritis, where resulting hypergastrinemia would be considered appropriate. Normal gastric histology, a low gastric pH, and inappropriately elevated gastrin level would be consistent with a type 2 gNET.

With type 2 gNETs further localization of a causative gastrinoma may be warranted with cross-sectional and/or functional imaging. Finally, because type 3 gNETs are not gastrin driven, fasting gastrin levels in these cases are typically normal.

If a type 1 gNET is suspected, endoscopic ultrasonography (EUS) can be considered to look for depth of invasion and lymph nodes in larger tumors (>1–2 cm), but is not necessary if less than 1 cm.[28] If a type 2 gNET is suspected, the duodenum should be carefully inspected for a duodenal gastrinoma given the concern for Zollinger-Ellison syndrome.[33] In these cases, EUS as well as cross-sectional/functional imaging are also performed to look for a gastrinoma in the gastrinoma triangle (duodenal sweep, porta hepatis, and pancreatic head/body). If a type 3 NET is suspected, EUS should be performed to assess for depth of invasion and the presence of lymph nodes.[33] In addition, with type 3 NETs, patients should undergo cross-sectional and functional imaging.

Duodenal and Ampullary

Presentation

Duodenal and ampullary NETs (dNETs) make up a small minority of NETs originating from the small intestine with 90% of dNETs being located in the first or second part of the duodenum.[9,10,37] Among dNETs, ampullary lesions have a higher risk of metastasis and worse survival compared with those arising from other areas of the duodenum.[38] There are 4 distinct types of NETs that can originate in the duodenum including gastrinoma, somatostatinoma, gangliocytic paragangliomas, and nonfunctioning dNETs.[39] Most dNETs are nonfunctional, and therefore these tumors are often incidentally discovered on EGD being performed for other indications[40]; however, dNETs can also present with clinical syndromes. Ampullary dNETs may present with jaundice if there is biliary obstruction. Gastrinomas are the most frequent functional dNET (27% to 58% of cases) and are associated with Zollinger-Ellison syndrome, which can present with abdominal pain and diarrhea, as well as severe esophagitis and peptic ulcer disease.[41] Somatostatinomas can also arise in the duodenum, often localizing in the periampullary region, and can present with clinical symptoms including weight loss and abdominal pain, as well as in some cases diabetes mellitus, steatorrhea and diarrhea, and cholelithiasis.[42]

Diagnosis

dNETs are often diagnosed incidentally on EGD. However, dNETs may be inaccessible with a standard upper endoscope, especially if they are located in the third or fourth portion of the duodenum or in the periampullary region. These tumors usually appear as small solitary lesions, except in the case of gastrinomas, which may appear as multiple lesions.[35] dNETs have an increased rate of lymph node metastases, even when small in size, with a 2003 study showing that 11% of dNETs less than or equal to 5 mm in size had lymph node metastases.[43] Therefore EUS as well as cross-sectional and functional imaging are important to properly stage dNETs. If the tumor has not invaded the muscularis propria, is less than 1 cm in size, and there is no evidence of lymph node involvement, endoscopic resection may be appropriate (discussed later).[44] If there is suspicion for a gastrinoma or somatostatinoma additional laboratory workup is also indicated.

Pancreatic

Presentation

pNETs (pNETs) are most commonly identified incidentally on an imaging study as most pNETs are nonfunctional and asymptomatic. However, some pNETs are functional (such as insulinoma and gastrinoma) and can present with a variety of clinical syndromes as noted in **Table 1**. Additionally a small subset of pNETs arise in the context of rare genetic syndromes including multiple endocrine neoplasia type 1 (MEN1) syndrome (previously referred to as Wermer syndrome), von Hippel-Lindau syndrome, neurofibromatosis type 1, and tuberous sclerosis.[45] MEN1 syndrome, which is also associated with parathyroid and pituitary tumors, is the most common cause of familial pNETs, with 30% to 80% of patients with MEN1 developing a pNET during their lifetime, with these tumors often being multifocal.[45]

Diagnosis

pNETs are often detected as an incidental lesion found on CT or MRI; however, histologic confirmation is typically made by EUS-guided fine-needle aspiration (FNA) or fine-needle biopsy (FNB). EUS can also be used to mark a pNET for easier intraoperative identification.[46,47] Although histologic confirmation is not always required for pNET diagnosis, EUS may be better than CT for detection of small pNETs, and therefore, may still have utility in the preoperative setting.[48–50] Finally, as part of pNET diagnosis, it is important to consider whether germline genetic testing is warranted, because management of pNETs arising in the setting of a genetic syndrome such as MEN1 is often different from that of sporadic pNETs.

Jejunal and Ileal

Presentation

The postduodenal small bowel is a common site for GEP-NETs to develop; and of the small bowel, the ileum is the most common site, especially the distal 100 cm.[9,10,51] Jejunal and ileal NETs often present with advanced disease because they are rarely found incidentally, unlike other luminal GEP-NETs. The most common method whereby ileal NETs are incidentally identified is through routine intubation of the terminal ileum during colonoscopy.[52] Presenting symptoms of jejunal and ileal NETs (which are often metastatic at the time of presentation) can include abdominal pain as well as the symptoms of carcinoid syndrome.[18] Postduodenal small bowel NETs are in fact the most common cause of carcinoid syndrome. In addition, jejunal and ileal NETs can induce fibrosis in the mesentery, which can lead to small bowel obstruction as well as intestinal ischemia.[53,54]

Diagnosis

Endoscopically, jejunal and ileal NETs appear as small, sessile, or polypoid lesions with a smooth surface and often a normal-appearing mucosal layer. Because jejunal and ileal NETs often present with metastatic disease, initial diagnosis is often made with biopsy of a metastatic lesion. Subsequent localization of the primary tumor in the small intestine can be very challenging. Functional imaging with a ^{68}Ga-DOTA-TATE PET-CT scan can identify the primary tumor in many cases of jejunal and ileal NETs, after which patients will often proceed to surgical resection.[55] In cases of metastatic NET where a primary tumor is not identified on functional imaging, there should be a high level of suspicion for a jejunal or ileal NET. In this situation, use of video capsule endoscopy (VCE) or balloon-assisted enteroscopy (BAE) may be helpful for localizing a postduodenal NET primary before proceeding with more invasive exploratory surgery.[56] VCE has been shown to successfully detect small bowel tumors, although the yield is rather low, and the sensitivity and specificity is less than that of surgery.[57–61] One obvious disadvantage to VCE is the inability to obtain histology, necessitating either surgery or a BAE to histologically diagnose an observed lesion. BAE can also be used to identify small bowel NETs and has the advantage of allowing concurrent tissue sampling; however, whether VCE or BAE is superior for detection of jejunal and ileal NETs remains uncertain with conflicting studies to date.[62–64] Jejunal and ileal NETs may also present with multifocal primary lesions, although interestingly, as a recent tumor genome sequencing study suggested, these lesions may be clonally independent.[51,65]

Colorectal and Appendiceal

Presentation
Among colorectal NETs, rectal NETs are more prevalent and more commonly benign when compared with NETs arising from the rest of the colon.[66,67] Many of these NETs are actually found incidentally on colonoscopy performed for other indications. Colorectal NETs can present with nonspecific abdominal symptoms such as abdominal pain, bloating, changes in bowel habits, weakness, and bleeding, but rarely with carcinoid syndrome. Colonic NETs present symptomatically more often than rectal NETs, and those presenting symptomatically are metastatic in approximately 40% of cases.[68] Appendiceal NETs are often identified incidentally on imaging or on postoperative histologic examination after an appendectomy for appendicitis. Rarely, appendiceal NETs can metastasize and lead to systemic symptoms such as abdominal pain, GI bleeding, or bowel obstruction. Metastasis and systemic symptoms are rarely seen with appendiceal NETs less than 2 cm.[69]

Diagnosis
Diagnosis of a colorectal NET is typically made during colonoscopy, although in some instances, there may be cross-sectional imaging suggesting a colonic mass beforehand. During colonoscopy, colorectal NETs appear as yellowish smooth, round, polypoid lesions, most commonly occurring within 5 to 10 cm from the anal verge.[67,70] There may also be central mucosal depression or ulceration, which increases risk of advanced, nonlocalized disease.[71] Patients with rectal NETs can undergo EUS to determine size, depth of invasion, and lymph node involvement, with the accuracy of EUS in determining these characteristics shown in multiple studies.[72,73] The decision to perform further staging of rectal NETs should depend on EUS findings and histology, and is discussed in the management of localized gastroenteropancreatic neuroendocrine tumors section - colorectal and appendiceal subsection. Patients with colonic NETs should undergo imaging if there is any concern for more advanced disease given the preference for surgical management in these patients.

Appendiceal NETs are typically diagnosed histologically after examination of a resection specimen, most frequently an appendectomy. A diagnosis of an appendiceal NET less than 1 cm with clean resection margins does not merit further studies. If an appendiceal NET is 1 to 2 cm with clear margins on resection, one-time imaging with CT or MRI is recommended to rule out lymph node involvement per the European Neuroendocrine Tumor Society (ENETS) guidelines, but not per National Comprehensive Cancer Network (NCCN) guidelines.[11,74] If margins are not clear with a 1 to 2 cm appendiceal NET and for all appendiceal NETs greater than > 2 cm, cross-sectional imaging should be performed with additional consideration of performing functional imaging.[11,74]

MANAGEMENT OF LOCALIZED GASTROENTEROPANCREATIC NEUROENDOCRINE TUMORS
Gastric

Management of gNETs has classically depended on the tumor subtype and depth of tumor invasion because these features were thought to be determinants of recurrence and survival. However, recent data have challenged that notion, showing that tumor size and grade may also be used in the management independent of gNET subtype.[75]

Type 1

The NCCN and ENETS guidelines largely agree on the endoscopic management of type 1 gNETs, where for tumors without invasion of the muscularis propria or metastasis, endoscopic mucosal resection (EMR) or endoscopic submucosal dissection (ESD) is recommended.[11,76,77] Endoscopic resection by ESD is preferable for tumors with submucosal invasion, which is often the case with type 1 and 2 gNETs, because it offers higher complete resection rates compared with EMR.[78] All type 1 gNETs that are 1 cm or greater in size should be endoscopically removed; however, there remains controversy about whether all small (<1 cm) type 1 gNETs should be removed or instead followed with continued endoscopic surveillance. For tumors greater than 2 cm, ESD offers a higher rate of complete resection.[79] In tumors with invasion beyond the submucosa or with lymph node metastasis, surgical resection is recommended. Treatment with somatostatin analogues (SSAs) is an option in patients with refractory disease or in those who are unable or unwilling to be managed endoscopically.[80,81] A newer gastrin/cholecystokinin-2 receptor antagonist, netazepide, is currently in clinical trials for treatment of type 1 gNETs after positive preliminary results.[82] Finally, in patients with refractory disease, surgical antrectomy is also an option to reduce gastrin, which is responsible for driving tumorigenesis, and subsequently lower recurrence risk of gNETs.[83] Regardless of the initial treatment strategy, surveillance upper endoscopy should be performed every 1 to 3 years, with shorter intervals being used for more extensive disease. Finally, because type 1 gNETs are associated with chronic autoimmune atrophic gastritis, vitamin B_{12} levels should be followed because B_{12} supplementation may be warranted.

Type 2

Management of type 2 gNETs, which are driven by gastrin production from gastrinomas, is directed at management of the gastrinomas and the gNETs. Similar to type 1 gNETs, prominent (1 cm or greater) type 2 gNETs can be resected endoscopically by EMR or ESD, especially when the primary gastrinoma is not resected.[11,76,77] Unlike type 1 gNETs, antrectomy will not be effective in suppressing growth of these gastrin-driven NETs; however, surgical removal of the causative gastrinoma may be considered, especially in patients without MEN1 syndrome. For patients with MEN1 syndrome, multifocal gastrinomas may be present and it may not be practical to remove all lesions. Medical treatment of type 2 gNETs with SSAs has also shown a benefit when the primary gastrinoma is not removed.[84] Furthermore, for patients without gastrinoma removal, high-dose PPI use will be required. Regardless of the treatment modality selected, once a diagnosis of a type 2 gNET is established, surveillance upper endoscopy should be performed every year.

Type 3

At present, type 3 gNETs should typically be managed through surgical resection given their more aggressive nature and higher rates of metastasis. Recent data, however, have challenged this surgery-first approach with the assertion that small (<1 cm), superficial, low-grade type 3 gNETs have lower risk, and therefore, endoscopic resection or limited surgical resection may be considered.[75,85] If endoscopic resection is considered, ESD is preferred over EMR. If a decision is made to manage a type 3 gNET with nonsurgical endoscopic resection, the patient will continue to need ongoing endoscopic surveillance, likely on at least a yearly basis.

Duodenal and Ampullary

All dNETs should be staged with cross-sectional imaging, and consideration of additional functional imaging and/or EUS should be individualized. All dNETs should undergo resection. Endoscopic resection with EMR or ESD is appropriate for all nonampullary dNETs less than 1 cm that are confined to the submucosal layer without metastatic disease.[77] Other endoscopic resection techniques that can be considered include ligation-assisted EMR as well as full-thickness endoscopic resection. Simpler polypectomy techniques such as forceps biopsy or cold and hot snare have been effective for small dNETs in a single-center series.[44,86] ESD allows for higher en bloc and histologic complete resection rates of dNETs compared with EMR or device-assisted EMR, but has a higher complication rate, including bleeding and perforation.[87] A recent study of endoscopic surveillance versus resection of small (<1 cm), grade 1, nonfunctioning, nonampullary dNETs did not have any tumor-related deaths, so it may also be reasonable to offer surveillance in select cases.[85]

There is less clarity for dNETs that are between 1 and 2 cm, in which case endoscopic or surgical resection (pancreaticoduodenectomy or duodenotomy with transduodenal local excision) are both considered feasible options, and this remains an area where additional study is needed.[77] For dNETs greater than 2 cm, if there is no evidence of distant metastatic disease, surgical resection should be considered.[77] These size-based recommendations result from data showing that the risk of lymph node or distant metastasis and recurrence is low in dNETs less than 1 cm, whereas there is reduced disease-specific survival in dNETs greater than 2 cm.[39,88–90] Although there are size-based management considerations for nonampullary dNETs, ampullary dNETs should all be managed surgically, regardless of their size.[77] Surgical resection should also be performed for all sporadic (ie, non-MEN1-associated) gastrinomas given improved cure rates in this specific population. However, surgery is not always recommended for gastrinomas arising in the setting of MEN1 syndrome.[91,92] For patients who undergo local resection of a dNET, endoscopic surveillance should be performed, although the interval for this monitoring remains uncertain. Initially after resection, endoscopic surveillance can be performed every 6 to 12 months, with consideration of an increased interval if no recurrence is identified.

Pancreatic

Management of pNETs depends on the subtype and functionality of the tumor, whether the pNET developed in the context of a high-risk genetic syndrome, and whether there is evidence of metastatic disease. Unlike other GEP-NETs, there is currently no role for endoscopy in the treatment of pNETs. However, EUS can be useful for staging and tissue acquisition either via FNA or FNB. Per a recent North American Neuroendocrine Tumor Society (NANETS) consensus statement, sporadic functional pNETs that are both localized and biochemically confirmed should undergo surgical resection, even when small in size, given the clinical significance of their associated syndromes and increased malignant potential.[48] Likewise, localized nonfunctional pNETs greater than 2 cm in size should also always undergo surgical resection per ENETS, NCCN, and NANETS recommendations.[11,48,93,94] There is no consensus on the optimal management approach of nonfunctional pNETs less than 2 cm in size, with disagreement about whether surgical resection or observation is best. A meta-analysis of 327 patients under surveillance with a pNET (with a range of different sizes) showed that 14% eventually underwent resection, but there were no deaths in the surveillance group.[95] On the other hand, a study of 300 patients with pNETs less than 2 cm from the National Cancer Database showed an 82.2%

5-year survival in patients who underwent resection and a 34.3% in those who did not.[96] Furthermore, a study of 392 patients who had surgical resection for pNETs less than 2 cm suggested that pNETs between 1.5 cm and 2 cm had a significantly higher chance of lymph node metastasis, suggesting that the cutoff for surveillance versus surgery may fall somewhere between 1 and 2 cm.[97] For low-grade, nonfunctional pNETs less than 2 cm that are not treated surgically, surveillance imaging every 6 to 12 months should be performed, with consideration of surgery if there is a 5 mm or greater increase in size during surveillance, or if the pNET surpasses 2 cm in size.[98]

Jejunal/Ileal

The management of localized NETs of the jejunum and ileum is surgical resection. At this time, there is no role for endoscopic resection in the treatment of jejunal and ileal NETs. However, VCE or BAE may be used to locate a NET of the jejunum or ileum, and BAE may also be used to facilitate a tissue diagnosis. As noted earlier, because NETs of the jejunum or ileum are often multifocal, manually inspecting the bowel during laparotomy to ensure that all NETs are resected is important. Postoperatively, these patients receive follow-up imaging to monitor for recurrence, but there is no role for endoscopy in follow-up.[99]

Colorectal and Appendiceal

For nonrectal colonic NETs that are greater than or equal to 2 cm in size, there is consensus that surgical resection is the favored treatment approach.[11,100] However, there remains controversy about how to manage nonrectal colonic NETs less than 2 cm in size. For this subset, ENETS recommends endoscopic resection so long as margins are clear, there is no invasion of the muscularis propria, and the NET is grade 1 or 2.[100] However, NCCN differs, and recommends surgical resection for all nonrectal colonic NETs.[11] Patients undergoing endoscopic resection of a nonrectal colonic NET will need regular endoscopic surveillance to monitor for recurrence.

Rectal NETs should also be completely resected, which has been proved to be superior to observation.[101] Given the more indolent nature of rectal NETs when compared with colonic NETs, staging imaging is not always required, especially if a small (<1 cm), low-grade, incidentally discovered rectal NET is completely resected during colonoscopy. However, there is some evidence that even presumed low-risk rectal NETs are capable of lymph node metastasis, with a recent study demonstrating that 25% of rectal NETs less than or equal to 10 mm had nodal involvement, leading to the investigators' proposal to stage all rectal NETs greater than 4 mm.[102] Staging can be performed with EUS, after which grade 1/2 rectal NETs less than 1 cm without invasion of the muscularis propria (ie, T1 lesion) can undergo endoscopic resection with EMR or ESD, which has been demonstrated to be effective when compared with surgical resection.[71,103] ESD is preferred over EMR if there is suspicion for submucosal invasion.[79] The data are less clear on whether endoscopic excision or surgical excision (which can be performed via a transanal approach) is the best management for localized rectal NETs between 1 and 2 cm. One study of 239 patients in Japan showed no local recurrence, a complication rate less than 4%, and only a 2.5% metastasis rate following ESD, suggesting that endoscopic management is a reasonable option.[104] For rectal NETs greater than 2 cm, those that have lymph node involvement, and those with grade 3 histology, radical surgical resection should be performed. However, a recent retrospective analysis of 178 patients from the National Cancer Database with rectal NETs greater than 2 cm showed similar survival between patients who underwent local excision and radical surgery. This indicates that there may be a subset of patients with NETs greater than 2 cm who may be able to be treated with less invasive surgery without compromising survival.[105]

After resection, grade 1/2 rectal NETs less than 1 cm with clean resection margins do not need follow-up. If margins are indeterminate, endoscopic evaluation should be repeated in 6 to 12 months for grade 1 rectal NETs, whereas more definitive resection should be attempted for grade 2 rectal NETs.[11] After local resection of a rectal NET 1 to 2 cm in size, patients should undergo EUS or MRI within 6 to 12 months postresection.[11,100]

Management of appendiceal NETs is surgical, and there is no routine role for endoscopy. Appendiceal NETs greater than 2 cm should typically be treated with a right hemicolectomy. However, for appendiceal NETs less than 2 cm in size with clear margins, without deep tissue invasion, and without concerning histologic features, appendectomy alone is sufficient for management.

MANAGEMENT OF ADVANCED GASTROENTEROPANCREATIC NEUROENDOCRINE TUMORS

Although this review has been primarily devoted to the diagnosis and management of localized GEP-NETs, the authors briefly discuss some of the other treatments available for advanced GEP-NETs. There are multiple comprehensive reviews that cover management of advanced GEP-NETs in more detail.[106,107]

Somatostatin Analogues

Most GEP-NETs express high levels of somatostatin receptors (SSTRs), and as such, this unique property has been used in treatment. The first SSA, octreotide, has been in use since the 1980s initially as a treatment of carcinoid syndrome, with later data showing improvement in survival in both functional and nonfunctional metastatic GEP-NETs.[108,109] Lanreotide is another SSA that also increases progression-free survival (PFS) in metastatic low-grade GEP-NETs.[110] Both octreotide and lanreotide are well-tolerated and administered as long-acting injectables, and are generally used as early-line treatments for metastatic GEP-NETs.

Surgery

Resection of the primary tumor in metastatic GEP-NETs has been an area of ongoing controversy. However, a recent study showed that primary GEP-NET resection was associated with prolonged survival.[111] Surgical resection can also be used to debulk metastatic disease, especially with extensive hepatic metastases, which has also been shown to prolong survival in select cases.[112]

Liver-Directed Therapies

GEP-NETs typically metastasize to the liver, and patients with extensive hepatic metastatic disease may benefit from liver-directed therapies including transarterial embolization (TAE), transarterial chemoembolization (TACE), or transarterial radioembolization (TARE). Although one retrospective analysis did show improved long-term survival in patients undergoing TACE, currently there are no clear data supporting one type of liver-directed therapy over others. This question is being investigated by the ongoing Randomized Embolization Trial for Neuroendocrine Tumor Metastases to the Liver (RETNET) study.[113,114] Liver-directed therapies do have risks, including hepatotoxicity, and there is ongoing work examining combining liver-directed therapy with systemic therapy.[115,116]

Peptide Receptor Radionuclide Therapy

Peptide receptor radionuclide therapy (PRRT) exploits the high proportion of SSTRs on the surface of GEP-NETs for therapeutic benefit. Although PRRT has been used for years in Europe, it was not until ^{177}Lu-DOTATATE was approved by the US Food and Drug Administration in 2018 for SSTR-positive GEP-NETs, based on the favorable results from the Neuroendocrine Tumors Therapy (NETTER-1) trial, that PRRT became widely available in the United States.[117] Real-world data have alluded to small bowel NETs having better response to PRRT than pNETs; however, it remains to be determined how to optimally incorporate PRRT among other modalities into the treatment of NETs.[118–120] PRRT is also associated with systemic toxicities that require close monitoring, including hematologic, renal, and hepatic toxicities.[121,122]

Targeted Therapies, Chemotherapy, and Immunotherapy

There are several targeted agents used in the treatment of GEP-NETs including mechanistic target of rapamycin (mTOR) inhibitors as well as tyrosine kinase inhibitors. Everolimus, which is an mTOR inhibitor, has been shown to prolong PFS in nonfunctional NETs of the GI tract and lung and has received FDA approval for this indication.[123,124] Sunitinib, a multireceptor tyrosine kinase inhibitor, has shown improved PFS in pNETs, and has received FDA approval for this indication.[125] Multiple other tyrosine kinase inhibitors are currently being investigated in clinical trials, including cabozantinib, lenvatinib, surufatinib, pazopanib, and axitinib, with these studies reviewed in-depth elsewhere.[106,107] Cytotoxic chemotherapy can also be considered in pNETs and in some refractory bowel NETs, the specifics of which are beyond the scope of this review.[11]

SPECIAL CONSIDERATIONS FOR MANAGEMENT OF FUNCTIONAL GASTROENTEROPANCREATIC NEUROENDOCRINE TUMORS

In addition to treating disease burden, patients with functional GEP-NETs may also need additional treatments to aid in control of their symptoms.

Functional Pancreatic Neuroendocrine Tumors

The foundation of controlling hormone production in patients with functional pNETS is treatment with a SSA. Additional treatments may be indicated, however, depending on the specific type of tumor and associated hormone that is produced. Patients with a gastrinoma should be treated with high-dose PPIs to suppress their gastrin-driven hypersecretion of acid. Continuation of PPI therapy in these individuals is important under all circumstances, which should be made clear to the patient and all of their treating providers. Patients with insulinomas who have not undergone curative resection can be treated with lifestyle modifications such as frequent small feedings, and when refractory, can be treated with glucose infusions as well as diaxozide.[126] Patients with VIPomas causing symptoms that are difficult to control can be treated with alpha-interferon, which has demonstrated a significant antisecretory effect in these patients.[126] Patients with ACTHomas can be treated with metyrapone and ketoconazole for the hormone excess.[126]

Carcinoid Syndrome

Carcinoid syndrome commonly manifests with diarrhea and flushing. The diarrhea from carcinoid syndrome can oftentimes be exceedingly difficult to manage. Dietary modifications, with frequent small meals and avoidance of aged cheeses and fermented foods with high amine content are generally advised to help with symptoms, although there is no robust evidence for this practice.[127] Use of SSAs such as octreotide or lanreotide can be effective in controlling diarrhea symptoms. In addition, empirical trials of bile acid sequestrants or antidiarrheals such as diphenoxylate and loperamide can be considered.[127] However, if SSA treatment is not effective for controlling carcinoid syndrome-related diarrhea, telotristat ethyl can be used. Telotristat ethyl is an inhibitor of tryptophan hydroxylase, the rate-limiting step in the synthesis of serotonin, and multiple clinical trials have shown its effectiveness in reducing diarrhea from carcinoid syndrome.[128,129] Although telotristat ethyl has been primarily studied with respect to diarrhea, it may also help with other symptoms of carcinoid syndrome, with patients on telotristat ethyl showing improved clinical outcomes.[130]

SUMMARY

GEP-NETs are a heterogeneous group of tumors that can be classified by their location, grade, functionality, and stage, with management varying based on these different elements. Given the increasing incidence of GEP-NETs, it is important for all medical practitioners to have a basic understanding of the principles of GEP-NET diagnosis and management, especially gastroenterologists, who will either encounter these tumors incidentally or will be intimately involved in the diagnosis and/or management of these patients.

CLINICS CARE POINTS

- The incidence of gastroenteropancreatic neuroendocrine tumors (GEP-NETs) is increasing, and these tumors are increasingly being identified incidentally in clinical practice.
- GEP-NETs are typically classified by their location, grade, stage, and functionality. GEP-NET classification has significant implications for subsequent tumor management.
- Diagnosis and management of GEP-NETs requires a multidisciplinary team of medical professionals, of which gastroenterologists are an important part.
- Endoscopy is critical in the diagnosis, management, and/or surveillance of GEP-NETs.

DISCLOSURE

C.J. Fernandes, G. Leung, and B.W. Katona: No relevant disclosures. J. R. Eads: Bristol Meyers Squibb (employment, stock—spouse); Janssen (employment—spouse); Advanced Accelerator Applications (advisory board); Ipsen (advisory board).

REFERENCES

1. Yao JC, Hassan M, Phan A, et al. One hundred years after "carcinoid": epidemiology of and prognostic factors for neuroendocrine tumors in 35,825 cases in the United States. J Clin Oncol 2008;26(18):3063–72.
2. Dasari A, Shen C, Halperin D, et al. Trends in the incidence, prevalence, and survival outcomes in patients with neuroendocrine tumors in the United States. JAMA Oncol 2017;3(10):1335–42.
3. Hemminki K, Li X. Incidence trends and risk factors of carcinoid tumors: a nationwide epidemiologic study from Sweden. Cancer 2001;92(8):2204–10.
4. Hauso O, Gustafsson BI, Kidd M, et al. Neuroendocrine tumor epidemiology: contrasting Norway and North America. Cancer 2008;113(10):2655–64.

5. Hallet J, Law CHL, Cukier M, et al. Exploring the rising incidence of neuroendocrine tumors: a population-based analysis of epidemiology, metastatic presentation, and outcomes. Cancer 2015;121(4):589–97.

6. Broder MS, Cai B, Chang E, et al. Incidence and prevalence of neuroendocrine tumors of the lung: analysis of a US commercial insurance claims database. BMC Pulm Med 2018;18:135.

7. Xu Z, Wang L, Dai S, et al. Epidemiologic trends of and factors associated with overall survival for patients with gastroenteropancreatic neuroendocrine tumors in the United States. JAMA Netw Open 2021;4(9):e2124750.

8. Das S, Dasari A. Epidemiology, incidence, and prevalence of neuroendocrine neoplasms: are there global differences? Curr Oncol Rep 2021;23(4):43.

9. Modlin IM, Lye KD, Kidd M. A 5-decade analysis of 13,715 carcinoid tumors. Cancer 2003;97(4):934–59.

10. Sackstein PE, O'Neil DS, Neugut AI, et al. Epidemiologic trends in neuroendocrine tumors: an examination of incidence rates and survival of specific patient subgroups over the past 20 years. Semin Oncol 2018;45(4):249–58.

11. National Comprehensive Cancer Network. Neuroendocrine and adrenal tumors. Version 4 2021. Available at: https://www.nccn.org/professionals/physician_gls/pdf/neuroendocrine.pdf. Accessed December 6, 2021.

12. Nagtegaal ID, Odze RD, Klimstra D, et al. The 2019 WHO classification of tumours of the digestive system. Histopathology 2020;76(2):182–8.

13. Özaslan E, Demir S, Karaca H, et al. Evaluation of the concordance between the stage of the disease and Ki-67 proliferation index in gastroenteropancreatic neuroendocrine tumors. Eur J Gastroenterol Hepatol 2016;28(7):836–41.

14. Yachida S, Vakiani E, White CM, et al. Small cell and large cell neuroendocrine carcinomas of the pancreas are genetically similar and distinct from well-differentiated pancreatic neuroendocrine tumors. Am J Surg Pathol 2012;36(2):173–84.

15. Dasari A, Mehta K, Byers LA, et al. Comparative study of lung and extrapulmonary poorly differentiated neuroendocrine carcinomas: A SEER database analysis of 162,983 cases. Cancer 2018;124(4):807–15.

16. Sorbye H, Strosberg J, Baudin E, et al. Gastroenteropancreatic high-grade neuroendocrine carcinoma. Cancer 2014;120(18):2814–23.

17. Kasumova GG, Tabatabaie O, Eskander MF, et al. National rise of primary pancreatic carcinoid tumors: comparison to functional and non-functional pancreatic neuroendocrine tumors. J Am Coll Surg 2017;224(6):1057–64.

18. Ito T, Lee L, Jensen RT. Carcinoid-syndrome: recent advances, current status and controversies. Curr Opin Endocrinol Diabetes Obes 2018;25(1):22–35.

19. Bhattacharyya S, Toumpanakis C, Caplin ME, et al. Analysis of 150 patients with carcinoid syndrome seen in a single year at one institution in the first decade of the twenty-first century. Am J Cardiol 2008;101(3):378–81.

20. Halperin DM, Shen C, Dasari A, et al. Frequency of carcinoid syndrome at neuroendocrine tumour diagnosis: a population-based study. Lancet Oncol 2017;18(4):525–34.

21. Zavras N, Schizas D, Machairas N, et al. Carcinoid syndrome from a carcinoid tumor of the pancreas without liver metastases: a case report and literature review. Oncol Lett 2017;13(4):2373–6.

22. Datta S, Williams N, Suortamo S, et al. Carcinoid syndrome from small bowel endocrine carcinoma in the absence of hepatic metastasis. Age Ageing 2011;40(6):760–2.

23. Datta J, Merchant NB. Terminal ileal carcinoid tumor without hepatic or extrahepatic metastasis causing carcinoid syndrome. Am Surg 2013;79(4):439–41.
24. Sonnet S, Wiesner W. Flush symptoms caused by a mesenteric carcinoid without liver metastases. JBR-BTR 2002;85(5):254–6.
25. Scherübl H. Rectal carcinoids are on the rise: early detection by screening endoscopy. Endoscopy 2009;41(2):162–5.
26. Deppen SA, Blume J, Bobbey AJ, et al. 68Ga-DOTATATE compared with 111In-DTPA-octreotide and conventional imaging for pulmonary and gastroenteropancreatic neuroendocrine tumors: a systematic review and meta-analysis. J Nucl Med Off Publ Soc Nucl Med 2016;57(6):872–8.
27. Pfeifer A, Knigge U, Binderup T, et al. 64Cu-DOTATATE PET for neuroendocrine tumors: a prospective head-to-head comparison with 111In-DTPA-octreotide in 112 patients. J Nucl Med Off Publ Soc Nucl Med 2015;56(6):847–54.
28. Gluckman CR, Metz DC. Gastric neuroendocrine tumors (Carcinoids). Curr Gastroenterol Rep 2019;21(4):13.
29. Rindi G, Luinetti O, Cornaggia M, et al. Three subtypes of gastric argyrophil carcinoid and the gastric neuroendocrine carcinoma: a clinicopathologic study. Gastroenterology 1993;104(4):994–1006.
30. Nandy N, Hanson JA, Strickland RG, et al. Solitary gastric carcinoid tumor associated with long-term use of omeprazole: a case report and review of the literature. Dig Dis Sci 2016;61(3):708–12.
31. Cavalcoli F, Zilli A, Conte D, et al. Gastric neuroendocrine neoplasms and proton pump inhibitors: fact or coincidence? Scand J Gastroenterol 2015;50(11):1397–403.
32. Giudici F, Cavalli T, Giusti F, et al. Natural history of MEN1 GEP-NET: single-center experience after a long follow-up. World J Surg 2017;41(9):2312–23.
33. Chin JL, O'Toole D. Diagnosis and management of upper gastrointestinal neuroendocrine tumors. Clin Endosc 2017;50(6):520–9.
34. Sato Y. Endoscopic diagnosis and management of type I neuroendocrine tumors. World J Gastrointest Endosc 2015;7(4):346–53.
35. Sato Y, Hashimoto S, Mizuno KI, et al. Management of gastric and duodenal neuroendocrine tumors. World J Gastroenterol 2016;22(30):6817–28.
36. Lundell L, Vieth M, Gibson F, et al. Systematic review: the effects of long-term proton pump inhibitor use on serum gastrin levels and gastric histology. Aliment Pharmacol Ther 2015;42(6):649–63.
37. Barat M, Dohan A, Dautry R, et al. Mass-forming lesions of the duodenum: a pictorial review. Diagn Interv Imaging 2017;98(10):663–75.
38. Randle RW, Ahmed S, Newman NA, et al. Clinical outcomes for neuroendocrine tumors of the duodenum and ampulla of Vater: a population-based study. J Gastrointest Surg 2014;18(2):354–62.
39. Vanoli A, La Rosa S, Klersy C, et al. Four neuroendocrine tumor types and neuroendocrine carcinoma of the duodenum: analysis of 203 cases. Neuroendocrinology 2017;104(2):112–25.
40. Gonzalez RS. Diagnosis and management of gastrointestinal neuroendocrine neoplasms. Surg Pathol Clin 2020;13(3):377–97.
41. Hoffmann KM, Furukawa M, Jensen RT. Duodenal neuroendocrine tumors: classification, functional syndromes, diagnosis and medical treatment. Best Pract Res Clin Gastroenterol 2005;19(5):675–97.
42. Krejs GJ, Orci L, Conlon JM, et al. Somatostatinoma syndrome. Biochemical, morphologic and clinical features. N Engl J Med 1979;301(6):285–92.

43. Soga J. Endocrinocarcinomas (carcinoids and their variants) of the duodenum. An evaluation of 927 cases. J Exp Clin Cancer Res CR 2003;22(3):349–63.

44. Yoon JY, Kumta NA, Kim MK. The role of endoscopy in small bowel neuroendocrine tumors. Clin Endosc 2021;54(6):818–24.

45. Pea A, Hruban RH, Wood LD. Genetics of pancreatic neuroendocrine tumors: implications for the clinic. Expert Rev Gastroenterol Hepatol 2015;9(11): 1407–19.

46. Lennon AM, Newman N, Makary MA, et al. EUS-guided tattooing before laparoscopic distal pancreatic resection (with video). Gastrointest Endosc 2010;72(5): 1089–94.

47. Di Leo M, Poliani L, Rahal D, et al. Pancreatic neuroendocrine tumours: the role of endoscopic ultrasound biopsy in diagnosis and grading based on the WHO 2017 classification. Dig Dis Basel Switz 2019;37(4):325–33.

48. Howe JR, Merchant NB, Conrad C, et al. The North American neuroendocrine tumor society consensus paper on the surgical management of pancreatic neuroendocrine tumors. Pancreas 2020;49(1):1–33.

49. Khashab MA, Yong E, Lennon AM, et al. EUS is still superior to multidetector computerized tomography for detection of pancreatic neuroendocrine tumors. Gastrointest Endosc 2011;73(4):691–6.

50. James PD, Tsolakis AV, Zhang M, et al. Incremental benefit of preoperative EUS for the detection of pancreatic neuroendocrine tumors: a meta-analysis. Gastrointest Endosc 2015;81(4):848–56.e1.

51. Keck KJ, Maxwell JE, Utria AF, et al. The distal predilection of small bowel neuroendocrine tumors. Ann Surg Oncol 2018;25(11):3207–13.

52. Zakaria A, Alnimer L, Byrd G, et al. Asymptomatic Ileal Neuroendocrine "Carcinoid" Tumor Incidentally Diagnosed on Colorectal Cancer Screening Colonoscopy: does Routine TI Intubation Matter? Case Rep Gastrointest Med 2021; 2021:6620036.

53. Warner TF, O'Reilly G, Lee GA. Mesenteric occlusive lesion and ileal carcinoids. Cancer 1979;44(2):758–62.

54. Anthony PP. Gangrene of the small intestine–a complication of argentaffin carcinoma. Br J Surg 1970;57(2):118–22.

55. Skoura E, Michopoulou S, Mohmaduvesh M, et al. The Impact of 68Ga-DOTATATE PET/CT imaging on management of patients with neuroendocrine tumors: experience from a national referral center in the United Kingdom. J Nucl Med Off Publ Soc Nucl Med 2016;57(1):34–40.

56. Wang SC, Parekh JR, Zuraek MB, et al. Identification of unknown primary tumors in patients with neuroendocrine liver metastases. Arch Surg 2010;145(3): 276–80.

57. Rondonotti E, Pennazio M, Toth E, et al. Small-bowel neoplasms in patients undergoing video capsule endoscopy: a multicenter European study. Endoscopy 2008;40(6):488–95.

58. Cobrin GM, Pittman RH, Lewis BS. Increased diagnostic yield of small bowel tumors with capsule endoscopy. Cancer 2006;107(1):22–7.

59. Bailey AA, Debinski HS, Appleyard MN, et al. Diagnosis and outcome of small bowel tumors found by capsule endoscopy: a three-center Australian experience. Am J Gastroenterol 2006;101(10):2237–43.

60. Furnari M, Buda A, Delconte G, et al. The role of wireless capsule endoscopy (WCE) in the detection of occult primary neuroendocrine tumors. J Gastrointest Liver Dis 2017;26(2):151–6.

61. Frilling A, Smith G, Clift AK, et al. Capsule endoscopy to detect primary tumour site in metastatic neuroendocrine tumours. Dig Liver Dis 2014;46(11):1038–42.

62. Bellutti M, Fry LC, Schmitt J, et al. Detection of neuroendocrine tumors of the small bowel by double balloon enteroscopy. Dig Dis Sci 2009;54(5):1050–8.

63. Manguso N, Gangi A, Johnson J, et al. The role of pre-operative imaging and double balloon enteroscopy in the surgical management of small bowel neuro-endocrine tumors: Is it necessary? J Surg Oncol 2018;117(2):207–12.

64. Ethun CG, Postlewait LM, Baptiste GG, et al. Small bowel neuroendocrine tu-mors: a critical analysis of diagnostic work-up and operative approach. J Surg Oncol 2016;114(6):671–6.

65. Elias E, Ardalan A, Lindberg M, et al. Independent somatic evolution underlies clustered neuroendocrine tumors in the human small intestine. Nat Commun 2021;12(1):6367.

66. Broecker JS, Ethun CG, Postlewait LM, et al. Colon and rectal neuroendocrine tumors: are they really one disease? A single-institution experience over 15 years. Am Surg 2018;84(5):717–26.

67. Ramage JK, De Herder WW, Delle Fave G, et al. ENETS consensus guidelines update for colorectal neuroendocrine neoplasms. Neuroendocrinology 2016; 103(2):139–43.

68. Crocetti E, Paci E. Malignant carcinoids in the USA, SEER 1992-1999. An epide-miological study with 6830 cases. Eur J Cancer Prev 2003;12(3):191–4.

69. Moertel CG, Weiland LH, Nagorney DM, et al. Carcinoid tumor of the appendix: treatment and prognosis. N Engl J Med 1987;317(27):1699–701.

70. Chablaney S, Zator ZA, Kumta NA. Diagnosis and management of rectal neuro-endocrine tumors. Clin Endosc 2017;50(6):530–6.

71. Park CH, Cheon JH, Kim JO, et al. Criteria for decision making after endoscopic resection of well-differentiated rectal carcinoids with regard to potential lymphatic spread. Endoscopy 2011;43(9):790–5.

72. Ishii N, Horiki N, Itoh T, et al. Endoscopic submucosal dissection and preoper-ative assessment with endoscopic ultrasonography for the treatment of rectal carcinoid tumors. Surg Endosc 2010;24(6):1413–9.

73. Kobayashi K, Katsumata T, Yoshizawa S, et al. Indications of endoscopic poly-pectomy for rectal carcinoid tumors and clinical usefulness of endoscopic ultra-sonography. Dis Colon Rectum 2005;48(2):285–91.

74. Pape UF, Perren A, Niederle B, et al. ENETS Consensus Guidelines for the man-agement of patients with neuroendocrine neoplasms from the jejuno-ileum and the appendix including goblet cell carcinomas. Neuroendocrinology 2012;95(2): 135–56.

75. Hanna A, Kim-Kiselak C, Tang R, et al. Gastric neuroendocrine tumors: reap-praisal of type in predicting outcome. Ann Surg Oncol 2021;28(13):8838–46.

76. Delle Fave G, O'Toole D, Sundin A, et al. ENETS consensus guidelines update for gastroduodenal neuroendocrine neoplasms. Neuroendocrinology 2016; 103(2):119–24.

77. Delle Fave G, Kwekkeboom DJ, Van Cutsem E, et al. ENETS Consensus Guide-lines for the management of patients with gastroduodenal neoplasms. Neuroen-docrinology 2012;95(2):74–87.

78. Kim HH, Kim GH, Kim JH, et al. The efficacy of endoscopic submucosal dissec-tion of type I gastric carcinoid tumors compared with conventional endoscopic mucosal resection. Gastroenterol Res Pract 2014;2014:253860.

79. Pimentel-Nunes P, Dinis-Ribeiro M, Ponchon T, et al. Endoscopic submucosal dissection: European Society of Gastrointestinal Endoscopy (ESGE) Guideline. Endoscopy 2015;47(9):829–54.
80. Massironi S, Zilli A, Fanetti I, et al. Intermittent treatment of recurrent type-1 gastric carcinoids with somatostatin analogues in patients with chronic autoimmune atrophic gastritis. Dig Liver Dis 2015;47(11):978–83.
81. Jianu CS, Fossmark R, Syversen U, et al. Five-year follow-up of patients treated for 1 year with octreotide long-acting release for enterochromaffin-like cell carcinoids. Scand J Gastroenterol 2011;46(4):456–63.
82. Boyce M, Moore AR, Sagatun L, et al. Netazepide, a gastrin/cholecystokinin-2 receptor antagonist, can eradicate gastric neuroendocrine tumours in patients with autoimmune chronic atrophic gastritis. Br J Clin Pharmacol 2017;83(3):466–75.
83. Jenny HE, Ogando PA, Fujitani K, et al. Laparoscopic antrectomy: a safe and definitive treatment in managing type 1 gastric carcinoids. Am J Surg 2016;211(4):778–82.
84. Tomassetti P, Migliori M, Caletti GC, et al. Treatment of type II gastric carcinoid tumors with somatostatin analogues. N Engl J Med 2000;343(8):551–4.
85. Exarchou K, Moore AR, Smart HL, et al. A "watch and wait" strategy involving regular endoscopic surveillance is safe for many patients with small, sporadic, grade 1, non-ampullary, non-functioning duodenal neuroendocrine tumours. Neuroendocrinology 2021;111(8):764–74.
86. Mahmud N, Tomizawa Y, Stashek K, et al. Endoscopic resection of duodenal carcinoid tumors: a single center comparison between simple polypectomy and endoscopic mucosal resection. Pancreas 2019;48(1):60–5.
87. Kim GH, Kim JI, Jeon SW, et al. Endoscopic resection for duodenal carcinoid tumors: a multicenter, retrospective study. J Gastroenterol Hepatol 2014;29(2):318–24.
88. Lee SW, Sung JK, Cho YS, et al. Comparisons of therapeutic outcomes in patients with nonampullary duodenal neuroendocrine tumors (NADNETs): a multicenter retrospective study. Medicine (Baltimore) 2019;98(26):e16154.
89. Park SG, Lee BE, Kim GH, et al. Risk factors for lymph node metastasis in duodenal neuroendocrine tumors: a retrospective, single-center study. Medicine (Baltimore) 2019;98(23):e15885.
90. Hatta W, Koike T, Iijima K, et al. The risk factors for metastasis in non-ampullary duodenal neuroendocrine tumors measuring 20 mm or less in diameter. Digestion 2017;95(3):201–9.
91. Norton JA, Alexander HR, Fraker DL, et al. Does the use of routine duodenotomy (DUODX) affect rate of cure, development of liver metastases, or survival in patients with Zollinger-Ellison syndrome? Ann Surg 2004;239(5):617–25.
92. Yates CJ, Newey PJ, Thakker RV. Challenges and controversies in management of pancreatic neuroendocrine tumours in patients with MEN1. Lancet Diabetes Endocrinol 2015;3(11):895–905.
93. Jensen RT, Cadiot G, Brandi ML, et al. ENETS Consensus Guidelines for the Management of Patients with Digestive Neuroendocrine Neoplasms: Functional Pancreatic Endocrine Tumor Syndromes. Neuroendocrinology 2012;95(2):98–119.
94. Falconi M, Bartsch DK, Eriksson B, et al. ENETS Consensus Guidelines for the management of patients with digestive neuroendocrine neoplasms of the digestive system: well-differentiated pancreatic non-functioning tumors. Neuroendocrinology 2012;95(2):120–34.

95. Partelli S, Cirocchi R, Crippa S, et al. Systematic review of active surveillance versus surgical management of asymptomatic small non-functioning pancreatic neuroendocrine neoplasms. Br J Surg 2017;104(1):34–41.

96. Sharpe SM, In H, Winchester DJ, et al. Surgical resection provides an overall survival benefit for patients with small pancreatic neuroendocrine tumors. J Gastrointest Surg 2015;19(1):117–23 [discussion: 123].

97. Dong DH, Zhang XF, Poultsides G, et al. Impact of tumor size and nodal status on recurrence of nonfunctional pancreatic neuroendocrine tumors ≤2 cm after curative resection: a multi-institutional study of 392 cases. J Surg Oncol 2019; 120(7):1071–9.

98. Falconi M, Eriksson B, Kaltsas G, et al. ENETS consensus guidelines update for the management of patients with functional pancreatic neuroendocrine tumors and non-functional pancreatic neuroendocrine tumors. Neuroendocrinology 2016;103(2):153–71.

99. Strosberg JR, Halfdanarson TR, Bellizzi AM, et al. The North American neuroendocrine tumor society consensus guidelines for surveillance and medical management of midgut neuroendocrine tumors. Pancreas 2017;46(6):707–14.

100. Caplin M, Sundin A, Nillson O, et al. ENETS Consensus Guidelines for the management of patients with digestive neuroendocrine neoplasms: colorectal neuroendocrine neoplasms. Neuroendocrinology 2012;95(2):88–97.

101. Zhao B, Hollandsworth HM, Lopez NE, et al. Outcomes for a large cohort of patients with rectal neuroendocrine tumors: an analysis of the national cancer database. J Gastrointest Surg 2021;25(2):484–91.

102. O'Neill S, Haji A, Ryan S, et al. Nodal metastases in small rectal neuroendocrine tumours. Colorectal Dis 2021;23(12):3173–9.

103. Kwaan MR, Goldberg JE, Bleday R. Rectal carcinoid tumors: review of results after endoscopic and surgical therapy. Arch Surg 2008;143(5):471–5.

104. Chen T, Yao LQ, Xu MD, et al. Efficacy and safety of endoscopic submucosal dissection for colorectal carcinoids. Clin Gastroenterol Hepatol 2016;14(4): 575–81.

105. Izquierdo KM, Humphries MD, Farkas LM. Size criteria is not sufficient in selecting patients for local excision versus radical excision for rectal neuroendocrine tumors >2 cm: a national cancer database analysis. Dis Colon Rectum 2021; 64(4):399–408.

106. Das S, Dasari A. Novel therapeutics for patients with well-differentiated gastroenteropancreatic neuroendocrine tumors. Ther Adv Med Oncol 2021;13.

107. Perez K, Chan J. Treatment of gastroenteropancreatic neuroendocrine tumors. Surg Pathol Clin 2019;12(4):1045–53.

108. Kvols LK, Moertel CG, O'Connell MJ, et al. Treatment of the malignant carcinoid syndrome. Evaluation of a long-acting somatostatin analogue. N Engl J Med 1986;315(11):663–6.

109. Rinke A, Müller HH, Schade-Brittinger C, et al. Placebo-controlled, double-blind, prospective, randomized study on the effect of octreotide LAR in the control of tumor growth in patients with metastatic neuroendocrine midgut tumors: a report from the PROMID Study Group. J Clin Oncol 2009;27(28):4656–63.

110. Caplin ME, Pavel M, Ćwikła JB, et al. Lanreotide in metastatic enteropancreatic neuroendocrine tumors. N Engl J Med 2014;371(3):224–33.

111. Tierney JF, Chivukula SV, Wang X, et al. Resection of primary tumor may prolong survival in metastatic gastroenteropancreatic neuroendocrine tumors. Surgery 2019;165(3):644–51.

112. Mayo SC, de Jong MC, Pulitano C, et al. Surgical management of hepatic neuro-endocrine tumor metastasis: results from an international multi-institutional analysis. Ann Surg Oncol 2010;17(12):3129–36.
113. Do Minh D, Chapiro J, Gorodetski B, et al. Intra-arterial therapy of neuroendocrine tumour liver metastases: comparing conventional TACE, drug-eluting beads TACE and yttrium-90 radioembolisation as treatment options using a propensity score analysis model. Eur Radiol 2017;27(12):4995–5005.
114. Chen JX, Wileyto EP, Soulen MC. Randomized embolization trial for neuroendocrine tumor metastases to the liver (RETNET): study protocol for a randomized controlled trial. Trials 2018;19(1):390.
115. Currie BM, Nadolski G, Mondschein J, et al. Chronic hepatotoxicity in patients with metastatic neuroendocrine tumor: transarterial chemoembolization versus transarterial radioembolization. J Vasc Interv Radiol 2020;31(10):1627–35.
116. Soulen MC, van Houten D, Teitelbaum UR, et al. Safety and feasibility of integrating yttrium-90 radioembolization with capecitabine-temozolomide for grade 2 liver-dominant metastatic neuroendocrine tumors. Pancreas 2018;47(8):980–4.
117. Strosberg J, El-Haddad G, Wolin E, et al. Phase 3 trial of 177Lu-dotatate for midgut neuroendocrine tumors. N Engl J Med 2017;376(2):125–35.
118. Kipnis ST, Hung M, Kumar S, et al. Laboratory, clinical, and survival outcomes associated with peptide receptor radionuclide therapy in patients with gastroenteropancreatic neuroendocrine tumors. JAMA Netw Open 2021;4(3):e212274.
119. Yordanova A, Wicharz MM, Mayer K, et al. The role of adding somatostatin analogues to peptide receptor radionuclide therapy as a combination and maintenance therapy. Clin Cancer Res 2018;24(19):4672–9.
120. Ballal S, Yadav MP, Damle NA, et al. Concomitant 177Lu-DOTATATE and capecitabine therapy in patients with advanced neuroendocrine tumors: a long-term-outcome, toxicity, survival, and quality-of-life study. Clin Nucl Med 2017;42(11):e457–66.
121. Heckert JM, Kipnis ST, Kumar S, et al. Abnormal pretreatment liver function tests are associated with discontinuation of peptide receptor radionuclide therapy in a U.S.-based neuroendocrine tumor cohort. Oncologist 2020;25(7):572–8.
122. Katona BW, Roccaro GA, Soulen MC, et al. Efficacy of peptide receptor radionuclide therapy in a united states-based cohort of metastatic neuroendocrine tumor patients: single-institution retrospective analysis. Pancreas 2017;46(9):1121–6.
123. Yao JC, Shah MH, Ito T, et al. Everolimus for advanced pancreatic neuroendocrine tumors. N Engl J Med 2011;364(6):514–23.
124. Yao JC, Fazio N, Singh S, et al. Everolimus for the treatment of advanced, nonfunctional neuroendocrine tumours of the lung or gastrointestinal tract (RADIANT-4): a randomised, placebo-controlled, phase 3 study. Lancet Lond Engl 2016;387(10022):968–77.
125. Raymond E, Dahan L, Raoul JL, et al. Sunitinib malate for the treatment of pancreatic neuroendocrine tumors. N Engl J Med 2011;364(6):501–13.
126. Oberg K. Management of functional neuroendocrine tumors of the pancreas. Gland Surg 2018;7(1):20–7.
127. Naraev BG, Halland M, Halperin DM, et al. Management of diarrhea in patients with carcinoid syndrome. Pancreas 2019;48(8):961–72.
128. Kulke MH, Hörsch D, Caplin ME, et al. Telotristat Ethyl, a Tryptophan Hydroxylase Inhibitor for the Treatment of Carcinoid Syndrome. J Clin Oncol 2017;35(1):14–23.

129. Kulke MH, O'Dorisio T, Phan A, et al. Telotristat etiprate, a novel serotonin synthesis inhibitor, in patients with carcinoid syndrome and diarrhea not adequately controlled by octreotide. Endocr Relat Cancer 2014;21(5):705–14.
130. Metz DC, Liu E, Joish VN, et al. Survival and clinical outcomes with telotristat ethyl in patients with carcinoid syndrome. Cancer Manag Res 2020;12: 9713–9.

Cancer in Inflammatory Bowel Disease

Adam S. Faye, MD, MS[1], Ariela K. Holmer, MD[1], Jordan E. Axelrad, MD, MPH*

KEYWORDS

- Inflammatory bowel disease • Crohn disease • Ulcerative colitis • Cancer
- Colorectal neoplasia • Dysplasia

KEY POINTS

- Individuals with inflammatory bowel diseases (IBD) are at an increased risk of developing intestinal neoplasia—particularly colorectal neoplasia, small bowel adenocarcinoma, intestinal lymphoma, and anal cancer—as a consequence of chronic intestinal inflammation.
- Individuals with IBD are also at risk for extraintestinal malignancies, such as cholangiocarcinoma, skin cancer, hematologic malignancies, genitourinary cancer, cervical cancer, and prostate cancer, thought to be a consequence of immunosuppressive therapies and an underlying inflammatory state.
- Colorectal cancer surveillance with colonoscopy using high-definition white light endoscopy should commence 8 to 10 years after IBD diagnosis among patients with significant colonic involvement (beyond the rectum) and continue at an interval of 1 to 3 years based on patient- and disease-related factors.
- If invisible dysplasia is identified, referral to an expert in IBD surveillance using chromoendoscopy is required.

INTRODUCTION

Inflammatory bowel diseases (IBD), comprising Crohn disease (CD) and ulcerative colitis (UC), are chronic inflammatory conditions of the gastrointestinal tract driven by inappropriate immune responses to an altered gut microbiome in genetically susceptible individuals.[1] IBD affects at least 0.4% of Europeans and North Americans, with a rising prevalence worldwide.[2–4]

Individuals with IBD are at an increased risk of developing intestinal neoplasia—particularly colorectal neoplasia (CRN), including colorectal dysplasia and colorectal

Grant support: J.E. Axelrad and A.S. Faye receive research support from the Crohn's and Colitis Foundation, J.E. Axelrad also receives research support from the Judith & Stewart Colton Center for Autoimmunity, the New York Crohn's and Colitis Organization, and the NIH NIDDK K23DK124570.
Inflammatory Bowel Disease Center at NYU Langone Health, 305 East 33rd Street, Lower Level, New York, NY 10016, USA
[1] Co-first authors.
* Corresponding author.
E-mail address: Jordan.Axelrad@nyulangone.org

cancer (CRC)—as a consequence of chronic colonic inflammation.[5-7] Others include small bowel adenocarcinoma, intestinal lymphoma, and anal cancer. In addition to cancers common in the general population, patients with IBD have also been shown to be at increased risk of developing extraintestinal malignancies, thought to be a consequence of immunosuppressive therapies and an underlying inflammatory state, including cholangiocarcinoma, skin cancer, hematologic malignancies, genitourinary (GU) cancer, cervical cancer, and prostate cancer. The focus of this review is to summarize (1) the risk of cancer in patients with IBD, (2) the diagnosis and management of CRN in IBD, and (3) the management of patients with IBD and active or recent cancer.

CANCER RISK AMONG PATIENTS WITH INFLAMMATORY BOWEL DISEASES
Colorectal Cancer

One of the most common malignancies in patients with IBD is CRC and is often the result of ongoing inflammation. Although prior studies have reported a risk of more than 15% after 30 years of active colonic disease, more recent estimates have shown a declining risk.[8,9] In a recent meta-analysis of population-based cohort studies, patients with IBD were estimated to have a 1%, 2%, and 5% risk of CRC after 10, 20, and greater than 20 years from initial IBD diagnosis, respectively.[10,11] It should be noted, however, that despite the decreasing rate of CRC, the incidence rate for early cancers has been increasing.[12] This is likely the result of a shift in the management of colonic dysplasia, with many being managed endoscopically rather than by colectomy. This may lead to a higher number of dysplastic areas being incompletely or partially resected, increasing the risk of progression to early-stage CRC. Despite this, 10-year survival rates remain high at almost 80%, with other studies showing no difference in outcomes when comparing IBD-associated and sporadic CRCs.[12,13]

Clinicians should also be aware that active colitis can increase the risk of multifocal dysplasia. Among a cohort of UC patients diagnosed with CRC, more than one-third had synchronous CRC or dysplasia at a distant site at time of colectomy.[12] This emphasizes the importance of close dysplasia surveillance and reinforces the need for endoscopic healing as outlined in the STRIDE-II guidelines.[14]

In addition to length of time with IBD, and extent of colonic disease, there are additional risk factors that increase the risk of CRC among patients with IBD. This includes (1) cumulative inflammation (calculated by summing the endoscopic disease severity at each surveillance endoscopy), which increases the likelihood of CRC more than two-fold for each 10-unit increase in score[15,16]; (2) the presence of concomitant primary sclerosing cholangitis (PSC), which on meta-analysis increased the odds of colorectal dysplasia and cancer more than three-fold when compared with patients with IBD who do not have PSC[17]; and (3) family history of CRC, which based upon a population-based cohort study of 19,876 individuals showed that a positive family history increased the risk of developing CRC more than two-fold among patients with IBD.[18,19] It should also be noted that patients with older-onset IBD are not at higher risk for developing CRC as compared with patients who have younger-onset IBD.[20]

Small Bowel Adenocarcinoma

Individuals who have CD with small bowel involvement are also at higher risk for small bowel adenocarcinoma. Although estimates have suggested an almost 20-fold increase in the likelihood of small bowel adenocarcinoma among patients with CD, the absolute risk remains very low (3 in 10,000 person-years).[21] In a more recent Denmark population-based study, analogous results were seen, as patients with CD had a higher likelihood of both small bowel adenocarcinomas (standardized incidence ratio [SIR] 14.38) and neuroendocrine tumors (SIR 6.83), but a low overall incidence (0.15%).[22] In a Surveillance, Epidemiology and End Results Medicare database study, the relative risk (RR) appeared similar in older individuals with CD, as patients aged 67 years and older had a 12-fold increase in risk of small bowel adenocarcinoma as compared with older adults without CD, although prevalence was reportedly higher at 1.6%.[23]

Regarding risk factors, small studies have suggested a higher risk of small bowel adenocarcinoma among men, tobacco users, those who have long-standing CD, penetrating CD, or prior small bowel resection, or as a result of therapy for CD.[22,24–26] These findings, however, are limited by small sample size.[27] In a recent, larger, population-based study of 47,370 patients with CD, identifiable risk factors for small bowel adenocarcinoma included those newly diagnosed, childhood-onset, ileal, and stricturing CD.[28]

Intestinal Lymphoma

In a large cross-sectional analysis of individuals living in Switzerland with IBD, intestinal lymphoma occurred at a rate of 48.3 cases per 100,000 patient-years (PY). Although this represents a two- to three-fold increase as compared with the general population (18 cases per 100,000 PY), similar to small bowel adenocarcinoma, the absolute risk remains low.[29] Furthermore, these intestinal lymphomas are predominantly B-cell non-Hodgkin lymphoma and are often associated with the presence of Epstein-Barr virus.[7,30] Furthermore, intestinal lymphomas occur more often in men, in patients with ongoing intestinal inflammation, and in patients who have had CD for more than 8 years.[7]

Anal Cancer

Similar to small intestinal adenocarcinoma and intestinal lymphoma, the absolute risk of anal cancer among patients with CD, although higher than the general population, remains low. One such risk factor for the development of anal squamous cell carcinoma is the presence of human papillomavirus.[31] In a recent study from the CESAME database, the incidence of anal squamous cell carcinoma was 2.6 per 10,000 PY among patients with IBD with anal or perianal lesions, as compared with 0.8 per 10,000 PY among patients with IBD without anal or perianal lesions.[32] In addition to human papillomavirus, longstanding perianal fistulizing disease has been shown to increase the risk of both anal squamous cell carcinoma and adenocarcinoma, with an incidence of 3.8 per 10,000 PY.[32]

Extraintestinal Malignancies

In addition to intestinal-related malignancies as described above, patients with IBD are also at risk for extraintestinal malignancies. Cholangiocarcinoma is 4 times more likely to occur in patients with IBD as compared with patients without IBD. In a Danish national cohort study assessing this, the incidence of cholangiocarcinoma was found to be 7.6 per 100,000 PY among patients with IBD as compared with 1.9 per 100,000 PY among controls.[33] Although not completely understood, this risk is predominantly driven by the concomitant presence of PSC, as patients with PSC have more than a 150-fold higher risk for developing cholangiocarcinoma compared with individuals without PSC.[34] This equates to a 5% to 10% lifetime risk of developing cholangiocarcinoma and often portends a poor prognosis once diagnosed.[7,34,35]

Skin cancer, including both nonmelanoma and melanoma skin cancer, is the most common cancer in the United States, with an estimated 5.4 million individuals affected.[36] This risk is higher among patients with IBD and is thought to be in part from the use of immunosuppressive therapy. Analogous to the increased risk of non-melanoma skin cancer seen in the transplant population, a similar increased risk is seen among patients with IBD who are using thiopurines. In a study of 108,579 patients with IBD, thiopurine use was associated with an almost two-fold increase in the development of nonmelanoma skin cancer.[37] In addition, ongoing thiopurine use may increase the risk of recurrent nonmelanoma skin cancer. In a recent retrospective Veterans Health Administration study, patients who had a prior basal cell carcinoma were more likely to have recurrence of disease in the setting of continued thiopurine use.[38] This increased risk of skin cancer is thought to persist even after discontinuation of thiopurines, emphasizing the importance of annual dermatologic examinations in patients with IBD, particularly if they are on thiopurines.[39]

Among patients using anti-tumor necrosis factor (anti-TNF) therapy, the increased risk of skin cancer seems to be predominantly melanoma in origin. In the above study looking at 108,579 patients with IBD, exposure to anti-TNF therapy increased the likelihood of developing melanoma by almost two-fold.[37] This, however, is in contrast to a prior nationwide study in Denmark that found no association between anti-TNF therapy and the development of melanoma.[40] In order to further elucidate this issue, a recent meta-analysis was performed that showed no significant difference in risk of melanoma among patients treated with biologics as compared with patients treated with nonbiologic therapies.[41] Regardless of anti-TNF use, however, all patients with IBD should receive yearly dermatologic examinations, as certain studies have even shown an increased risk of melanoma among patients with IBD not on biologic therapy.[42]

Nonintestinal lymphoma is another risk associated with IBD-related therapy, and more specifically with thiopurine use. In a recent meta-analysis, the SIR of lymphoma among patients with IBD treated with thiopurines ranged from 2.8 to 9.2.[43] The *absolute* risk was highest among older individuals (1:354 per PY), whereas the highest *relative* risk was among individuals under the age of 30 years (SIR 7.0).[43] Although most of these lymphomas are B cell in origin, men under the age of 35 years are also at risk for hepatosplenic T-cell lymphoma. This often results from long-term use of thiopurines, is often fatal, and requires close monitoring if used in this setting.[44] Although data surrounding the use of ani-TNF and development of lymphoma have been conflicting, more recent studies have suggested no increased risk associated with anti-TNF monotherapy.[45–48]

GU cancer is another malignancy that has been shown to be associated with thiopurine use among patients with IBD. More specifically, in the CESAME cohort, 16 of 19,486 (0.08%) patients developed kidney and/or bladder cancer, with those using thiopurines having a 2.8 times higher risk as compared with individuals not using thiopurines.[49] These results are analogous to a population-based study in Denmark, which showed that use of azathioprine among patients with IBD was associated with a 2.8 times higher rate of developing urinary tract cancer.[50] Additional risk factors for the development of GU cancer among patients with IBD include male sex and older age.[49]

In addition to GU cancer, there have also been recent data suggesting a link between IBD and prostate cancer. In a recent retrospective single-center study of 10,000 men, the incidence of prostate cancer was 4.4% among those who had IBD as compared with 0.65% among those who did not have IBD (hazard ratio [HR], 4.8).[51] In a prospective study of UK biobank samples, prostate cancer appeared to be associated with the presence of UC (HR, 1.47), but not CD.[52] Although further research is needed to make more definitive conclusions, preliminary laboratory-based work has shown an association between ongoing intestinal inflammation and the development of protumorigenic states in the prostate, suggesting a biologically plausible link.[53]

In a nationwide cohort study, similar results were seen when assessing rates of cervical cancer in women with and without IBD. Notably, women with UC and CD had a higher risk for cervical cancer development both before and after diagnosis of their IBD.[54] These results were confirmed in a recent multicenter Dutch prospective cohort study, where women with IBD were noted to be at a 1.3 times higher risk for developing high-grade dysplasia (HGD) and/or cervical cancer as compared with female-matched controls without IBD.[55] Additional risk factors included smoking and the presence of ileocolonic or upper gastrointestinal disease, which also increased the risk of cervical dysplasia and cancer 1.8 to 3 times, respectively.[55]

COLORECTAL CANCER SURVEILLANCE AND DYSPLASIA MANAGEMENT

Endoscopic surveillance programs for CRC, which are endorsed by all major gastroenterology and oncology societies, are based on indirect evidence of benefit.[56–63]

Generally, US guidelines recommend that CRN surveillance commence 8 to 10 years after diagnosis among patients with significant colonic involvement (beyond the rectum) and continue at an interval of 1 to 3 years based on patient- and disease-related factors. Among patients with colonic IBD who are diagnosed with PSC, colonoscopy should be performed at the time of PSC diagnosis with annual surveillance thereafter. Among patients without concomitant PSC, the interval for surveillance varies by society, with some recommending specific intervals based on risk stratification according to patient- and disease-related clinical characteristics.[64,65] Among patients with a first-degree relative with CRC, the initial examination should occur 10 years before age of CRC in the first-degree relative or after 8 years of IBD, whichever occurs first. Patients with isolated IBD proctitis do not require regular surveillance, unless there is proximal disease extension. Ileoanal pouch surveillance should be performed at least annually in those at high risk for developing CRN (PSC or previous CRN), as well as in those with persistent moderate to severe pouchitis and/or prepouch ileitis. In those patients at lower risk with a pouch, surveillance intervals should be individualized.

Quality metrics for colonoscopic surveillance in IBD reflect CRC screening and surveillance recommendations in the general population with some additional considerations, including the use of image-enhancing techniques, such as chromoendoscopy (CE).[59,60,63–67] It is recommended that surveillance examinations be performed by an experienced gastroenterologist specialized in IBD when disease is in remission and with adequate bowel preparation. Even with active disease, the identification of low-grade dysplasia (LGD), HGD, and CRC is still reliable with interobserver agreement. In quiescent disease, a large field of pseudopolyps, scars, or impassable strictures that compromise surveillance should prompt discussion of colectomy. Despite guidelines and quality metrics, widespread adherence to recommended surveillance techniques remains low.[68–71]

Based on updated guidance, standard of care for surveillance using high-definition white light endoscopy (HD-WLE) should include 4 nontargeted random biopsies every 10 cm from flat mucosa in areas previously affected by colitis, and placed in separate jars with the goal of detecting subtle or "invisible" dysplasia.[63] Additional biopsies should be taken from areas of prior dysplasia or poor mucosal visibility. However, CE has substantially improved dysplasia detection and brought into question whether "invisible" dysplasia is a true entity.[72,73] Application of dye CE (DCE) during colonoscopy with indigo carmine or methylene blue improves the visualization of subtle lesions in areas of adequate bowel preparation, minimal pseudopolyps, and endoscopically quiescent disease. A meta-analysis of 6 studies including 1358 patients with IBD undergoing surveillance with DCE (n = 670) or HD-WLE (n = 688) found that more dysplasia was identified with DCE compared with HD-WLE (19% vs 9%, $P = .08$).[74] However, a randomized controlled trial comparing HD-WLE with random biopsies (n = 102) with DCE with targeted biopsies (n = 108) showed no difference in dysplasia detection.[75] Virtual chromoendoscopy (VCE), such as narrow-band imaging, is an electronic imaging technology that provides mucosal contrast enhancement without the use of a dye. Studies evaluating the utility of VCE have not consistently demonstrated a higher yield of dysplasia detection.[66,76–78] A recent randomized controlled trial comparing VCE, DCE, and HD-WLE found that HD-WLE and VCE were noninferior to DCE,[79] and a follow-up meta-analysis of 11 randomized controlled trials comprising 1328 patients demonstrated that VCE performed similarly to DCE and HD-WLE with respect to dysplasia detection on a per-patient basis.[80]

Although CE is endorsed by multiple consensus recommendations,[63,66] the role of CE and random biopsies with HD-WLE is controversial, as the vast majority of neoplasia is accepted to be visible and CE adds to procedural time.[73,75,81–84] Although nontargeted biopsies are not required if CE is performed using HD-WLE, it should be considered for those at high risk of CRC, including patients with PSC, a personal history of dysplasia, or tubular-appearing colon suggestive of high cumulative inflammatory burden.[73] Currently, questions remain regarding which surveillance technique is superior for the group of patients with IBD and colonic involvement but no other risk factors for CRC: HD-WLE with random biopsies, HD-WLE with targeted biopsies, or HD-WLE with CE and targeted biopsies.

Dysplasia Types and Categories

The management of IBD-associated CRN is highly dependent on consistent definitions and characterization of lesions. Imprecise terminologies, such as dysplasia-associated lesion or mass, adenoma-associated lesion or mass, flat and raised dysplasia, were replaced by a modified Paris classification[85]—which has been classically applied to dysplastic lesions diagnosed in individuals without IBD—in an effort to more appropriately and consistently describe dysplastic lesions in individuals with IBD.[66] The SCENIC consensus statement recommended broad categorization of dysplasia as "visible," defined as a dysplastic lesion seen on endoscopy, and "invisible," defined as dysplasia diagnosed on histopathology from a nontargeted biopsy in the absence of a discrete lesion. The modified classification also included polypoid (≥2.5 mm) and nonpolypoid (<2.5 mm) lesions under the broader category of "visible" and further modified to include descriptors for visible dysplasia, including the presence of ulceration and the distinctness of the borders of the lesion.[86]

When a lesion concerning for dysplasia is identified on endoscopy, descriptors should include size, morphology (polypoid vs nonpolypoid), border (distinct vs indistinct), and features suggestive of submucosal invasion and invasiveness, such as depressed areas, ulceration, or nonlifting with injection.[66] A potentially resectable lesion should have discrete margins that are identifiable and would enable complete resection endoscopically. Biopsies should be obtained of the tissue surrounding the polyp to ensure that the surrounding tissue is free of dysplasia.

Dysplasia Management

The management of visible dysplasia in IBD is multidisciplinary. It requires confirmation by an expert IBD pathologist, therapeutic resection, medical management with risk factor modification, and surgical consultation with continued surveillance in the absence of colectomy (**Fig. 1**). The SCENIC consensus emphasized the importance of distinguishing polypoid from nonpolypoid (ie, flat) lesions, primarily owing to therapeutic and prognostic implications, as well as subsequent surveillance considerations.

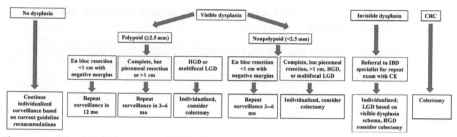

Fig. 1. HD-WLC for CRN screening/surveillance in an at-risk patient with colonic IBD. (Special considerations: concomitant PSC, history of CRN.)

Nonpolypoid lesions have a higher risk of progression to CRC compared with polypoid lesions.[87,88] In addition, histologic grade and focality impact prognosis and subsequent surveillance. For patients with en bloc resection of polypoid lesions less than 1 cm with confirmed negative margins, surveillance colonoscopy is recommended at 12 months.[66] For lesions removed piecemeal or with size greater than 1 cm, surveillance colonoscopy should be performed within 3 to 6 months, with the shorter interval favored for HGD.[66] Progression to HGD or CRC following complete resection of unifocal LGD is rare, whereas multifocal LGD carries substantial risk.[72,09-91] The management following complete resection of a visible lesion with HGD is controversial, and the decision of continuing shorter interval surveillance should be made on a case-by-case basis.[66,67,92] Compared with polypoid lesions, the course of nonpolypoid lesions following endoscopic resection is not well defined. In patients with complete endoscopic resection of nonpolypoid dysplasia, ongoing surveillance is suggested rather than colectomy with intervals similar to those recommended for polypoid dysplasia and with similar alterations according to histology and other factors. Surgical referral should still be discussed given the higher risk of incomplete resection of nonpolypoid lesions with a corresponding higher rate of recurrence and progression to HGD/CRC compared with polypoid lesions.[93]

If invisible dysplasia is identified and confirmed by a second pathologist with IBD expertise, timely referral to an expert in IBD surveillance using CE with HD-WLE is required. If no lesions are identified, random biopsies should be repeated. If LGD is detected randomly, surveillance should be performed every 3 to 6 months; however, surgery should still be discussed with patients given the significant risk of progressing to HGD/CRC.[93] In patients with PSC and LGD, there is a much lower threshold for colectomy given the significantly higher risk of progression. If HGD is detected on random biopsies, a repeat examination should be performed by an endoscopist experienced in IBD dysplasia detection and resection using HD-WLE with CE, and if no resectable lesions are identified, colectomy is indicated.

The success of endoscopic resection relies on the achievement of en bloc resection with negative margins. Endoscopic resection techniques include mucosal resection and submucosal dissection, with the latter having only limited data in the IBD population.[94-96] If endoscopic resection cannot be reliably achieved, then surgery may be indicated, with the surgery of choice being colectomy in UC or segmental resection versus colectomy in Crohn colitis depending on disease involvement. Other indications for surgery include any dysplasia in a patient with PSC, a personal history of CRC, severe pseudopolyposis or stricture limiting adequate quality surveillance, or multifocal dysplasia.[97]

Finally, optimal disease control with effective medical therapy is critical to minimizing an individual's lifetime risk of developing CRC.

MANAGEMENT OF PATIENTS WITH INFLAMMATORY BOWEL DISEASES WITH ACTIVE OR RECENT CANCER

With a rapidly growing aging population, the medical management of patients with IBD and active or recent cancer will become increasingly more important.[98] The effect of cancer treatment on underlying IBD disease activity and the risk of cancer progression or recurrence with IBD-directed immunosuppressive therapy are unique concerns in this patient population.

Impact of Cancer Treatment on Inflammatory Bowel Diseases Management

The treatment of extraintestinal cancers can impact the underlying course of IBD, as immunosuppressive therapy is used in the management of both cancer and IBD. In a retrospective study of 84 IBD patients diagnosed with cancer, 67% of patients with active IBD achieved remission during their cancer treatment course.[99] Of these, 90% received treatment with cytotoxic chemotherapy, suggesting a protective effect on intestinal inflammation. Furthermore, 90% of these patients *remained* in remission at 5 years, indicating a durable benefit to cytotoxic chemotherapy in patients with concomitant IBD. Conversely, hormonal therapy alone or in combination with cytotoxic chemotherapy was associated with an increased risk of IBD relapse (HR, 11.04; 95% confidence interval [CI], 1.22 to 99.85 and 9.7; 95% CI, 1.16 to 81.08 respectively).

The effect of hormonal deprivation therapy on the disease course of IBD was further examined in a multicenter study of 447 patients with either breast or prostate cancer and IBD. Of 400 patients with inactive IBD, 28% experienced disease relapse, and hormonal therapy alone or in combination with cytotoxic chemotherapy was significantly associated with risk of IBD flare (HR, 2.00; 95% CI, 1.21–3.29 and 1.86; CI, 95% CI, 1.01–3.43, respectively).[100] Of those in remission, only 42% of patients receiving hormone compared with 75% receiving cytotoxic chemotherapy remained in remission on follow-up (250 months). In patients with active IBD, no significant risk factors for achieving remission were identified.

Consistent hormone replacement therapy in postmenopausal patients with IBD was found to provide a significant protective effect on IBD disease activity, likely attributed to the anti-inflammatory properties of estrogen.[101] However, in premenopausal women, others describe an increased risk of developing IBD, specifically CD, with exposure to oral contraceptives.[102] Although further evidence is needed to clarify the impact of hormonal therapy on the development and disease course of IBD, patients diagnosed with cancers that are commonly treated with hormone deprivation therapy may be at increased risk for IBD disease reactivation and should be closely followed by a gastroenterologist.

In terms of IBD management, oncologists commonly defer to a gastroenterologist regarding guidance on IBD-directed immunosuppressive therapy. This underscores the importance of understanding the interplay between IBD disease activity and specific cancer treatment types, as well as maintaining close communication with the oncologist throughout the cancer treatment course.

Impact of Inflammatory Bowel Diseases Therapies on Active Cancer

Although there is considerable evidence for the risk of malignancy associated with immunosuppressive therapy in patients with IBD, less is known regarding the risk in those with active cancer. Pivotal randomized control trials and long-term safety registries have few to no data on patients with IBD with active cancer, and smaller observational studies have commonly excluded patients with active cancer.[45,103,104]

Recently, a retrospective, multicenter study evaluating the safety of IBD-directed immunosuppressive therapy in patients with active and recent prior cancer found similar rates of cancer progression in patients exposed to TNF-α antagonists versus non-TNF biologics versus immunomodulator monotherapy.[105] Of 107 patients with active cancer (72% solid tumor, 400 PY follow-up), 19 patients had progression of cancer and 20 were hospitalized for serious infection. After adjusting for age, type of active cancer, and immunomodulator status, there was no difference in the risk of cancer progression (HR, 1.55; 95% CI, 0.48–5.03), mortality (HR, 2.74; 95% CI, 0.25–30.5), and serious infections (HR, 1.90; 95% CI, 0.15–24.0) between TNF-α antagonists versus non-TNF biologics.

Similar to IBD, checkpoint inhibitor colitis is also commonly treated with biologics, such as TNF-α antagonists and anti-integrins. Immune therapies, such as cytotoxic T-lymphocyte-associated protein 4 (CTLA-4), programmed cell death protein 1 (PD-1), and programmed death-ligand 1 (PD-L1) inhibitors, have improved outcomes for patients with non–small cell lung cancer and melanoma, however are associated with an increased risk of diarrhea and colitis.[106,107] In a meta-analysis of 10 studies evaluating the gastrointestinal toxicities associated with immune checkpoint inhibitors, the RR of all-grade diarrhea and colitis was 1.64 (95% CI, 1.19–2.26; $P = .002$) and 10.35 (95% CI, 5.78–18.53; $P<.00001$), respectively.[108] Although there are no prospective clinical trials to guide management of checkpoint inhibitor colitis, both infliximab and vedolizumab are used in patients who are steroid refractory.[109] Treatment with infliximab has been associated with faster symptom improvement and shorter duration of steroid use.[110] Compared with infliximab, treatment with vedolizumab has led to shorter duration of steroid exposure (35 vs 50 days; $P<.001$), fewer hospitalizations (16% vs 28%; $P = .005$), and shorter length of hospital stay (median 10.5 vs 13.5 days; $P = .043$); however, treatment resulted in a longer time to clinical response (17.5 vs 13 days; $P = .012$).[111]

In patients with underlying IBD, treatment with immune checkpoint inhibitors can increase the risk of relapse in IBD and need for biologic therapy. In a meta-analysis of 12 studies consisting of 193 patients with IBD, treatment with immune checkpoint inhibitors led to IBD relapse in 40% of patients with at least one-third requiring biologics.[112] CTLA-4 inhibitors were associated with a higher risk of relapse compared with PD-1 and PD-L1 inhibitors. As a greater proportion of patients with cancer receive immunotherapy in the near future, further data on predictive biomarkers, therapeutic drug monitoring, and long-term safety of biologics are needed to optimize management in patients with checkpoint inhibitor colitis.

Impact of Inflammatory Bowel Diseases Therapies on Prior Cancer

Patients with IBD with a history of cancer may be at risk for developing a new or recurrent cancer. Evidence-based recommendations for the management of IBD-directed immunosuppressive therapy in patients with prior cancer remain limited, although steadily increasing. Given the known risks of lymphoma and other malignancies associated with immunosuppressants, there may be concern that IBD-directed therapy increases the risk of cancer recurrence.[113] However, recent retrospective data have not corroborated this increased risk. In a multicenter study from the New York Crohn's and Colitis Organization, the investigators evaluated the risk of new or recurrent cancer in patients with a prior history of cancer, with exposure to either TNF-α antagonists, antimetabolites, combination therapy, or no treatment. Of 333 patients, 90 (27%) patients developed an incident cancer. There was no difference in the risk of incident cancer or time to recurrent cancer between TNF-α antagonists versus antimetabolites versus combination therapy versus no treatment (incidence rate per 100 PY = 2.46 vs 5.75 vs 3.63 vs 5.40, respectively).[114] Similarly, in a meta-analysis of 16 retrospective studies, including more than 11,700 patients with immune-mediated diseases and a prior history of cancer, there was no significant difference in the rates of cancer recurrence in patients receiving anti-TNF therapy, immunomodulators, or no immunosuppression (33.8 per 1000 PY vs 36.2 per 1000 PY vs 37.5 per 1000 PY).[115]

Vedolizumab, a gut-selective $\alpha4\beta7$ integrin inhibitor, is considered to be less immunosuppressive with an overall favorable safety profile, and has recently been evaluated in patients with prior malignancy.[116] Vedamurthy and colleagues[117] compared the risk of new or recurrent cancers in patients with IBD treated with vedolizumab (96 patients) compared with TNF-α antagonists (184 patients) compared with no treatment (183 patients) after an index cancer diagnosis. After adjusting for confounders, there was no increase in the risk of new or recurrent cancer in patients exposed to vedolizumab versus TNF-α antagonists versus no therapy (HR, 1.38; 95% CI, 0.38–1.36 vs HR, 1.03; 95% CI, 0.65–1.64, respectively). These data suggest that, overall, treatment with TNF-α antagonists or vedolizumab is not associated with an increased risk of cancer recurrence or development of a new incident cancer, and the initiation or continuation of IBD-directed therapy should be based on disease extent, severity, and oncologic treatment plan.

Prospective studies on the risks of immunosuppressive therapy will be highly informative when managing patients with IBD and cancer. The ongoing SAPPHIRE registry is currently examining the risks of cancer recurrence in patients with IBD exposed to immunosuppression compared with those not exposed to immunosuppression.[118] In preliminary data, 231 patients with IBD and an index cancer were evaluated (48% men, median age 54 years, 47% solid tumor cancers). Of these, 23% of patients was exposed to immunomodulators, 31% was exposed to TNF-α antagonists, 28% was exposed to vedolizumab, 14% was exposed to ustekinumab, and 39% was exposed to no immunosuppression. On follow-up, exposure to biologics or immunomodulators was not associated with an increased risk of new or recurrent cancer when compared with no therapy (6.2 per 100 PY; RR, 4.6; 95% CI, 0.84–25; 5.9 per 100 PY; RR, 3.3, 95% CI, 0.94–11.58; 3.0 per 100 PY, respectively). Exposure to combination therapy with a biologic plus immunomodulator was however associated with an increased risk of new or recurrent cancer (14.4 per 100 PY; RR, 6.1; 95% CI, 1.7–22).

SUMMARY AND FUTURE DIRECTIONS

Patients with IBD are at an increased risk of cancer secondary to long-standing intestinal inflammation and secondary to immunosuppressive therapies. As the population of patients with IBD ages, there is an increasing risk of cancer development. Many of these patients will require cancer treatment, and many will require further treatment for their IBD. Much remains unknown regarding the interaction between IBD, medications for IBD, and cancer treatment, as well as the risk of cancer recurrence in patients with IBD and a history of cancer.

Overall, data are lacking regarding specific cancers, treatments, and risk of recurrence under varying medications for IBD. More data from prospective registries, such as SAPPHIRE,[118] will permit the development of evidence-based, quantitative risk-benefit models, including cancer and IBD-related variables to assist clinicians in managing this complex patient population.

CLINICS CARE POINTS

- In addition to cancers common in the general population, patients with IBD have also been shown to be at increased risk of developing intestinal and extraintestinal malignancies.

- The identification of cancer in a patient with IBD requires close collaboration with the treating gastroenterologist and oncologist.

DISCLOSURE

J.E. Axelrad reports receiving research grants from BioFire Diagnostics; consultancy fees or honorarium from BioFire Diagnostics, Janssen, Pfizer, Abbvie, and BMS; and holds US Patent 2012/0052124A1 and no other conflicts of interest. A.K. Holmer reports consultancy fees or honorarium from Pfizer.

REFERENCES

1. Kaser A, Zeissig S, Blumberg RS. Inflammatory bowel disease. Annu Rev Immunol 2010;28:573–621.
2. Ng SC, Shi HY, Hamidi N, et al. Worldwide incidence and prevalence of inflammatory bowel disease in the 21st century: a systematic review of population-based studies. Lancet 2017;390:2769–78.
3. Kaplan GG. The global burden of IBD: from 2015 to 2025. Nat Rev Gastroenterol Hepatol 2015;12:720–7.
4. Molodecky NA, Soon IS, Rabi DM, et al. Increasing incidence and prevalence of the inflammatory bowel diseases with time, based on systematic review. Gastroenterology 2012;142:46–54.e42 [quiz: e30].
5. Rutter MD, Saunders BP, Wilkinson KH, et al. Thirty-year analysis of a colonoscopic surveillance program for neoplasia in ulcerative colitis. Gastroenterology 2006;130:1030–8.
6. Ullman TA, Itzkowitz SH. Intestinal inflammation and cancer. Gastroenterology 2011;140:1807–16.
7. Beaugerie L, Itzkowitz SH. Cancers complicating inflammatory bowel disease. N Engl J Med 2015;372:1441–52.
8. Eaden JA, Abrams KR, Mayberry JF. The risk of colorectal cancer in ulcerative colitis: a meta-analysis. Gut 2001;48:526–35.
9. Axelrad JE, Lichtiger S, Yajnik V. Inflammatory bowel disease and cancer: The role of inflammation, immunosuppression, and cancer treatment. World J Gastroenterol 2016;22:4794–801.
10. Bernstein CN, Blanchard JF, Kliewer E, et al. Cancer risk in patients with inflammatory bowel disease: a population-based study. Cancer 2001;91:854–62.
11. Lutgens MWMD, van Oijen MGH, van der Heijden GJMG, et al. Declining risk of colorectal cancer in inflammatory bowel disease: an updated meta-analysis of population-based cohort studies. Inflamm Bowel Dis 2013;19:789–99.
12. Choi C-HR, Rutter MD, Askari A, et al. Forty-Year Analysis of Colonoscopic Surveillance Program for Neoplasia in Ulcerative Colitis: An Updated Overview. Am J Gastroenterol 2015;110:1022–34.
13. Reynolds IS, O'Toole A, Deasy J, et al. A meta-analysis of the clinicopathological characteristics and survival outcomes of inflammatory bowel disease associated colorectal cancer. Int J Colorectal Dis 2017;32:443–51.

14. Turner D, Ricciuto A, Lewis A, et al. STRIDE-II: An Update on the Selecting Therapeutic Targets in Inflammatory Bowel Disease (STRIDE) Initiative of the International Organization for the Study of IBD (IOIBD): Determining Therapeutic Goals for Treat-to-Target strategies in IBD. Gastroenterology 2021;160:1570–83.

15. Rutter M, Saunders B, Wilkinson K, et al. Severity of inflammation is a risk factor for colorectal neoplasia in ulcerative colitis. Gastroenterology 2004;126:451–9.

16. Choi C-HR, Al Bakir I, Ding N-SJ, et al. Cumulative burden of inflammation predicts colorectal neoplasia risk in ulcerative colitis: a large single-centre study. Gut 2019;68:414–22.

17. Zheng H-H, Jiang X-L. Increased risk of colorectal neoplasia in patients with primary sclerosing cholangitis and inflammatory bowel disease: a meta-analysis of 16 observational studies. Eur J Gastroenterol Hepatol 2016;28:383–90.

18. Askling J, Dickman PW, Karlén P, et al. Family history as a risk factor for colorectal cancer in inflammatory bowel disease. Gastroenterology 2001;120:1356–62.

19. Cleveland NK, Rubin DT. Cancer prevention in patients with inflammatory bowel disease. Pract Gastroenterol 2021;45:12–28.

20. Cheddani H, Dauchet L, Fumery M, et al. Cancer in Elderly Onset Inflammatory Bowel Disease: A Population-Based Study. Am J Gastroenterol 2016;111:1428–36.

21. Laukoetter MG, Mennigen R, Hannig CM, et al. Intestinal cancer risk in Crohn's disease: a meta-analysis. J Gastrointest Surg 2011;15:576–83.

22. Bojesen RD, Riis LB, Høgdall E, et al. Inflammatory Bowel Disease and Small Bowel Cancer Risk, Clinical Characteristics, and Histopathology: A Population-Based Study. Clin Gastroenterol Hepatol 2017;15:1900–7.e2.

23. Shaukat A, Virnig DJ, Howard D, et al. Crohn's disease and small bowel adenocarcinoma: a population-based case-control study. Cancer Epidemiol Biomarkers Prev 2011;20:1120–3.

24. Palascak-Juif V, Bouvier AM, Cosnes J, et al. Small bowel adenocarcinoma in patients with Crohn's disease compared with small bowel adenocarcinoma de novo. Inflamm Bowel Dis 2005;11:828–32.

25. Lashner BA. Risk factors for small bowel cancer in Crohn's disease. Dig Dis Sci 1992;37:1179–84.

26. Chen CC, Neugut AI, Rotterdam H. Risk factors for adenocarcinomas and malignant carcinoids of the small intestine: preliminary findings. Cancer Epidemiol Biomarkers Prev 1994;3:205–7.

27. Cahill C, Gordon PH, Petrucci A, et al. Small bowel adenocarcinoma and Crohn's disease: any further ahead than 50 years ago? World J Gastroenterol 2014;20:11486–95.

28. Axelrad JE, Olén O, Sachs MC, et al. Inflammatory bowel disease and risk of small bowel cancer: a binational population-based cohort study from Denmark and Sweden. Gut 2021;70(2):297–308.

29. Scharl S, Barthel C, Rossel J-B, et al. Malignancies in Inflammatory Bowel Disease: Frequency, Incidence and Risk Factors-Results from the Swiss IBD Cohort Study. Am J Gastroenterol 2019;114:116–26.

30. Sokol H, Beaugerie L, Maynadié M, et al. Excess primary intestinal lymphoproliferative disorders in patients with inflammatory bowel disease. Inflamm Bowel Dis 2012;18:2063–71.

31. Ruel J, Ko HM, Roda G, et al. Anal neoplasia in inflammatory bowel disease is associated with HPV and perianal disease. Clin Transl Gastroenterol 2016;7:e148.

32. Beaugerie L, Carrat F, Nahon S, et al. High Risk of Anal and Rectal Cancer in Patients With Anal and/or Perianal Crohn's Disease. Clin Gastroenterol Hepatol 2018;16:892–9.e2.

33. Erichsen R, Jepsen P, Vilstrup H, et al. Incidence and prognosis of cholangio-carcinoma in Danish patients with and without inflammatory bowel disease: a national cohort study, 1978-2003. Eur J Epidemiol 2009;24:513–20.

34. Singh S, Talwalkar JA. Primary sclerosing cholangitis: diagnosis, prognosis, and management. Clin Gastroenterol Hepatol 2013;11:898–907.

35. Burak K, Angulo P, Pasha TM, et al. Incidence and risk factors for cholangiocar-cinoma in primary sclerosing cholangitis. Am J Gastroenterol 2004;99:523–6.

36. Rogers HW, Weinstock MA, Feldman SR, et al. Incidence estimate of nonmela-noma skin cancer (keratinocyte carcinomas) in the U.S. population, 2012. JAMA Dermatol 2015;151:1081–6.

37. Long MD, Martin CF, Pipkin CA, et al. Risk of melanoma and nonmelanoma skin cancer among patients with inflammatory bowel disease. Gastroenterology 2012;143:390–9.e1.

38. Khan N, Patel D, Trivedi C, et al. Repeated occurrences of basal cell cancer in patients with inflammatory bowel disease treated with immunosuppressive med-ications. Am J Gastroenterol 2020;115:1246–52.

39. Peyrin-Biroulet L, Khosrotehrani K, Carrat F, et al. Increased risk for nonmela-noma skin cancers in patients who receive thiopurines for inflammatory bowel disease. Gastroenterology 2011;141:1621–16228.e1.

40. Nyboe Andersen N, Pasternak B, Basit S, et al. Association between tumor ne-crosis factor-α antagonists and risk of cancer in patients with inflammatory bowel disease. JAMA 2014;311:2406–13.

41. Esse S, Mason KJ, Green AC, et al. Melanoma Risk in Patients Treated With Bio-logic Therapy for Common Inflammatory Diseases: A Systematic Review and Meta-analysis. JAMA Dermatol 2020;156:787–94.

42. Singh S, Nagpal SJS, Murad MH, et al. Inflammatory bowel disease is associ-ated with an increased risk of melanoma: a systematic review and meta-anal-ysis. Clin Gastroenterol Hepatol 2014;12:210–8.

43. Kotlyar DS, Lewis JD, Beaugerie L, et al. Risk of lymphoma in patients with in-flammatory bowel disease treated with azathioprine and 6-mercaptopurine: a meta-analysis. Clin Gastroenterol Hepatol 2015;13:847–58.e4 [quiz: e48].

44. Kotlyar DS, Osterman MT, Diamond RH, et al. A systematic review of factors that contribute to hepatosplenic T-cell lymphoma in patients with inflammatory bowel disease. Clin Gastroenterol Hepatol 2011;9:36–41.e1.

45. Lemaitre M, Kirchgesner J, Rudnichi A, et al. Association between use of thio-purines or tumor necrosis factor antagonists alone or in combination and risk of lymphoma in patients with inflammatory bowel disease. JAMA 2017;318:1679–86.

46. Yang C, Huang J, Huang X, et al. Risk of Lymphoma in Patients With Inflamma-tory Bowel Disease Treated With Anti-tumour Necrosis Factor Alpha Agents: A Systematic Review and Meta-analysis. J Crohns Colitis 2018;12:1042–52.

47. Dahmus J, Rosario M, Clarke K. Risk of Lymphoma Associated with Anti-TNF Therapy in Patients with Inflammatory Bowel Disease: Implications for Therapy. Clin Exp Gastroenterol 2020;13:339–50.

48. Osterman MT, Sandborn WJ, Colombel J-F, et al. Increased risk of malignancy with adalimumab combination therapy, compared with monotherapy, for Crohn's disease. Gastroenterology 2014;146:941–9.

49. Bourrier A, Carrat F, Colombel JF, et al. Excess risk of urinary tract cancers in patients receiving thiopurines for inflammatory bowel disease: a prospective observational cohort study. Aliment Pharmacol Ther 2016;43:252–61.
50. Pasternak B, Svanström H, Schmiegelow K, et al. Use of azathioprine and the risk of cancer in inflammatory bowel disease. Am J Epidemiol 2013;177:1296–305.
51. Burns JA, Weiner AB, Catalona WJ, et al. Inflammatory bowel disease and the risk of prostate cancer. Eur Urol 2019;75:846–52.
52. Meyers TJ, Weiner AB, Graff RE, et al. Association between inflammatory bowel disease and prostate cancer: A large-scale, prospective, population-based study. Int J Cancer 2020;147:2735–42.
53. Desai AS, Sagar V, Lysy B, et al. Inflammatory bowel disease induces inflammatory and pre-neoplastic changes in the prostate. Prostate Cancer Prostatic Dis 2021. https://doi.org/10.1038/s41391-021-00392-7.
54. Rungoe C, Simonsen J, Riis L, et al. Inflammatory bowel disease and cervical neoplasia: a population-based nationwide cohort study. Clin Gastroenterol Hepatol 2015;13:693–700.e1.
55. Goetgebuer RL, Kreijne JE, Aitken CA, et al. Increased Risk of High-grade Cervical Neoplasia in Women with Inflammatory Bowel Disease: A Case-controlled Cohort Study. J Crohns Colitis 2021;15:1464–73.
56. Farraye FA, Odze RD, Eaden J, et al. AGA medical position statement on the diagnosis and management of colorectal neoplasia in inflammatory bowel disease. Gastroenterology 2010;138:738–45.
57. Cairns SR, Scholefield JH, Steele RJ, et al. Guidelines for colorectal cancer screening and surveillance in moderate and high risk groups (update from 2002). Gut 2010;59:666–89.
58. Annese V, Daperno M, Rutter MD, et al. European evidence based consensus for endoscopy in inflammatory bowel disease. J Crohns Colitis 2013;7:982–1018.
59. Kornbluth A, Sachar DB. Practice Parameters Committee of the American College of Gastroenterology. Ulcerative colitis practice guidelines in adults: American College Of Gastroenterology, Practice Parameters Committee. Am J Gastroenterol 2010;105:501–23 [quiz: 524].
60. American Society for Gastrointestinal Endoscopy Standards of Practice Committee, Shergill AK, Lightdale JR, et al. The role of endoscopy in inflammatory bowel disease. Gastrointest Endosc 2015;81:1101–11021.e1.
61. Lutgens MWMD, Oldenburg B, Siersema PD, et al. Colonoscopic surveillance improves survival after colorectal cancer diagnosis in inflammatory bowel disease. Br J Cancer 2009;101:1671–5.
62. Choi PM, Nugent FW, Schoetz DJ, et al. Colonoscopic surveillance reduces mortality from colorectal cancer in ulcerative colitis. Gastroenterology 1993;105:418–24.
63. Murthy SK, Feuerstein JD, Nguyen GC, et al. AGA clinical practice update on endoscopic surveillance and management of colorectal dysplasia in inflammatory bowel diseases: expert review. Gastroenterology 2021;161:1043–51.e4.
64. Eaden JA, Mayberry JF, British Society for Gastroenterology, et al. Guidelines for screening and surveillance of asymptomatic colorectal cancer in patients with inflammatory bowel disease. Gut 2002;51(Suppl 5):V10–2.
65. Harbord M, Eliakim R, Bettenworth D, et al. Corrigendum: Third European Evidence-based Consensus on Diagnosis and Management of Ulcerative Colitis. Part 2: Current Management. J Crohns Colitis 2017;11:1512.

66. Laine L, Kaltenbach T, Barkun A, et al. SCENIC international consensus statement on surveillance and management of dysplasia in inflammatory bowel disease. Gastrointest Endosc 2015;81:489–501.e26.
67. Annese V, Beaugerie L, Egan L, et al. European Evidence-based Consensus: Inflammatory Bowel Disease and Malignancies. J Crohns Colitis 2015;9:945–65.
68. Gearry RB, Wakeman CJ, Barclay ML, et al. Surveillance for dysplasia in patients with inflammatory bowel disease: a national survey of colonoscopic practice in New Zealand. Dis Colon Rectum 2004;47:314–22.
69. Kaplan GG, Heitman SJ, Hilsden RJ, et al. Population-based analysis of practices and costs of surveillance for colonic dysplasia in patients with primary sclerosing cholangitis and colitis. Inflamm Bowel Dis 2007;13:1401–7.
70. Eaden JA, Ward BA, Mayberry JF. How gastroenterologists screen for colonic cancer in ulcerative colitis: an analysis of performance. Gastrointest Endosc 2000;51:123–8.
71. Rijn AF van, Fockens P, Siersema PD, et al. Adherence to surveillance guidelines for dysplasia and colorectal carcinoma in ulcerative and Crohn's colitis patients in the Netherlands. World J Gastroenterol 2009;15:226.
72. Ten Hove JR, Mooiweer E, van der Meulen de Jong AE, et al. Clinical implications of low grade dysplasia found during inflammatory bowel disease surveillance: a retrospective study comparing chromoendoscopy and white-light endoscopy. Endoscopy 2017;49:161–8.
73. Moussata D, Allez M, Cazals-Hatem D, et al. Are random biopsies still useful for the detection of neoplasia in patients with IBD undergoing surveillance colonoscopy with chromoendoscopy? Gut 2018;67:616–24.
74. Jegadeesan R, Desai M, Sundararajan T, et al. P172 chromoendoscopy versus high definition white light endoscopy for dysplasia detection in patients with inflammatory bowel disease: a systematic review and meta-analysis. Gastroenterology 2018;154:S93.
75. Yang D-H, Park SJ, Kim H-S, et al. High-Definition Chromoendoscopy Versus High-Definition White Light Colonoscopy for Neoplasia Surveillance in Ulcerative Colitis: A Randomized Controlled Trial. Am J Gastroenterol 2019;114:1642–8.
76. Dekker E, van den Broek FJ, Reitsma JB, et al. Narrow-band imaging compared with conventional colonoscopy for the detection of dysplasia in patients with longstanding ulcerative colitis. Endoscopy 2007;39:216–21.
77. Pellisé M, López-Cerón M, Rodríguez de Miguel C, et al. Narrow-band imaging as an alternative to chromoendoscopy for the detection of dysplasia in longstanding inflammatory bowel disease: a prospective, randomized, crossover study. Gastrointest Endosc 2011;74:840–8.
78. Ignjatovic A, Tozer P, Grant K, et al. Outcome of benign strictures in ulcerative colitis. Gut 2011;60:A221–2.
79. Iacucci M, Kaplan GG, Panaccione R, et al. A randomized trial comparing high definition colonoscopy alone with high definition dye spraying and electronic virtual chromoendoscopy for detection of colonic neoplastic lesions during IBD surveillance colonoscopy. Am J Gastroenterol 2018;113:225–34.
80. El-Dallal M, Chen Y, Lin Q, et al. Meta-analysis of Virtual-based Chromoendoscopy Compared With Dye-spraying Chromoendoscopy Standard and High-definition White Light Endoscopy in Patients With Inflammatory Bowel Disease at Increased Risk of Colon Cancer. Inflamm Bowel Dis 2020;26:1319–29.
81. Iannone A, Ruospo M, Wong G, et al. Chromoendoscopy for surveillance in ulcerative colitis and Crohn's disease: A systematic review of randomized trials. Clin Gastroenterol Hepatol 2017;15:1684–97.e11.

82. Rubin DT, Ananthakrishnan AN, Siegel CA, et al. ACG clinical guideline: ulcerative colitis in adults. Am J Gastroenterol 2019;114:384–413.

83. van den Broek FJC, Stokkers PCF, Reitsma JB, et al. Random biopsies taken during colonoscopic surveillance of patients with longstanding ulcerative colitis: low yield and absence of clinical consequences. Am J Gastroenterol 2014;109: 715–22.

84. Rubin DT, Rothe JA, Hetzel JT, et al. Are dysplasia and colorectal cancer endoscopically visible in patients with ulcerative colitis? Gastrointest Endosc 2007; 65:998–1004.

85. Anon. The Paris endoscopic classification of superficial neoplastic lesions: esophagus, stomach, and colon: November 30 to December 1, 2002. Gastrointest Endosc 2003;58:S3–43.

86. Endoscopic Classification Review Group. Update on the Paris classification of superficial neoplastic lesions in the digestive tract. Endoscopy 2005;37:570–8.

87. Wanders LK, Dekker E, Pullens B, et al. Cancer risk after resection of polypoid dysplasia in patients with longstanding ulcerative colitis: a meta-analysis. Clin Gastroenterol Hepatol 2014;12:756–64.

88. Voorham QJM, Rondagh EJA, Knol DL, et al. Tracking the molecular features of nonpolypoid colorectal neoplasms: a systematic review and meta-analysis. Am J Gastroenterol 2013;108:1042–56.

89. Pekow JR, Hetzel JT, Rothe JA, et al. Outcome after surveillance of low-grade and indefinite dysplasia in patients with ulcerative colitis. Inflamm Bowel Dis 2010;16:1352–6.

90. Navaneethan U, Jegadeesan R, Gutierrez NG, et al. Progression of low-grade dysplasia to advanced neoplasia based on the location and morphology of dysplasia in ulcerative colitis patients with extensive colitis under colonoscopic surveillance. J Crohns Colitis 2013;7:e684–91.

91. Zisman TL, Bronner MP, Rulyak S, et al. Prospective study of the progression of low-grade dysplasia in ulcerative colitis using current cancer surveillance guidelines. Inflamm Bowel Dis 2012;18:2240–6.

92. ASGE Standards of Practice Committee, Evans JA, Chandrasekhara V, et al. The role of endoscopy in the management of premalignant and malignant conditions of the stomach. Gastrointest Endosc 2015;82:1–8.

93. Choi CR, Ignjatovic-Wilson A, Askari A, et al. Low-grade dysplasia in ulcerative colitis: risk factors for developing high-grade dysplasia or colorectal cancer. Am J Gastroenterol 2015;110:1461–71 [quiz: 1472].

94. Iacopini F, Saito Y, Yamada M, et al. Curative endoscopic submucosal dissection of large nonpolypoid superficial neoplasms in ulcerative colitis (with videos). Gastrointest Endosc 2015;82:734–8.

95. Suzuki N, Toyonaga T, East JE. Endoscopic submucosal dissection of colitis-related dysplasia. Endoscopy 2017;49:1237–42.

96. Kinoshita S, Uraoka T, Nishizawa T, et al. The role of colorectal endoscopic submucosal dissection in patients with ulcerative colitis. Gastrointest Endosc 2018; 87:1079–84.

97. Itzkowitz SH, Present DH. Crohn's and Colitis Foundation of America Colon Cancer in IBD Study Group. Consensus conference: Colorectal cancer screening and surveillance in inflammatory bowel disease. Inflamm Bowel Dis 2005;11: 314–21.

98. Faye AS, Colombel J-F. Aging and IBD: A new challenge for clinicians and researchers. Inflamm Bowel Dis 2022;28:126–32.

99. Axelrad JE, Fowler SA, Friedman S, et al. Effects of cancer treatment on inflammatory bowel disease remission and reactivation. Clin Gastroenterol Hepatol 2012;10:1021–7.e1.

100. Axelrad JE, Bazarbashi A, Zhou J, et al. Hormone therapy for cancer is a risk factor for relapse of inflammatory bowel diseases. Clin Gastroenterol Hepatol 2020;18:872–80.e1.

101. Kane SV, Reddy D. Hormonal replacement therapy after menopause is protective of disease activity in women with inflammatory bowel disease. Am J Gastroenterol 2008;103:1193–6.

102. Cornish JA, Tan E, Simillis C, et al. The risk of oral contraceptives in the etiology of inflammatory bowel disease: a meta-analysis. Am J Gastroenterol 2008;103: 2394–400.

103. D'Haens G, Reinisch W, Panaccione R, et al. Lymphoma Risk and Overall Safety Profile of Adalimumab in Patients With Crohn's Disease With up to 6 Years of Follow-Up in the Pyramid Registry. Am J Gastroenterol 2018;113: 872–82.

104. Rutgeerts P, Sandborn WJ, Feagan BG, et al. Infliximab for induction and maintenance therapy for ulcerative colitis. N Engl J Med 2005;353:2462–76.

105. Holmer AK, Luo J, Park S, et al. S697 Comparative Safety of Biologic Agents in Patients With Inflammatory Bowel Disease with Active or Recent Malignancy: A Multi-Center Cohort Study. Am J Gastroenterol 2021;116:S316.

106. Bellaguarda E, Hanauer S. Checkpoint Inhibitor-Induced Colitis. Am J Gastroenterol 2020;115:202–10.

107. Ribas A, Hamid O, Daud A, et al. Association of pembrolizumab with tumor response and survival among patients with advanced melanoma. JAMA 2016; 315:1600–9.

108. Abdel-Rahman O, ElHalawani H, Fouad M. Risk of gastrointestinal complications in cancer patients treated with immune checkpoint inhibitors: a meta-analysis. Immunotherapy 2015;7:1213–27.

109. Dougan M, Wang Y, Rubio-Tapia A, et al. AGA clinical practice update on diagnosis and management of immune checkpoint inhibitor colitis and hepatitis: expert review. Gastroenterology 2021;160:1384–93.

110. Johnson DH, Zobniw CM, Trinh VA, et al. Infliximab associated with faster symptom resolution compared with corticosteroids alone for the management of immune-related enterocolitis. J Immunother Cancer 2018;6:103.

111. Zou F, Faleck D, Thomas A, et al. Efficacy and safety of vedolizumab and infliximab treatment for immune-mediated diarrhea and colitis in patients with cancer: a two-center observational study. J Immunother Cancer 2021; 9:e003277.

112. Meserve J, Facciorusso A, Holmer AK, et al. Systematic review with meta-analysis: safety and tolerability of immune checkpoint inhibitors in patients with pre-existing inflammatory bowel diseases. Aliment Pharmacol Ther 2021; 53:374–82.

113. Holmer A, Singh S. Overall and comparative safety of biologic and immunosuppressive therapy in inflammatory bowel diseases. Expert Rev Clin Immunol 2019;15:969–79.

114. Axelrad J, Bernheim O, Colombel J-F, et al. Risk of New or Recurrent Cancer in Patients With Inflammatory Bowel Disease and Previous Cancer Exposed to Immunosuppressive and Anti-Tumor Necrosis Factor Agents. Clin Gastroenterol Hepatol 2016;14:58–64.

115. Shelton E, Laharie D, Scott FI, et al. Cancer Recurrence Following Immune-Suppressive Therapies in Patients With Immune-Mediated Diseases: A Systematic Review and Meta-analysis. Gastroenterology 2016; 151:97–109.e4.
116. Meserve J, Aniwan S, Koliani-Pace JL, et al. Retrospective analysis of safety of vedolizumab in patients with inflammatory bowel diseases. Clin Gastroenterol Hepatol 2019;17:1533–40.e2.
117. Vedamurthy A, Gangasani N, Ananthakrishnan AN. Vedolizumab or tumor necrosis factor antagonist use and risk of new or recurrent cancer in patients with inflammatory bowel disease with prior malignancy: A retrospective cohort study. Clin Gastroenterol Hepatol 2022;20:88–95.
118. Axelrad JE, Colombel JF, Scherl EJ, et al. Fr514 the sapphire registry: safety of immunosuppression in a prospective cohort of inflammatory bowel disease patients with a history of cancer. Gastroenterology 2021;160:S340.

The Microbiome in Gastrointestinal Cancers

Michael G. White, MD, MSc[a], Jennifer A. Wargo, MD, MMSc[a,b],*

KEYWORDS

- Microbiome • Tumor microenvironment • Colorectal adenocarcinoma
- Gastric adenocarcinoma • Pancreatic ductal adenocarcinoma

KEY POINTS

- The gut microbiome and host immune system are in a dynamic homeostasis whose alterations have been associated with the development and progression of a variety of malignancies.
- The tumoral microbiome plays a role in the tumor microenvironment modulating immune responses to tumors and has the potential to affect the pharmacodynamics of some cytotoxic therapies.
- Further work is needed to delineate mechanisms behind these observations and translate them to clinical benefit for patients.

INTRODUCTION

Not long after the introduction of the germ theory of disease by Louis Pasteur and Robert Koch, Izmar Isidor Boas and Bruno Oppler began to describe bacteria within the luminal contents of the stomach of patients with gastric cancer and specific species that were notably absent from the contents of healthy controls. This noted "colonization" of the stomach with bacteria was thought to potentially relate to physiologic changes within the stomach itself associated with carcinogenesis.[1] Given the inherent limitations of the time, however, these associations could only be made through microscopic evaluation of stomach or stool contents or by culturing these contents within various media—leading to notable biases in observations and clouding more in-depth study. A century later, we are continuing to discover and describe the role of bacteria in cancer initiation, progression, and evasion of contemporary therapeutics (cytotoxic chemotherapy, immunotherapy, and radiation therapy). In the last

[a] Department of Surgical Oncology, The University of Texas MD Anderson Cancer Center, 1515 Holcombe Boulevard, Unit 1484, Houston, TX 77030, USA; [b] Department of Genomic Medicine, The University of Texas MD Anderson Cancer Center, 1515 Holcombe Boulevard, Unit 1484, Houston, TX 77030, USA
* Corresponding author. Department of Genomic Medicine, The University of Texas MD Anderson Cancer Center, 1515 Holcombe Boulevard, Unit 1484, Houston, TX 77030.
E-mail address: jwargo@mdanderson.org

Gastroenterol Clin N Am 51 (2022) 667–680
https://doi.org/10.1016/j.gtc.2022.06.007
0889-8553/22/© 2022 Elsevier Inc. All rights reserved.

3 decades, with the introduction and popularization of next-generation sequencing (NGS) technologies, an omics-based approach to the microbiome has led to a vastly more comprehensive and detailed descriptions of human microbiology and downstream insights into their role in gastrointestinal (GI) malignancies outlined here.

Although several hypotheses have been suggested across disease histologies, the role of bacterial or viral species in the development of GI malignancies continues to be elucidated. To date, several viruses and bacteria including *Helicobacter pylori,* hepatitis B and C, HIV human papillomavirus, Epstein–Barr virus, human herpesvirus type 8, human T-cell lymphotropic virus type 1, *Opisthorchis viverrini, Clonorchis sinensis*, and *Schistosoma haematobium* have been clearly linked to carcinogenesis.[2] These microbes, and others under active study, are thought to affect cancer outcomes through alterations of metabolomic pathways, induced changes in the host immune system, and alterations in the pharmacokinetics of anticancer agents. Beyond the epidemiologic or culture-based systems of study, the contemporary hypotheses of the role of microbes in these systems are heavily dependent on accurate descriptions of the host immune system and the tumor microenvironment.

The introduction of NGS techniques was a disruptor in microbial research. Using NGS techniques, it is now possible to definitely and precisely describe the microbial compositions of gut luminal contents, tumors, healthy tissues, and circulating plasma. One of the earliest of these techniques sequences the RNA from the 16s ribosomal component of the 30s ribosomal subunit of prokaryotic species. These RNA can be sequenced using NGS technology to provide the rapid and accurate identification of bacterial species. In addition, several software packages have recently been developed to identify bacterial, viral, or fungal sequence reads in transcriptomic, exomic, and genomic sequencing of human tissue. Classically discarded as a quality control step in standard human sequencing, these tools leverage discarded raw sequence reads aligned to microbial sequences or various bacterial taxa or viruses.

Importantly, these observations describe a point in time of a complex system and are independent of culture growth kinetics or other microbial factors that were inherent biases in years passed. Simultaneously, recognition of the importance of the immune system in cancer surveillance and suppression has been increasingly appreciated in the last decade. This has led to the description of a critical axis that exists between the host microbiome, immune system, and cancer-specific outcomes. Ultimately, as the importance of these bacterial and viral species throughout the body is understood, therapeutics leveraging these observations to improve care is being developed, providing the opportunity for these advances in knowledge to improve patient outcomes.

Here, we review work demonstrating a variety of associations between GI malignancies (gastric, pancreatic, and colorectal adenocarcinoma [CRC]) and the gut and tumoral microbiome. We also review the role these microbes play in evasion of therapeutics targeting these cancers. Last, hypotheses and early data supporting the mechanistic underpinnings of these associations are described. Understanding of these factors is critical to leveraging work associating microbial changes with disease to tailor dietary or novel targeted therapies to improve health across the spectrum of malignant disease.

THE MICROBIOME AND CARCINOGENESIS

The host microbiome has long been considered a potential contributing factor to the development of a variety of malignancies. To date, several bacteria and viruses have been clearly delineated as contributing to carcinogenesis. These contributions occur through direct cytotoxic effects disrupting autophagy and apoptosis pathways as well as modulating oncogenic signaling pathways. Observed effects vary by bacterial taxa and cancer histology of interest. Moreover, beyond individual taxa associations, broader microbial community level shifts have the potential to modulate cancer risk via microbial metabolites and the overall health of the gut-immune axis.

Colon Polyps and the Microbiome

A CRC is classically thought of as the progression of normal colonic epithelium to polyp formation through progressive cellular changes that eventually lead to an adenoma and continued cellular alterations resulting in the CRC. Microbes have been shown to correlate both with CRC and their precursor polyps. At the polyp stage, these tissues have been noted to have higher rates of proteobacteria as well as lower rates of bacteroidetes when compared with healthy colonic tissue.[3] In studying the gut microbiome of patients with colon polyps, a general bacterial dysbiosis as well as fungal signatures of the ascomycota/basidiomycota ratio was noted along with the increased proportions of opportunistic fungi *Trichosporon* and *Malassezia*.[4,5] Although these correlations are intriguing, a causal role of these gut microbiomes in CRC development has, to date, only been suggested in murine models via the administration of stool from patients with CRC leading to higher rates of high-grade dysplasia and polyp formation.[6] Furthermore, the impact of the gut microbiome on the host immune system was reflected in upregulation of inflammatory pathways and intestinal recruitment of T-helper-1 (Th1) and Th17 cells. Lastly, in animal models with induced colorectal carcinogenesis, germ-free rats grew fewer and smaller tumors when compared with rats with conventional gut microbiota suggesting a critical role of the microbiome in formation of colonic polyps.[6]

Colorectal Adenocarcinoma and the Gut Microbiome

CRC is the third most commonly diagnosed malignancy worldwide and the third most common cause of cancer-related mortality. It has been associated with diets high in red meat, low-fiber diets, alcohol consumption, smoking, and obesity. Importantly, CRC has been rising in incidence (especially in younger populations) and hypothesized to have a potential link to environmental exposures given this recent and sudden rise. Moreover, several studies are underway to correlate this increase in incidence with the gut microbiome given its strong link to environmental exposure and potentially with CRC development.

The flora of the gut under normal physiologic conditions varies from proximal to distal and is reflective of one's exposome—their location, diet, medications, and other lifestyle factors.[7] These changes are reflected in enzymatic activity, pH, and fermentation of luminal contents. The resulting changes are reflected in various genera of bacteria being abundant within the GI tract and colon. Beyond red meat, epidemiologic associations have been made with high-fat diets which have been shown to increase sulfate-reducing bacteria. These bacteria are critical to the transformation of primary to secondary bile acids shown be potentially related to carcinogenesis.[8] Conversely, butyric acid and short-chain fatty acids (generated from fermented fiber) have been shown to be protective of CRC development.[9] The role of metabolites has also been shown to affect the function of p53, converting it from a tumor suppressor to oncogene depending on the levels of luminal gallic acid.[10] These well-described associations between CRC and diet have therefore led to intensive study of the role of the gut microbiome in the development of CRC.[11] Various reports have suggested the most abundant geni of bacteria to be *Bacteroides*, *Prevotella*, and *Ruminococcus* in

CRC patients.[12] Importantly, markers of a "healthy" microbiome remain elusive, although markers of carcinogenesis and dysregulation are increasingly well described.

As noted in other malignancies, the gut microbiome and metabolome have been shown to correlate with colorectal cancer in a stage-specific manner.[13,14] In the case of CRC, *Fusobacterium nucleatum*, and *Solobacterium moorei* were present in higher abundance in patients with later-stage CRC. *Bacteroides fragilis* and colibactin-producing *Escherichia coli* have also been associated with CRC and have been suggested to play a potential causal role in initiation and progression of these tumors.[15–18]

It has been demonstrated that *B fragilis* enterotoxin plays a multifactorial role in oncogenesis. This enterotoxin's mechanism is similar to colibactin produced by *E coli*[19,20] and has the ability to induce direct DNA damage via reactive oxygen species. This then leads to the Th17 recruitment which produces IL-17 and downstream NF-κB (Nuclear factor kappa-light-chain-enhancer of activated B cells) signaling as well as E-cadherin, β-catenin, and STAT3 (Signal transducer and activator of transcription 3).[21,22] This induces a pro-inflammatory setting stimulating IL-8, TGFβ (Transforming growth factor beta), C5a (complement component 5a), leukotriene B4, and growth-related oncogene-α, featuring immature myeloid cells that lead to an oncogenic microenvironment favoring cancer initiation and progression.[15,23,24] At the same time, *B fragilis* enterotoxin plays a role breaking down mucus overlying the colonic epithelial cells allowing for the adhesion of *B fragilis* and other opportunistic species.[25]

At a more global level, the administration of stool from patients with CRC was able to induce higher rates of dysplasia and polyp formation suggesting a causal role of the gut microbiome in colorectal cancer initiation.[6] Beyond direct invasion, toxin production, and DNA damage, the effect of the immune system is significant with the host immune system recognizing various microbial markers. Recognition of these microbe-associated molecular patterns (MAMPs) leads to the activation of NOD (nucleotide-binding oligomerization domain)-like receptors and Toll-like receptors (TLRs) that lead to the regulation of inflammatory pathways and the proliferation of various immune compartments.[26–28] In particular, TLR2 has been suggested to play a role suppressing local immune response and leading to protection of the colonic epithelium.[29–31] The importance of the interface between host systemic immunity and the gut microbiome in these observed effects was demonstrated in animal models of CRC carcinogenesis, germ-free rats grew fewer and smaller tumors than those with a common gut microbiota.[32]

Gastric Adenocarcinoma and the Gut Microbiome

Gastric cancer is the fourth most common cancer worldwide and the second most common cause of cancer-related death. Chronic *H pylori* infection has been associated with the development of peptic ulcer disease and gastric adenocarcinoma.

Gastric adenocarcinoma development has been correlated with both local gastric luminal contents[33] and the colonic gut microbiome.[34] In the case of luminal contents, the most robustly described is the case of *H pylori* that has been clearly and mechanistically associated with the development of peptic ulcer disease. Intriguingly, the association between *H pylori* infection and gastric cancer risk was shown to be strongly associated with patient ancestry in a cohort of Colombian patients.[35] Although those with Amerindian ancestry were at a high risk of gastric cancer in the setting of *H pylori* infection, it was relatively benign in a cohort of those with African ancestry suggesting germline risk is strongly intertwined with this risk profile.

The demonstrated mechanism behind the development of gastric adenocarcinoma secondary to *H pylori* infection is the injection of cytotoxin-associated gene A (CagA) and vacuolating toxin A (VacA) into gastric epithelial cells. In the case of CagA, this leads to the loss of cell polarity, induction of inflammation (interferon-γ, TNF [Tumor necrosis factor]-α, IL-1, IL-1β, IL-6, IL-7, IL-8, IL-10, and IL-18), disruption of epithelial junctions, and oncogenic signaling initiation (ERK/MAPK [extracellular signal-regulated kinases/mitogen-activated protein kinase], PI3K/Akt [Phosphoinositide 3-kinase/Protein kinase], NF-jB, Wnt [Wingless-related]/β-catenin, Ras [Rat sarcoma virus], sonic hedgehog, and STAT3) that induce an oncologic inflammatory milieu.[36–38] In addition, VacA induces vacuolation and autophagy of epithelial cells, increased MAP kinase activity, VEGF (Vascular endothelial growth factor), and Wnt/β-catenin.[39–43]

Aside from the specific associations and mechanism behind H pylori carcinogenesis, more global dysbiosis has been noted in the gastric luminal contents of these patients. These changes have been noted to change across stages of development and progression of gastric adenocarcinoma. This work has identified overall compositional changes in gastric luminal contents as well as enrichments of P stomatis (Peptostreptococcus stomatis), Dialister pneumosintes, S exigua (Slackia exigua), Parvimonas micra, and Streptococcus anginosus.[33]

Beyond these local associations of gastric luminal contents and local effect, the role of the gut microbiome in gastric cancer carcinogenesis has been elucidated recently. Specifically, Clostridium and Fusobacterium species have been noted in higher abundance in patients with gastric cancer as compared with the general population.[44] These findings were further validated along with a more comprehensive report of differential abundance in patients with gastric cancer described by Zhang and colleagues.[34] In the representative of the translational potential of this work, both Lactobacillus and Megasphaera were found to be potentially useful as markers for gastric adenocarcinoma detection. These associations must be taken in light of the significant work in other disease histologies and associations between colonic gut flora and disease initiation and progression. Further work will ultimately be needed to define whether these associations are correlative or causal.

Pancreatic Adenocarcinoma and the Gut Microbiome

Pancreatic cancer is the 12th most common cancer worldwide and the 7th cause of cancer-related death. It has an almost inherently poor prognosis with a median survival of 9 months. It is associated with smoking, obesity, alcohol, chronic pancreatitis, and type 2 diabetes.

Epidemiologic data have intriguingly linked periodontal disease with pancreatic ductal adenocarcinoma (PDAC) incidence across several cohort studies with a wide range of reported risks.[45–49] Given these associations, directed analyses of the oral microbiomes of patients with pancreatic cancer and healthy controls demonstrated alterations in a variety of bacterial species including Neisseria elongate, Streptococcus mitis, Fusobacterium, Leptotrichia, Firmicutes, and Porphyromonas. These were shown to be differentially abundant between groups of cases and controls.[50–54] Intriguingly, one of these studies also noted circulating antibodies to these oral bacteria correlated with risk of PDAC.[54]

Similar to previously described associations in colorectal and gastric cancer, it has been noted that there are differential abundances of bacteria in fecal samples of patients with PDAC as compared with healthy controls. This is perhaps not surprising given the critical role the colonic gut microbiome plays in normal pancreas physiology.[55] To date, however, this has only been completed in a single study demonstrating an increase in proteobacteria in PDAC and a depletion in short-chain fatty acid synthesis association modules, with an increase in modules associated with bacterial virulence.[56] Ultimately, validation and further study is needed to solidify these observations and study any potential causal role of the gut microbiome in PDAC.

Although minimal data exist for associations between the colonic microbiome and PDAC, there are correlative trials associating gastric H pylori infection with PDAC—although these are significantly confounded by lifestyle factors such as smoking and obesity.[57] The proposed mechanism lies behind the upregulation of KRAS, mutated in the majority of PDAC, by H pylori.[58] In addition, H pylori has the potential to upregulate Bcl-xL (B-cell lymphoma-extra large), MCL-1 (Induced myeloid leukemia cell differentiation protein), surviving, c-myc (Myelocytomatosis), and cyclin D1 which all have the potential to contribute to PDAC carcinogenesis.[59–61]

As described in CRC, the role of MAMPs in PDAC has been preliminarily studied as well. The induction of the immune system via MAMPs has been shown to lead to pancreatitis and potentially progress to pancreatic cancer.[62,63] Although F nucleatum, as in CRC, is also a negative prognostic factor in PDAC.[64] Finally, the taste receptor 2 member 38 (T2R38) has been shown to be expressed in PDAC. Moreover, Pseudomonas aeruginosa is a T2R38 ligand that has been shown to lead to invasion and metastasis via ABCB1.[65]

THE MICROBIOME IN DISEASE PROGRESSION

Beyond cancer initiation and carcinogenesis, bacteria have the potential to induce metastatic spread. These effects are possible both in the disruption of vascular barriers that may initially confine malignancies and alterations in the immune system both globally and locally that diminish its routine immune surveillance functions that act to suppress metastatic spread. For clinicians caring for solid tumors such as the GI malignancies reviewed here, this is a particularly critical step in disease progression as this classically represents the point at which patients move from being curable to incurable. As such, the potential future role of the microbiome in prognosis, surveillance, and therapy is immense.

Colorectal Adenocarcinoma

Beyond gut microbial associations, the specific bacterial taxa previously mentioned (F nucleatum) is oftentimes found within colorectal cancers themselves. These observations suggest a potential role in carcinogenesis for a subset of patients with colorectal cancer.[66–71] Beyond associations with colorectal cancer, a specific phenotype seems to be associated with F nucleatum positive CRC. These tumors are predominantly right sided and associated with an overall poor prognosis.[72–75] In the case of F nucleatum positive rectal cancer, clearance of tumoral F nucleatum is associated with improved recurrence free survival as compared with those that remain positive post-neoadjuvant chemoradiotherapy, demonstrating tumoral levels to be a modifiable risk factor that has the potential to improve cancer-specific outcomes. Although numerous groups have posited hypotheses as to the mechanisms behind these observations, the role of F nucleatum in carcinogenesis is likely multifactorial.

Of these hypotheses, the role of Fap2 (fusobacterial Gal-GalNAc-binding lectin), a virulent epithelial adhesin, is often suggested as a potential mechanism to explain these observations. Fap2 permits adhesion to a CRC polysaccharide and generates a FadA (Fusobacterium Adhesions Gene A) adhesion complex capable of stimulating Wnt/β-catenin, leading to the increased expression of oncogenic and inflammatory responses.[76–78] Treatment of murine models of CRC with F nucleatum was able to mimic similar transcriptional and inflammatory pathways seen clinically.[68,79] Furthermore, incubation of CRC cell lines with *F nucleatum* before injection into mice led to increased growth rates of incubated cell lines as compared with control.[76,80]

As detailed above, several bacterial taxa have been implicated in the development of CRC. Beyond these associations, overlapping and unique species also play a role in the progression of disease. In the case of *F nucleatum*, murine models of colorectal cancer liver metastasis have been shown to show a less virulent phenotype with the eradication of *F nucleatum* from the murine gut.[81] Interestingly, these tumors that are *F nucleatum* positive have *F nucleatum* present in positive lymph nodes as well as liver metastases, further strengthening the potential association between its presence and disease progression and metastasis.[81]

Similarly, the development of metastasis via disruption of the vascular barrier and formation or a pre-metastatic niche has been shown to be driven, in murine models by gut bacteria (potentially *E coli* C17). Moreover, circulating markers of gut vascular permeability (plasmalemma vesicle-associated protein-1) were shown to correlate with outcomes in clinical specimens and again be diminished with eradication of gut bacteria.[82–86]

Pancreatic Adenocarcinoma

Apart from limited data describing the role of the gut microbiome in pancreatic cancer, there has been a significant body of work recently describing the role of the tumoral microbiome's role in the microenvironment of PDAC. In the case of PDAC, the tumoral microbiome seems to play two distinct roles—in the modulation of immune response as measured by T-cell activation[87–89] and in the inactivation of common cytotoxic agents such as gemcitabine.[90] Importantly, these observations are tied to outcomes of patients with PDAC, as long-term survivorship was associated with a more diverse tumor microbiome, specific bacterial taxa (*Saccharopolyspora*, *Pseudoxanthomonas*, and *Streptomyces*), and a more robust microbially driven immune response in the tumor microenvironment.

THE MICROBIOME AND RESPONSE TO THERAPY

Intriguingly, a variety of bacterial species have been shown to alter response to various therapeutics. In the case of immune checkpoint blockade (ICB), this is somewhat expected given the known significant impact the gut microbiome has on modulating the host immune system. A similar effect has been seen locally as well, with the tumor microbiome modulating response to immunotherapies. Lastly, the degradation of cytotoxic therapies by tumoral bacterial have been shown to by decrease in the efficacy of cytotoxic chemotherapy. These initial findings lay the groundwork for the potential of microbial modulation to augment other therapies—as has been seen in the case of fecal transplantation inducing response to ICB in melanoma.[91]

Colorectal Adenocarcinoma

A subset of colorectal cancers, microsatellite mismatch repair deficient, are known to be responsive to the ICB.[92] Response to ICB, however, is not uniform. Similar to other histologies, this heterogeneity has been hypothesized to, at least partially, correlate with specific gut microbial communities and changes.[93] Studies quantifying this association and overlap with gut signatures predictive of response in other histologies, however, are ongoing in the setting of promising preclinical models.[94]

Although microbial markers of response to checkpoint blockade are actively being studied, markers of response to cytotoxic therapies are increasingly well described. In the case of *F nucleatum*, previously associated with carcinogenesis, it has also been associated with chemoresistance in CRC.[14,74] This induced chemoresistance has been noted with both oxaliplatin and 5-FU via the activation of autophagy pathways and innate immune signaling via TLR4 and MyD88.[74] These effects were shown to be abrogated in preclinical models via the modulation of the gut microbiome with antibiotic therapy, again suggesting a causal rather than correlative association.[95]

Pancreatic Adenocarcinoma

As previously noted, bacteria within PDAC tumors have the ability to inactive cytotoxic agents such as gemcitabine. These initial analyses importantly provide insights in prognostication while also suggesting potential future novel treatment strategies. Moreover, unique neoantigen properties of long-term survivors noted by Balachandran and colleagues demonstrate circulating levels of MUC16 (CA125) and T-cell reactivity are associated with survival and that their loss is associated with relapse.[87] Pushalkar and colleagues were able to demonstrate the tumoral microbiome acts to suppress monocytic cellular differentiation that leads to T-cell anergy.[88] These mechanistic associations are important keys as the correlative versus causal role of the microbiome continues to be delineated while also allowing for more directed hypothesis generation in other disease sites.

SUMMARY

As outlined above, the interplay between the gut and tumoral microbiome, host immune responses, carcinogenesis, and evasion of therapeutics is a complex system with significant cross-talk between these interrelated variables. Although these associations begin to be deconvoluted, the perennial question in microbiome research exists between causation and correlation. Hypotheses exist for several specific bacteria, and we see overlap between taxa or pathway associations with various disease histologies—short-chain fatty acids, H pylori, and F nucleatum are clear examples of this. Moreover, with the initiation of clinical trials modulating the microbiome through fecal transplantation, prebiotics, or other novel methods, of these associated mechanisms will be tested with continued rigor and continue to provide further insights.

Microbial modulation via phase I studies of fecal transplantation in melanoma patients demonstrated the potential efficacy of gut microbial alteration in optimizing responses to therapy.[91,96] This work provided clear insight that fecal transplantation was able to increase tumor immune infiltrates and induce response in 30% to 40% of otherwise checkpoint blockade refractory patients. Although these findings were noted in cutaneous malignancies, these therapies have the potential to improve outcomes in checkpoint responsive GI malignancies and warrants study in cytotoxic therapies. In the case of fecal transplant technologies, inherent difficulties in scalability are likely insurmountable on a population level. These studies, however, importantly inform the development of directed microbial modulation as well as dietary and prebiotic modulation of the gut microbiome.

An increasing interest in the use of changes in diet and/or the use prebiotics (nondigestible agents used to promote beneficial microbes) has driven directed work studying the potential benefits of these agents in improving response to various therapies. Dietary associations with various malignancies have long been described, such as associations between red meat intake and colorectal cancer.[11] In this case, however, the use of nutritional supplements such as fiber[97] or soluble vitamins such as magnesium[98] has been shown to improve response with these dietary effects seen during their treatment window. This allows clinicians to make a more targeted and directed intervention beyond global dietary changes. Intriguingly, probiotics (ingested live bacteria) decrease gut microbial diversity and have been associated with worse outcomes in immunotherapy-treated patients.[97]

Perhaps the most immediate potential clinical application of the microbiome lies in the ability of gut, tumoral, or circulating microbes to act as screening or prognostic tests at population or individual levels. Recent analysis of the cancer genome atlas has shown histology and stage-specific circulating microbial signatures detectable across disease sites.[99] These microbes exist in tissue and/or blood oftentimes already collected as part of standard of care and could be queried through scalable targeted assays or can be sequenced as part of exploratory research protocols. Furthermore, with continued optimization of gut microbial collection techniques, patients can now submit stool samples remotely for 16s or whole-genome sequencing. The ability of these or other markers to augment current standard of care tests, however, remains unknown and will require independent study for each disease histology.

As the microbiome is increasingly recognized as critical to human health and normal immune function, its importance to malignant disease development, progression, and response to therapy is increasingly clear. Moving forward, clinical trials and careful prospective studies are needed to begin to integrate these findings into clinical practice. As the early adoption of various treatment modalities is initiated, it will be increasingly important to actively study these patients to further improve and learn from these early studies. Ultimately, the last decade has shown continued interest and momentum behind the study and utilization of microbial modulation to improve cancer care.

CLINICS CARE POINTS

- The gut microbiome is an emerging factor in the development and progression of gastrointestinal malignancies.
- While emerging therapeutics in benign disease such as refractory clostridium difficile infection are approaching approval in the United States, therapeutic and diagnostic strategies are still under development.
- Commercially available fecal profiling offer little insight into one's overall microbial health and their results should be interpreted with caution.

FUNDING

M.G.W. is supported by the National Institutes of Health (T32 CA 009599) and the MD Anderson Cancer Center support grant (P30 CA016672). J.A.W. is supported by the NIH (1 R01 CA219896-01A1), the Melanoma Research Alliance (4022024), the American Association for Cancer Research Stand Up To Cancer (SU2C-AACR-IRG-19-17) and the MD Anderson Cancer Center's Melanoma Moon Shots Program.

REFERENCES

1. Turck FB. The early diagnosis of carcinoma of the stomach, with the bacteriology of the stomach contents. J Am Med Assoc 1895;XXIV(11):404–6.
2. Plummer M, de Martel C, Vignat J, et al. Global burden of cancers attributable to infections in 2012: a synthetic analysis. Lancet Glob Health 2016;4(9):e609–16.
3. Dejea CM, Sears CL. Do biofilms confer a pro-carcinogenic state? Gut Microbes 2016;7(1):54–7.

4. Gao R, Kong C, Li H, et al. Dysbiosis signature of mycobiota in colon polyp and colorectal cancer. Eur J Clin Microbiol Infect Dis 2017;36(12):2457–68.

5. Hong BY, Ideta T, Lemos BS, et al. Characterization of Mucosal Dysbiosis of Early Colonic Neoplasia. NPJ Precis Oncol 2019;3:29.

6. Wong SH, Zhao L, Zhang X, et al. Gavage of Fecal Samples From Patients With Colorectal Cancer Promotes Intestinal Carcinogenesis in Germ-Free and Conventional Mice. Gastroenterology 2017;153(6):1621–33.e6.

7. Morad G, Helmink BA, Sharma P, et al. Hallmarks of response, resistance, and toxicity to immune checkpoint blockade. Cell 2021;184(21):5309–37.

8. Wells JE, Hylemon PB. Identification and characterization of a bile acid 7alpha-dehydroxylation operon in Clostridium sp. strain TO-931, a highly active 7alpha-dehydroxylating strain isolated from human feces. Appl Environ Microbiol 2000;66(3):1107–13.

9. Canani RB, Costanzo MD, Leone L, et al. Potential beneficial effects of butyrate in intestinal and extraintestinal diseases. World J Gastroenterol 2011;17(12):1519–28.

10. Kadosh E, Snir-Alkalay I, Venkatachalam A, et al. The gut microbiome switches mutant p53 from tumour-suppressive to oncogenic. Nature 2020;586(7827):133–8.

11. Larsson SC, Wolk A. Meat consumption and risk of colorectal cancer: a meta-analysis of prospective studies. Int J Cancer 2006;119(11):2657–64.

12. Hillman ET, Lu H, Yao T, et al. Microbial Ecology along the Gastrointestinal Tract. Microbes Environ 2017;32(4):300–13.

13. Nakatsu G, Li X, Zhou H, et al. Gut mucosal microbiome across stages of colorectal carcinogenesis. Nat Commun 2015;6:8727.

14. Yachida S, Mizutani S, Shiroma H, et al. Metagenomic and metabolomic analyses reveal distinct stage-specific phenotypes of the gut microbiota in colorectal cancer. Nat Med 2019;25(6):968–76.

15. Boleij A, Hechenbleikner EM, Goodwin AC, et al. The Bacteroides fragilis toxin gene is prevalent in the colon mucosa of colorectal cancer patients. Clin Infect Dis 2015;60(2):208–15.

16. Goodwin AC, Destefano Shields CE, Wu S, et al. Polyamine catabolism contributes to enterotoxigenic Bacteroides fragilis-induced colon tumorigenesis. Proc Natl Acad Sci U S A 2011;108(37):15354–9.

17. Arthur JC, Perez-Chanona E, Mühlbauer M, et al. Intestinal inflammation targets cancer-inducing activity of the microbiota. Science 2012;338(6103):120–3.

18. Bonnet M, Buc E, Sauvanet P, et al. Colonization of the human gut by E. coli and colorectal cancer risk. Clin Cancer Res 2014;20(4):859–67.

19. Tomkovich S, Yang Y, Winglee K, et al. Locoregional Effects of Microbiota in a Preclinical Model of Colon Carcinogenesis. Cancer Res 2017;77(10):2620–32.

20. Dalmasso G, Cougnoux A, Delmas J, et al. The bacterial genotoxin colibactin promotes colon tumor growth by modifying the tumor microenvironment. Gut Microbes 2014;5(5):675–80.

21. Wu S, Powell J, Mathioudakis N, et al. Bacteroides fragilis enterotoxin induces intestinal epithelial cell secretion of interleukin-8 through mitogen-activated protein kinases and a tyrosine kinase-regulated nuclear factor-kappaB pathway. Infect Immun 2004;72(10):5832–9.

22. Wu S, Rhee KJ, Albesiano E, et al. A human colonic commensal promotes colon tumorigenesis via activation of T helper type 17 T cell responses. Nat Med 2009;15(9):1016–22.

23. Toprak NU, Yagci A, Gulluoglu BM, et al. A possible role of Bacteroides fragilis enterotoxin in the aetiology of colorectal cancer. Clin Microbiol Infect 2006; 12(8):782–6.

24. Kim JM, Lee JY, Yoon YM, et al. Bacteroides fragilis enterotoxin induces cyclooxygenase-2 and fluid secretion in intestinal epithelial cells through NF-kappaB activation. Eur J Immunol 2006;36(9):2446–56.

25. Dejea CM, Fathi P, Craig JM, et al. Patients with familial adenomatous polyposis harbor colonic biofilms containing tumorigenic bacteria. Science 2018; 359(6375):592–7.

26. Fukata M, Abreu MT. TLR4 signalling in the intestine in health and disease. Biochem Soc Trans 2007;35(Pt 6):1473–8.

27. Rakoff-Nahoum S, Medzhitov R. Innate immune recognition of the indigenous microbial flora. Mucosal Immunol 2008;1(Suppl 1):S10–4.

28. Parlato M, Yeretssian G. NOD-like receptors in intestinal homeostasis and epithelial tissue repair. Int J Mol Sci 2014;15(6):9594–627.

29. Asquith M, Powrie F. An innately dangerous balancing act: intestinal homeostasis, inflammation, and colitis-associated cancer. J Exp Med 2010;207(8):1573–7.

30. Fukata M, Abreu MT. Microflora in colorectal cancer: a friend to fear. Nat Med 2010;16(6):639–41.

31. An J, Ha EM. Combination Therapy of Lactobacillus plantarum Supernatant and 5-Fluouracil Increases Chemosensitivity in Colorectal Cancer Cells. J Microbiol Biotechnol 2016;26(8):1490–503.

32. Vannucci L, Stepankova R, Kozakova H, et al. Colorectal carcinogenesis in germ-free and conventionally reared rats: different intestinal environments affect the systemic immunity. Int J Oncol 2008;32(3):609–17.

33. Coker OO, Dai Z, Nie Y, et al. Mucosal microbiome dysbiosis in gastric carcinogenesis. Gut 2018;67(6):1024–32.

34. Zhang Y, Shen J, Shi X, et al. Gut microbiome analysis as a predictive marker for the gastric cancer patients. Appl Microbiol Biotechnol 2021;105(2):803–14.

35. Kodaman N, Pazos A, Schneider BG, et al. Human and Helicobacter pylori coevolution shapes the risk of gastric disease. Proc Natl Acad Sci U S A 2014; 111(4):1455–60.

36. Noto JM, Peek RM Jr. The Helicobacter pylori cag Pathogenicity Island. Methods Mol Biol 2012;921:41–50.

37. Covacci A, Censini S, Bugnoli M, et al. Molecular characterization of the 128-kDa immunodominant antigen of Helicobacter pylori associated with cytotoxicity and duodenal ulcer. Proc Natl Acad Sci U S A 1993;90(12):5791–5.

38. Tummuru MK, Cover TL, Blaser MJ. Cloning and expression of a high-molecular-mass major antigen of Helicobacter pylori: evidence of linkage to cytotoxin production. Infect Immun 1993;61(5):1799–809.

39. Suzuki J, Ohnsihi H, Shibata H, et al. Dynamin is involved in human epithelial cell vacuolation caused by the Helicobacter pylori-produced cytotoxin VacA. J Clin Invest 2001;107(3):363–70.

40. Yahiro K, Akazawa Y, Nakano M, et al. Helicobacter pylori VacA induces apoptosis by accumulation of connexin 43 in autophagic vesicles via a Rac1/ERK-dependent pathway. Cell Death Discov 2015;1:15035.

41. Jain P, Luo ZQ, Blanke SR. Helicobacter pylori vacuolating cytotoxin A (VacA) engages the mitochondrial fission machinery to induce host cell death. Proc Natl Acad Sci U S A 2011;108(38):16032–7.

42. Ki MR, Lee HR, Goo MJ, et al. Differential regulation of ERK1/2 and p38 MAP kinases in VacA-induced apoptosis of gastric epithelial cells. Am J Physiol Gastrointest Liver Physiol 2008;294(3):G635–47.
43. Liu N, Zhou N, Chai N, et al. Helicobacter pylori promotes angiogenesis depending on Wnt/beta-catenin-mediated vascular endothelial growth factor via the cyclooxygenase-2 pathway in gastric cancer. BMC Cancer 2016;16:321.
44. Hsieh YY, Tung SY, Pan HY, et al. Increased Abundance of Clostridium and Fusobacterium in Gastric Microbiota of Patients with Gastric Cancer in Taiwan. Sci Rep 2018;8(1):158.
45. Hujoel PP, Drangsholt M, Spiekerman C, et al. An exploration of the periodontitis-cancer association. Ann Epidemiol 2003;13(5):312–6.
46. Ahn J, Segers S, Hayes RB. Periodontal disease, Porphyromonas gingivalis serum antibody levels and orodigestive cancer mortality. Carcinogenesis 2012; 33(5):1055–8.
47. Stolzenberg-Solomon RZ, Dodd KW, Blaser MJ, et al. Tooth loss, pancreatic cancer, and Helicobacter pylori. Am J Clin Nutr 2003;78(1):176–81.
48. Michaud DS, Kelsey KT, Papathanasiou E, et al. Periodontal disease and risk of all cancers among male never smokers: an updated analysis of the Health Professionals Follow-up Study. Ann Oncol 2016;27(5):941–7.
49. Michaud DS, Joshipura K, Giovannucci E, et al. A prospective study of periodontal disease and pancreatic cancer in US male health professionals. J Natl Cancer Inst 2007;99(2):171–5.
50. Farrell JJ, Zhang L, Zhou H, et al. Variations of oral microbiota are associated with pancreatic diseases including pancreatic cancer. Gut 2012;61(4):582–8.
51. Torres PJ, Fletcher EM, Gibbons SM, et al. Characterization of the salivary microbiome in patients with pancreatic cancer. Peerj 2015;3:e1373.
52. Fan X, Alekseyenko AV, Wu J, et al. Human oral microbiome and prospective risk for pancreatic cancer: a population-based nested case-control study. Gut 2018; 67(1):120–7.
53. Olson SH, Satagopan J, Xu Y, et al. The oral microbiota in patients with pancreatic cancer, patients with IPMNs, and controls: a pilot study. Cancer Causes Control 2017;28(9):959–69.
54. Michaud DS, Izard J, Wilhelm-Benartzi CS, et al. Plasma antibodies to oral bacteria and risk of pancreatic cancer in a large European prospective cohort study. Gut 2013;62(12):1764–70.
55. Thomas RM, Jobin C. Microbiota in pancreatic health and disease: the next frontier in microbiome research. Nat Rev Gastroenterol Hepatol 2020;17(1):53–64.
56. Zhou W, Zhang, Li Z, et al. The fecal microbiota of patients with pancreatic ductal adenocarcinoma and autoimmune pancreatitis characterized by metagenomic sequencing. J Transl Med 2021;19(1):215.
57. Rabelo-Goncalves EM, Roesler BM, Zeitune JM. Extragastric manifestations of Helicobacter pylori infection: Possible role of bacterium in liver and pancreas diseases. World J Hepatol 2015;7(30):2968–79.
58. Huang H, Daniluk J, Liu Y, et al. Oncogenic K-Ras requires activation for enhanced activity. Oncogene 2014;33(4):532–5.
59. Daniluk J, Liu Y, Deng D, et al. An NF-kappaB pathway-mediated positive feedback loop amplifies Ras activity to pathological levels in mice. J Clin Invest 2012; 122(4):1519–28.
60. Fukuda A, Wang SC, Morris JPt, et al. Stat3 and MMP7 contribute to pancreatic ductal adenocarcinoma initiation and progression. Cancer Cell 2011;19(4): 441–55.

61. Lesina M, Kurkowski MU, Ludes K, et al. Stat3/Socs3 activation by IL-6 trans-signaling promotes progression of pancreatic intraepithelial neoplasia and development of pancreatic cancer. Cancer Cell 2011;19(4):456–69.

62. Liu M, Peng J, Tai N, et al. Toll-like receptor 9 negatively regulates pancreatic islet beta cell growth and function in a mouse model of type 1 diabetes. Diabetologia 2018;61(11):2333–43.

63. Wang F, Jin R, Zou BB, et al. Activation of Toll-like receptor 7 regulates the expression of IFN-lambda1, p53, PTEN, VEGF, TIMP-1 and MMP-9 in pancreatic cancer cells. Mol Med Rep 2016;13(2):1807–12.

64. Mitsuhashi K, Nosho K, Sukawa Y, et al. Association of Fusobacterium species in pancreatic cancer tissues with molecular features and prognosis. Oncotarget 2015;6(9):7209–20.

65. Gaida MM, Mayer C, Dapunt U, et al. Expression of the bitter receptor T2R38 in pancreatic cancer: localization in lipid droplets and activation by a bacteria-derived quorum-sensing molecule. Oncotarget 2016;7(11):12623–32.

66. Castellarin M, Warren RL, Freeman JD, et al. Fusobacterium nucleatum infection is prevalent in human colorectal carcinoma. Genome Res 2012;22(2):299–306.

67. Kostic AD, Gevers D, Pedamallu CS, et al. Genomic analysis identifies association of Fusobacterium with colorectal carcinoma. Genome Res 2012;22(2):292–8.

68. Kostic AD, Chun E, Robertson L, et al. Fusobacterium nucleatum potentiates intestinal tumorigenesis and modulates the tumor-immune microenvironment. Cell Host Microbe 2013;14(2):207–15.

69. Ahn J, Sinha R, Pei Z, et al. Human gut microbiome and risk for colorectal cancer. J Natl Cancer Inst 2013;105(24):1907–11.

70. McCoy AN, Araújo-Pérez F, Azcárate-Peril A, et al. Fusobacterium is associated with colorectal adenomas. PLoS One 2013;8(1):e53653.

71. Warren RL, Freeman DJ, Pleasance S, et al. Co-occurrence of anaerobic bacteria in colorectal carcinomas. Microbiome 2013;1(1):16.

72. Mima K, Nishihara R, Qian ZR, et al. Fusobacterium nucleatum in colorectal carcinoma tissue and patient prognosis. Gut 2016;65(12):1973–80.

73. Flanagan L, Schmid J, Ebert M, et al. Fusobacterium nucleatum associates with stages of colorectal neoplasia development, colorectal cancer and disease outcome. Eur J Clin Microbiol Infect Dis 2014;33(8):1381–90.

74. Yu T, Guo F, Yu Y, et al. Fusobacterium nucleatum Promotes Chemoresistance to Colorectal Cancer by Modulating Autophagy. Cell 2017;170(3):548–63.e6.

75. Mima K, Cao Y, Chan AT, et al. Fusobacterium nucleatum in Colorectal Carcinoma Tissue According to Tumor Location. Clin Transl Gastroenterol 2016;7(11):e200.

76. Rubinstein MR, Wang X, Liu W, et al. Fusobacterium nucleatum promotes colorectal carcinogenesis by modulating E-cadherin/β-catenin signaling via its FadA adhesin. Cell Host Microbe 2013;14(2):195–206.

77. Ikegami A, Chung P, Han YW. Complementation of the fadA mutation in Fusobacterium nucleatum demonstrates that the surface-exposed adhesin promotes cellular invasion and placental colonization. Infect Immun 2009;77(7):3075–9.

78. Abed J, Emgård JE, Zamir G, et al. Fap2 Mediates Fusobacterium nucleatum Colorectal Adenocarcinoma Enrichment by Binding to Tumor-Expressed Gal-GalNAc. Cell Host Microbe 2016;20(2):215–25.

79. Yu YN, Yu TC, Zhao HJ, et al. Berberine may rescue Fusobacterium nucleatum-induced colorectal tumorigenesis by modulating the tumor microenvironment. Oncotarget 2015;6(31):32013–26.

80. Yang Y, Weng W, Peng J, et al. Fusobacterium nucleatum Increases Proliferation of Colorectal Cancer Cells and Tumor Development in Mice by Activating Toll-Like

Receptor 4 Signaling to Nuclear Factor-κB, and Up-regulating Expression of MicroRNA-21. Gastroenterology 2017;152(4):851–66.e4.

81. Bullman S, Pedamallu CS, Sicinska E, et al. Analysis of Fusobacterium persistence and antibiotic response in colorectal cancer. Science 2017;358(6369):1443–8.

82. Spadoni I, Pietrelli A, Pesole G, et al. Gene expression profile of endothelial cells during perturbation of the gut vascular barrier. Gut Microbes 2016;7(6):540–8.

83. Spadoni I, Zagato E, Bertocchi A, et al. A gut-vascular barrier controls the systemic dissemination of bacteria. Science 2015;350(6262):830–4.

84. Bertocchi A, Carloni S, Ravenda PS, et al. Gut vascular barrier impairment leads to intestinal bacteria dissemination and colorectal cancer metastasis to liver. Cancer Cell 2021;39(5):708–724 e1.

85. Costa-Silva B, Aiello NM, Ocean AJ, et al. Pancreatic cancer exosomes initiate pre-metastatic niche formation in the liver. Nat Cell Biol 2015;17(6):816–26.

86. Seubert B, Grünwald B, Kobuch J, et al. Tissue inhibitor of metalloproteinases (TIMP)-1 creates a premetastatic niche in the liver through SDF-1/CXCR4-dependent neutrophil recruitment in mice. Hepatology 2015;61(1):238–48.

87. Balachandran VP, Luksza M, Zhao JN, et al. Identification of unique neoantigen qualities in long-term survivors of pancreatic cancer. Nature 2017;551(7681):512–6.

88. Pushalkar S, Hundeyin M, Daley D, et al. The Pancreatic Cancer Microbiome Promotes Oncogenesis by Induction of Innate and Adaptive Immune Suppression. Cancer Discov 2018;8(4):403–16.

89. Riquelme E, Zhang Y, Zhang L, et al. Tumor Microbiome Diversity and Composition Influence Pancreatic Cancer Outcomes. Cell 2019;178(4):795–806.e2.

90. Geller LT, Barzily-Rokni M, Danino T, et al. Potential role of intratumor bacteria in mediating tumor resistance to the chemotherapeutic drug gemcitabine. Science 2017;357(6356):1156–60.

91. Baruch EN, Youngster I, Ben-Betzalel G, et al. Fecal microbiota transplant promotes response in immunotherapy-refractory melanoma patients. Science 2021;371(6529):602–9.

92. Overman MJ, McDermott R, Leach JL, et al. Nivolumab in patients with metastatic DNA mismatch repair-deficient or microsatellite instability-high colorectal cancer (CheckMate 142): an open-label, multicentre, phase 2 study. Lancet Oncol 2017;18(9):1182–91.

93. Helmink BA, Khan MAW, Hermann A, et al. The microbiome, cancer, and cancer therapy. Nat Med 2019;25(3):377–88.

94. Xu X, Lv J, Guo F, et al. Gut Microbiome Influences the Efficacy of PD-1 Antibody Immunotherapy on MSS-Type Colorectal Cancer via Metabolic Pathway. Front Microbiol 2020;11:814.

95. Iida N, Dzutsev A, Stewart CA, et al. Commensal bacteria control cancer response to therapy by modulating the tumor microenvironment. Science 2013;342(6161):967–70.

96. Davar D, Dzutsev AK, McCulloch JA, et al. Fecal microbiota transplant overcomes resistance to anti-PD-1 therapy in melanoma patients. Science 2021;371(6529):595–602.

97. Spencer CN, McQuade JL, Gopalakrishnan V, et al. Dietary fiber and probiotics influence the gut microbiome and melanoma immunotherapy response. Science 2021;374(6575):1632–40.

98. Lotscher J, Marti ILAA, Kirchhammer N, et al. Magnesium sensing via LFA-1 regulates CD8(+) T cell effector function. Cell 2022;185(4):585–602.e29.

99. Poore GD, Kopylova E, Zhu Q, et al. Microbiome analyses of blood and tissues suggest cancer diagnostic approach. Nature 2020;579(7800):567–74.

Moving?

Make sure your subscription moves with you!

To notify us of your new address, find your **Clinics Account Number** (located on your mailing label above your name), and contact customer service at:

Email: journalscustomerservice-usa@elsevier.com

800-654-2452 (subscribers in the U.S. & Canada)
314-447-8871 (subscribers outside of the U.S. & Canada)

Fax number: 314-447-8029

Elsevier Health Sciences Division
Subscription Customer Service
3251 Riverport Lane
Maryland Heights, MO 63043

*To ensure uninterrupted delivery of your subscription,
please notify us at least 4 weeks in advance of move.

Printed and bound by CPI Group (UK) Ltd, Croydon, CR0 4YY

03/10/2024

01040405-0005